Straight A's
in
Pediatric Nursing
Second Edition

 Wolters Kluwer | Lippincott Williams & Wilkins
Health

Philadelphia · Baltimore · New York · London
Buenos Aires · Hong Kong · Sydney · Tokyo

STAFF

Executive Publisher
Judith A. Schilling McCann, RN, MSN

Editorial Director
David Moreau

Clinical Director
Joan M. Robinson, RN, MSN

Art Director
Mary Ludwicki

Electronic Project Manager
John Macalino

Senior Managing Editor
Jaime Stockslager Buss, MSPH, ELS

Clinical Project Manager
Beverly Ann Tscheschlog, RN, BS

Editors
Sid Karpoff, Janeen Levine,
Gale Thompson

Clinical Editor
Bethany J. Hemphill, RN, CPNP

Copy Editors
Kimberly Bilotta (supervisor),
Scotti Cohn, Heather Ditch,
Jeannine Fielding, Amy Furman,
Lisa Stockslager, Dorothy P. Terry

Designers
Joseph J. Clark, Arlene Putterman

Digital Composition Services
Diane Paluba (manager),
Joyce Rossi Biletz, Donna S. Morris

Associate Manufacturing Manager
Beth J. Welsh

Editorial Assistants
Karen J. Kirk, Jeri O'Shea,
Linda K. Ruhf

Indexer
Barbara Hodgson

The clinical treatments described and recommended in this publication are based on research and consultation with nursing, medical, and legal authorities. To the best of our knowledge, these procedures reflect currently accepted practice. Nevertheless, they can't be considered absolute and universal recommendations. For individual applications, all recommendations must be considered in light of the patient's clinical condition and, before administration of new or infrequently used drugs, in light of the latest package-insert information. The authors and publisher disclaim any responsibility for any adverse effects resulting from the suggested procedures, from any undetected errors, or from the reader's misunderstanding of the text.

STRPED2E021109

Library of Congress
Cataloging-in-Publication Data

Straight A's in pediatric nursing.—2nd ed.
   p. ; cm.
   Includes bibliographical references and index.
   1. Pediatric nursing—Outlines, syllabi, etc. 2. Pediatric nursing—Examinations, questions, etc. I. Lippincott Williams & Wilkins.
   [DNLM: 1. Pediatric Nursing—Examination Questions. 2. Nursing Assessment—Examination Questions. 3. Nursing Care—Examination Questions. WY 18.2 S8963 2008]
   RJ245.S695 2008
   618.92'00231—dc22
ISBN-13: 978-1-58255-697-0 (alk. paper)
ISBN-10: 1-58255-697-0 (alk. paper)   2007030534

Contents

Advisory board

Contributors and consultants

Stephanie C. Butkus, RN, MSN, CPNP, IBCLC
Assistant Professor Division of Nursing
Kettering (Ohio) College of Medical Arts

Anita Carroll, RN, MSN, EdD
Instructor
West Texas A&M University School of Nursing
Canyon

Sherrill Conroy, RN, BN, MEd, DPHIL
Assistant Professor, Faculty of Nursing
University of Alberta
Edmonton, Alberta, Canada

Dana M. Etzel-Hardman, RN, BSN, CPN
Training and Education Specialist
Children's Hospital of Pittsburgh

Deborah Mayo, ARNP/CPNP, MSN, Captain (ret) U.S. Public Health Service
Pediatric Nurse Practitioner
Oklahoma State Department of Health
Logan County Health Department
Guthrie

Virginia Richardson, RN, DNS, CPNP
Coordinator of the Pediatric Nurse Practitioner Program
Associate Professor
Indiana University School of Nursing
Indianapolis

Nan C. Riedè, RN, MSN
Assistant Professor
Baptist College of Health Sciences
Memphis

Suzan C. Shane, RN, APN-P, EdD
Associate Professor
OSF St. Francis Medical Center College of Nursing
Peoria, Ill.

Janet Somlyay, MSN, CNS, CPNP, CNE
Clinical Nurse Specialist
Cheyenne (Wyo.) Regional Medical Center

Julee Waldrop, MS, FNP, PNP
Clinical Associate Professor, Director Newborn Nursery
The University of North Carolina
Chapel Hill

Jan Weust, RN, MSN
Nursing Faculty
Ivy Tech Community College
Terre Haute, Ind.

Robin R. Wilkerson, PhD, RN
Associate Professor & Assistant Dean of Undergraduate Program
University of Mississippi School of Nursing
Jackson

Kelly Witter, RN, MSN, CLC
Director
Great Oaks School of Practical Nursing
Cincinnati

How to use this book

S*traight A's* is a multivolume study guide series developed especially for nursing students. Each volume provides essential course material in a unique two-column design. The easy-to-read interior outline format offers a succinct review of key facts as presented in leading textbooks on the subject. The bulleted exterior columns provide only the most crucial information, allowing for quick, efficient review right before an important quiz or test.

Special features appear in every chapter to make information accessible and easy to remember. The **Pretest** helps the student identify topic areas that may require more study. **Learning objectives** encourage the student to evaluate knowledge before and after study. The **Chapter overview** highlights the chapter's major concepts. The **NCLEX checks** at the end of each chapter offer additional opportunities to review material and assess knowledge gained before moving on to new information.

Other features appear throughout the book to facilitate learning. **Clinical alerts** appear in color to bring the reader's attention to important, potentially life-threatening considerations that could affect patient care. **Time-out for teaching** highlights key areas to address when teaching patients. **Go with the flow** charts promote critical thinking. Finally, a Windows-based software program (see CD-ROM on inside back cover) poses more than 250 multiple-choice and alternate-format NCLEX-style questions to assess student knowledge.

The *Straight A's* volumes are designed as learning tools, not as primary information sources. When read conscientiously as a supplement to class attendance and textbook reading, *Straight A's* can enhance understanding and help improve test scores and final grades.

Foreword

As the number of children in the United States younger than age 21 increases annually, now representing more than 30% of the total population, it becomes more apparent that graduate nurses need to know about well-child health care, acute and chronic disease states in pediatric populations, and appropriate nursing interventions. Recognizing developmental stages, acquiring skills, and teaching families are critical in the care of children and require different skills sets than caring for adults. Nurses with a strong grasp of these important concepts are in a good position to help families deal with everyday situations, resulting in positive outcomes for their children. Unfortunately, clinical experiences in the care of children are commonly limited in nursing programs because most ill children are cared for in the home and hospital stays are short. Therefore, to be well prepared to care for these patients and their families and to have the knowledge needed to pass the NCLEX® examination, student nurses must rely on review books to study important content and practice answering questions.

Straight A's in Pediatric Nursing, Second Edition, is an excellent resource that can help nursing students and graduates study for pediatric nursing classes as well as prepare for the NCLEX. This one-of-a-kind book offers an easy-to-read, succinct synopsis of key concepts of pediatric nursing in two formats. The inner columns provide a quick review of essentials of pediatric nursing, whereas the outer columns provide only the key facts. Each system-focused chapter outlines common pediatric conditions, their causes and pathophysiology, common complications, assessment and diagnostic test findings, medical management, and nursing interventions.

Pretest questions and learning objectives at the start of every chapter prepare readers for what they need to know and help to identify areas of weakness. NCELX-style end-of-chapter questions, which include alternate-format types and rationales for correct and incorrect answer choices, gauge readers' comprehension of the content. Question categories are the same as those found on the NCLEX, so students become familiar with the testing areas. An accompanying CD offers more than 250 additional NCLEX-style questions to test knowledge of pediatric nursing care.

Providing safe, comprehensive care to infants, children, and adolescents is a challenge, even for experienced nurses. *Straight A's in Pediatric Nursing,* Second Edition, can help build the foundation necessary to provide that care to this important population.

Beth Richardson, DNS, RN, CPNP
Associate Professor and Coordinator
Pediatric Nurse Practitioner Program
Indiana University School of Nursing
Indianapolis

1

Nursing care during growth and development

PRETEST

1. Who developed the psychosocial theory of child development?

☐ 1. Lawrence Kohlberg

☐ 2. Sigmund Freud

☐ 3. Erik Erikson

☐ 4. Jean Piaget

CORRECT ANSWER: 3

2. What's the fourth stage of Erikson's five stages of childhood?

☐ 1. Industry versus inferiority

☐ 2. Identity versus role confusion

☐ 3. Trust versus mistrust

☐ 4. Initiative versus guilt

CORRECT ANSWER: 1

3. Which ages properly describe the neonatal period?

☐ 1. Birth to 14 days

☐ 2. Birth to 28 days

☐ 3. Birth to 168 days

☐ 4. Birth to 356 days

CORRECT ANSWER: 2

4. At what age does the posterior fontanel close?

☐ 1. 2 months

☐ 2. 6 months

☐ 3. 12 months

☐ 4. 18 months

CORRECT ANSWER: 1

5. At what age should a mother seek further evaluation if her child hasn't been successful at toilet training?

☐ 1. 18 months

☐ 2. 24 months

☐ 3. 3 years

☐ 4. 5 years

CORRECT ANSWER: 4

LEARNING OBJECTIVES

After studying this chapter, you should be able to:

● Discuss the major concepts associated with growth and development and describe their impact on pediatric nursing.

● Identify the physical, psychosocial, and cognitive developmental tasks for the child from birth through adolescence.

● Determine the child's nutritional and safety needs.

● Plan communication and other nursing interventions based on the child's needs and ability to comprehend.

● Discuss pain management interventions for the child.

● Identify interventions for accurately administering pediatric medications.

CHAPTER OVERVIEW

The concepts of growth and development are fundamental to the practice of pediatric nursing. Throughout the periods of child development, major milestones are accomplished. For each of these developmental periods, important aspects of care involving such topics as nutrition, language, safety, and discipline must be addressed. Special areas of concern related to communication, pain perception, and medication administration are essential for providing patient-specific nursing care.

PRINCIPLES OF PEDIATRIC NURSING

- **Patient population**
  - Children from birth through adolescence
  - Care spans the continuum from well-child care to illness and death
- **Intervention goals and considerations**
  - All interventions are family-centered; the child and family are treated as a unit
  - Interventions are geared toward helping the child and family unit attain, maintain, or regain optimal health
  - Health and development are affected by environment and heredity
  - Nursing interventions are guided primarily by the child's level of development and secondarily by chronological age

CONCEPTS OF GROWTH AND DEVELOPMENT

- **Definitions**
  - Growth implies an increase in size, such as height and weight, but doesn't necessarily include development
  - Development refers to the acquisition of skills and abilities that takes place throughout life
  - Parents need to be taught the normal growth and development parameters of children
- **Paths of progression**
  - From head to toe (cephalocaudally) — for example, head control precedes the ability to walk
  - From the trunk to the tips of the extremities (proximodistally) — for example, the neonate can move his arms and legs easily but can't pick up objects with his fingers
  - From the general to the specific (simple tasks are mastered before advancing to those that are more complex) — for example, progressing from crawling to walking to skipping

Progression of growth and development

- From head to toe (cephalocaudally)
- From trunk to tips of the extremities (proximodistally)
- From general to specific

Developmental stages

- Infancy
- Toddler-preschool
- School age
- Adolescence

Cognitive theory

- Piaget
- Describes successive stages of mental activity that occur during childhood
- Four stages

Four stages of cognitive development

- Sensorimotor (birth to age 2)
- Preoperational (ages 2 to 7)
- Concrete operational (ages 7 to 11)
- Formal operational thought (ages 12 to 15)

Developmental stages

- Growth follows an orderly, predictable (although variable) pattern during developmental periods
- Infancy—a period of rapid growth in which the head, especially the brain, grows faster than other tissues
- Toddler-preschool stage—a period of slow growth in which the trunk grows fastest
- School age—a period of slow growth in which the limbs grow fastest
- Adolescence—a period of rapid growth for the trunk, including the gonads and associated tissues

Environmental influences on growth and development

- Culture and socioeconomic status
  - Cultural environment determines a child's language and greatly influences his actions
  - Socioeconomic status may affect the child's access to medical care, housing, and nutrition—all of which can impact growth and development

Theories of growth and development

(see *Theories of growth and development*)

- Cognitive theory (Jean Piaget)
  - Mental activity occurs in successive stages during childhood
  - By successfully encountering new experiences, the child adapts and progresses to the next stage
  - The child incorporates new ideas, skills, and knowledge into familiar patterns of thought and action; when faced with a problem that's new or too complex to fit into his existing pattern of thought, the child accommodates, drawing on past experiences that are closest to his current problem to solve it
  - Development occurs in four stages; the child can't progress to a more advanced stage if he hasn't accomplished the one preceding it.
    - Sensorimotor stage (birth to age 2)—during this stage, the child progresses from reflex activity through simple repetitive behaviors to imitative behaviors
    - Preoperational stage (ages 2 to 7)—this stage is marked by egocentricity (the child can't comprehend a point of view different than his own); it's a time of magical thinking and increased ability to use symbols and language
    - Concrete operational stage (ages 7 to 11)—the child's thought processes become more logical and coherent; he can use inductive reasoning to solve problems but still can't think abstractly; he's less self-centered
    - Formal operational thought stage (ages 12 to 15)—this stage is characterized by adaptability and flexibility; the adolescent can

Theories of growth and development

The child development theories discussed in this chart shouldn't be compared directly because they measure different aspects of development. Erik Erikson's psychosocial-based theory is the most commonly accepted model for child development, although it can't be empirically tested.

AGE-GROUP	PSYCHO-SOCIAL THEORY	COGNITIVE THEORY	PSYCHO-SEXUAL THEORY	MORAL DEVELOPMENT
Infancy (birth to age 1)	Trust versus mistrust	Sensorimotor (birth to age 2)	Oral	Not applicable
Toddlerhood (ages 1 to 3)	Autonomy versus shame and doubt	Sensorimotor to preoperational	Anal	Preconventional
Preschool age (ages 3 to 6)	Initiative versus guilt	Preoperational (ages 2 to 7)	Phallic	Preconventional
School age (ages 6 to 12)	Industry versus inferiority	Concrete operational (ages 7 to 11)	Latency	Conventional
Adolescence (ages 12 to 19)	Identity versus role confusion	Formal operational thought (ages 12 to 15)	Genitalia	Postconventional

think abstractly, form logical conclusions from his observations, and establish and test hypotheses
- Psychosocial theory (Erik Erikson)
  - Major personality changes occur throughout an individual's life cycle
  - Passage from one stage to another depends on the use of skills acquired in the preceding stage; however, new situations may provide opportunities for learning to cope with deficits experienced in earlier stages
  - There are five childhood stages
    • Trust versus mistrust (birth to age 1) — the child develops trust as the primary caregiver meets his needs
    • Autonomy versus shame and doubt (ages 1 to 3) — the child learns to control his body functions and becomes increasingly independent, preferring to do things himself
    • Initiative versus guilt (ages 3 to 6) — the child learns about the world through play and develops a conscience
    • Industry versus inferiority (ages 6 to 12) — the child enjoys working on projects and with others and tends to follow rules; competition with others is keen, and forming social relationships takes on great importance

Psychosocial theory

- Erikson
- Describes major personality changes that occur throughout an individual's life
- Five stages

Erikson's five childhood stages

- Trust versus mistrust (birth to age 1)
- Autonomy versus shame and doubt (ages 1 to 3)
- Initiative versus guilt (ages 3 to 6)
- Industry versus inferiority (ages 6 to 12)
- Identity versus role confusion (ages 12 to 18)

Psychosexual theory

- Freud
- Explains that the human mind consists of the id, ego, and superego
- Five stages
- Oral stage (birth to age 1)
- Anal stage (ages 1 to 3)
- Phallic stage (ages 3 to 6)
- Latency period (ages 6 to 12)
- Genitalia stage (age 12 and older)

Moral development

- Kohlberg
- Explains how children develop sense of right and wrong
- Three levels

Kohlberg's levels of cognitive development

- Preconventional level of morality (ages 2 to 7)
- Conventional level of morality (ages 7 to 12)
- Postconventional autonomous level of morality (age 12 and older)

• Identity versus role confusion (ages 12 to 18) — changes in his body are taking place rapidly, and the child is preoccupied with how he looks and how others view him; while trying to meet the expectations of his peers, he's also trying to establish his own identity

- Psychosexual theory (Sigmund Freud)
  - The human mind (personality) consists of three major entities: the id (seeks immediate gratification), the ego (orients the individual to reality), and the superego (is responsible for the existence of a conscience and an individual's ideals)
  - Each stage must be mastered before the child can move on to the next stage
    • Oral stage (birth to age 1) — the child seeks pleasure through sucking, biting, and other oral activities
    • Anal stage (ages 1 to 3) — the child undergoes toilet training and learns to control his excreta
    • Phallic stage (ages 3 to 6) — the child is interested in his genitalia and various sensations and discovers the difference between boys and girls
    • Latency period (ages 6 to 12) — the child expands on traits developed in earlier stages and concentrates on playing and learning
    • Genitalia stage (age 12 and older) — the production of sex hormones becomes intense, and the reproductive system reaches maturation
- Moral development (Lawrence Kohlberg)
  - This theory addresses the way children develop a sense of right and wrong
  - There are three sequential levels of cognitive development
    • Preconventional level of morality (ages 2 to 7) — the child attempts to follow rules set by those in authority; he tries to adjust his behavior according to good, bad, right, and wrong
    • Conventional level of morality (ages 7 to 12) — the child seeks conformity and loyalty; he attempts to justify, support, and maintain the social order and follows fixed rules
    • Postconventional autonomous level of morality (age 12 and older) — the adolescent strives to construct a personal and functional value system independent of authority figures and his peers

ASSESSING AND MEASURING GROWTH AND DEVELOPMENT

● **Chronological age**
  • Years or months since birth date

● **Mental age**
  • Level of cognitive function
  • This determination is based on at least two types of intelligence tests administered over 6 months, with the child in optimal health

● **Bone age**
  • Radiographic studies of the tarsals and carpals indicate the degree of ossification
  • This measure is used for the child who's shorter or taller than chronological age suggests

● **Adjusted or corrected age**
  • Chronological age minus the number of weeks born prematurely
  • Used up to age 2

● **Developmental assessment**
  • Determines whether the child has achieved certain expected goals during a developmental stage
  • If an expected goal isn't achieved, the acquisition of subsequent skills may be delayed
  • Denver Developmental Screening Test (Denver II)
    – The test is designed for a child up to age 6
    – It measures gross motor, fine motor, language, and personal–social development; it doesn't measure intelligence
  • Other standardized screening tests in use include:
    – Parents Evaluation of Developmental Status (PEDS) for children ages 0 to 8; has 10 items and is accompanied by a decision pathway
    – Ages and Stages Questionnaire (ASQ) for children ages 0 to 5; measures development of communication, gross motor, fine motor, problem-solving, and personal (social) skills

Factors measured by Denver Developmental Screening Test

• Gross motor function
• Fine motor function
• Language
• Personal-social development

INFANT (BIRTH THROUGH AGE 1)

● **Neonatal period (birth to 28 days)**
  • Head and chest circumferences are relatively equal; head circumference may be up to ¾″ (2 cm) greater than the chest circumference
  • Head length is one-fourth total body length
  • Brain growth depends on myelinization
  • All behavior is under reflex control; extremities are flexed
  • Hearing and touch are well developed; a hearing screening is recommended for all neonates
  • Vision is poor; the neonate fixates momentarily on light
  • The neonate is stimulated by being held or rocked, listening to music, and watching a black-and-white mobile
  • When lying prone, the neonate can lift his head

Normal findings in neonates

• Pulse rate: 110 to 160 beats/minute
• Respiratory rate: 32 to 60 breaths/minute
• Blood pressure: 82/46 mm Hg

- Normal pulse rate ranges from 110 to 160 beats/minute (count the apical pulse for 1 minute)
- Normal respiratory rate ranges from 32 to 60 breaths/minute
    - Respiration is irregular and from the abdomen
    - The neonate is an obligate nose breather
- Average blood pressure is 82/46 mm Hg (use the correct size cuff: one and one-half times the diameter of the extremity, or no less than one-half and no greater than two-thirds the length of the part of the extremity being used)
- Temperature regulation is altered because of poorly developed sweating and shivering mechanisms
    - Limit exposure time during baths
    - When the neonate is wet or cold, cover his head
- Mortality is higher in the neonatal period than in any other growth stage

Ages 1 to 4 months
- The posterior fontanel closes (usually by age 2 months)
- The infant begins to hold up his head
- At ages 4 to 8 weeks, reflexes reach their peak, especially the sucking reflex, which affords nutrition, survival, and psychological pleasure
- At age 3 months, the most primitive reflexes begin to disappear except for the protective and postural reflexes (blink, parachute, cough, swallow, and gag reflexes), which remain for life
- The infant observes people's faces and watches mobiles (an appropriate toy for an infant younger than age 3 months)
- The infant develops binocular vision; the eyes can follow an object 180 degrees and any intermittent strabismus should be resolved by age 4 months
- The infant begins to put his hand to his mouth
- The infant reaches out voluntarily but uncoordinatedly
- The infant cries to express needs
- The infant's instinctual smile appears at age 2 months and the social smile, at age 3 months
    - The social smile is the infant's first social response
    - The social smile initiates social relationships, indicates memory traces, and signals the beginning of thought processes
- At age 4 months, the infant laughs in response to his environment
- The infant recognizes his parents' voices
- The infant sits in an infant seat
- The infant explores his feet

Ages 5 to 6 months
- Birth weight doubles
- The infant can sleep through the night with one or two naps a day

Protective and postural reflexes that remain for life

- Blink
- Parachute
- Cough
- Swallow
- Gag

Role of the infant's social smile

- Initiates social relationships
- Indicates memory traces
- Signals the beginning of thought processes

- The infant begins teething (lower central incisors appear first); this may result in increased drooling and irritability
- The infant rolls over from his stomach to his back
- When lying prone, the infant uses his arms to push his chest up and to push his body toward his feet (crawl)
- The infant voluntarily grasps and releases objects
- The infant transfers toys from one hand to the other
- The infant sits with support
- The infant cries when his parents leave; this is a normal sign of attachment
- The infant discerns one face from another and exhibits stranger anxiety (is wary of strangers and clings to or clutches his parents)
- The infant begins to exhibit comforting habits — sucks his thumb, rubs his ear, holds a blanket or stuffed toy, rocks
  - All these habits symbolize parents and security
  - Thumb sucking in infancy doesn't result in malocclusion of permanent teeth

● Ages 7 to 9 months
- The infant sits alone without assistance
- The infant creeps on his hands and knees with his belly off of the floor
- The infant stands and stays up by grasping for support
- The infant develops a pincer grasp, places everything in his mouth, and is, therefore, at high risk for aspirating objects
- The infant self-feeds crackers; the infant who's physically and emotionally ready can begin to be weaned to a cup
- The infant verbalizes all vowels and most consonants but speaks no intelligible words
- The infant begins to imitate the expressions of others
- The infant likes to look in the mirror
- The infant develops object permanence and searches for objects outside his perceptual field
- The infant understands the word "no"; discipline can begin

● Ages 10 to 12 months
- Birth weight triples, and birth length increases about 50%
- The infant cruises (takes side steps while holding on) at age 10 months, walks with support at age 11 months, and stands alone and takes his first steps at age 12 months
- The infant says "mama" and "dada" and responds to his own name at age 10 months; he can say about five words but understands many more at age 12 months
- The infant claps his hands, waves bye-bye, and enjoys rhythm games
- The infant enjoys books and toys to build with and knock over

TOP 6

Checks in infant assessment

1. Head and chest circumferences in neonate are relatively equal.
2. Neonate's behavior is controlled by reflexes.
3. At ages 1 to 4 months, posterior fontanel closes.
4. At ages 5 to 6 months, birth weight doubles and infant voluntarily grasps and releases objects and exhibits signs of attachment to parent.
5. At ages 7 to 9 months, infant searches for objects outside his perceptual field.
6. At ages 10 to 12 months, birth weight triples and birth length increases about 50%.

Helping parents choose a feeding method

The infant's family needs information to make the right feeding choice. Be sure to provide information about the following feeding method options.

BREAST-FEEDING

With exclusive breast-feeding, the mother has no bottles or nipples to wash and sterilize and no formula to buy. An allergic reaction is less likely, and milk is always available. Night feedings are more convenient because there's no bottle to prepare. The infant benefits from the frequent direct physical contact, and the mother may feel that she has a more intimate bond with her baby.

Breast pump

When breast-feeding is inconvenient, the mother may express her milk by hand or with a breast pump for later bottle-feeding. With this method, the infant still receives only breast milk, but another family member may give the feeding.

Partial breast-feeding

Combined breast- and bottle-feeding should be discouraged because it significantly diminishes lactation. The best supplemental bottle contains pumped breast milk.

FORMULA FEEDING

Although breast-feeding has its advantages, formula feeding is an acceptable alternative. Many mothers choose this method to allow fathers to share in feeding. Also, it may be indicated when maternal illness makes breast-feeding unsafe (as with human immunodeficiency virus infection).

- The infant explores everything by feeling, pushing, turning, pulling, biting, smelling, and testing for sound

● **Nutrition guidelines**
  - Review guidelines with the parents
  - Introduce foods in this sequence:
    – Begin with breast milk or iron-fortified infant formula (see *Helping parents choose a feeding method*)
      · Breast milk provides the best nutrition for the infant; the American Academy of Pediatrics (AAP) and the American Dietetic Association recommend breast-feeding exclusively for the first 4 to 6 months of life and then in combination with infant foods until age 1
      - Breast-feeding right after birth helps the uterus to contract and return to its former size and position
      - Breast milk contains the perfect balance of carbohydrates, proteins, and fats
      - It supplies essential nutrients in an easily digestible form
      - Breast milk is a rich source of linoleic acid (an essential fatty acid) and cholesterol, which are needed for brain development

Benefits of breast milk

- Contains the perfect balance of carbohydrates, proteins, and fats
- Supplies essential nutrients in an easily digestible form
- Contains linoleic acid and cholesterol, which are needed for brain development
- Contains immune factors that protect infants from infection

Solid foods and infant age

This table gives an overview of solid foods that are appropriate for a developing infant.

AGE	TYPE OF FOOD	RATIONALE
4 months	Rice cereal mixed with formula	Less likely than wheat to cause an allergic reaction
5 to 6 months	Strained vegetables and fruits	Vegetables offered before fruit because they may be more readily accepted
6 to 8 months	Finger foods (bananas, crackers)	Promotes self-feeding
7 to 8 months	Strained meats, cheese, yogurt, rice, noodles, pudding	Important source of iron and adds variety to diet
10 months	Mashed egg yolk (avoid whites until age 1); bite-sized cooked food	Decreased risk of choking; although infant chews well, avoid foods likely to cause choking
12 months	Foods from the adult table	Chopped or mashed according to infant's ability to chew

- It contains immune factors that protect infants from infection, such as antibodies (especially immunoglobulin A) and white blood cells
– Give the breast-fed infant an iron supplement after age 4 months because the iron received before birth is depleted
– Provide a diet adequate in vitamin D to avoid rickets; breast-fed infants should be supplemented with 200 international units of vitamin D per day before age 2 months; commercial formula already is fortified with vitamin D
– Ideally, don't give solid foods for the first 6 months
  · Before age 6 months, the GI tract tolerates solid foods poorly
  · Because of a strong extrusion reflex, the infant pushes food out of his mouth
  · The risk of food allergy development may increase
– Provide rice cereal as the first solid food, followed by any other cereal except wheat
– Give yellow and green vegetables next
– Provide noncitrus fruits, followed by citrus fruits after age 6 months
– Give the infant teething biscuits during teething period
– Provide foods with sufficient protein, such as meat, after age 6 months (see *Solid foods and infant age*)
– After age 12 months, switch from formula to regular whole milk
  · Don't give skim milk because fatty acids are needed for myelinization

TOP 4

Nutrition guidelines for infants

1. Breast milk is best for the infant.
2. Parents using formula should switch to whole-fat milk after age 12 months and continue until age 2.
3. Baby bottles shouldn't be propped.
4. Only one new food should be introduced at a time; wait 4 to 7 days between each new food.

• Whole milk should be continued until age 2, as recommended by the AAP
• Follow these rules for feeding:
  – Don't prop up a baby bottle; propping increases the risk of aspiration as well as the development of otitis media and tooth decay
  – Add a fluoride supplement at age 2 weeks (for those infants who are breast-fed or receive ready-to-feed formula exclusively or who live in areas where the local water supply isn't adequately fluoridated)
    • Fluoride is essential for building strong teeth
    • It also provides resistance to dental caries
  – Don't put food or cereal in a baby bottle
  – Introduce one new food at a time; wait 4 to 7 days before introducing a new food to determine the infant's tolerance to it and the potential for allergy

● Safety guidelines (review with the parents)

• Follow crib guidelines
• Keep crib rails fully up at all times
  – Cribs should be placed away from windows and curtain cords
  – Crib slats should be no more than 2″ (5.1 cm) apart
• Use car seats properly
  – Car seats are required by law in all states
  – Follow the manufacturer's directions for use
• Never leave the infant unattended on the dressing table or any other high place; keep a hand on an infant who's lying on an open surface
• Always support an infant's head
• Check the temperature (90° to 100° F [32.2° to 37.8° C]) and depth (2″ at most) of bath water; constantly hold the infant during a bath
• Check the temperature of formula and foods; they should feel lukewarm when a few drops are placed on the caregiver's skin, typically the inner wrist area
  – Don't warm formula, breast milk, or foods in the microwave; doing so may cause uneven heating, resulting in burns
  – Defrosting breast milk in the microwave may destroy its immune factors
  – Set the hot water heater to 120° F (48.9° C)
• Remove potentially harmful items (pins, dust balls, small objects, and plastic bags) from the infant's environment to avoid aspiration or suffocation
• Insert safety plugs in wall outlets; prevent access to electrical cords
• Use gates across stairways and other potentially dangerous areas
• Use of walkers should be discouraged
• Place infants supine for sleep to decrease the risk of sudden infant death syndrome
  – Use a firm sleep surface

Safety guidelines for infants

• Always keep crib rails fully up.
• Follow car seat manufacturer's directions for use.
• Don't leave an infant unattended on an open surface.
• Place infants supine for sleep.

Food safety guidelines

• Check the temperature of formula and foods; they should feel lukewarm to the inside of the caregiver's wrist.
• Don't warm breast milk, formula, or foods in the microwave; uneven heating may cause burns.
• Avoid defrosting breast milk in the microwave; such heat may destroy the milk's immune factors.

– Keep soft objects and loose bedding out of crib
– Pillows, quilts, sheepskins, and comforters should be kept out of infant's sleeping environment
• Avoid overheating; infant should be lightly clothed for sleep

TODDLER (AGES 1 TO 3)

● Introduction
• This is a period of slow growth, with a weight gain of 4 to 6 lb (1.8 to 2.7 kg) per year
• Growth is measured in height rather than length
• Normal pulse rate is 100 beats/minute
• Normal respiratory rate is 26 breaths/minute
• Normal blood pressure is 99/64 mm Hg
• Vision still isn't mature
• The anterior fontanel closes between ages 12 and 18 months

● Psychosocial development
• The toddler is egocentric
• The toddler follows wherever his parents go
  – Start playing peek-a-boo to develop trust
  – Progress to playing hide-and-seek to reinforce the idea that his parents will return
• Separation anxiety arises
  – The toddler sees bedtime as desertion
  – The toddler develops a fear of the dark
  – Separation anxiety demonstrates closeness between the toddler and his parents; the toddler screams and cries when his parents leave and then may sulk and engage in comfort measures
  – The parent who's leaving should say so and should promise to return
    • The parent should leave a personal item with the toddler
    • Prepare the parents for the toddler's reaction, and explain that this process promotes trust
• Transitional objects (blankets, bottles, comforting habits) represent the toddler's parents and security; as long as they don't impede daily functioning and social interactions, they aren't detrimental to mental health
• If the toddler is a head-banger or rocks in bed, ensure his safety but ignore the behavior
• The toddler may engage in solitary play and have little interaction with others; this progresses to parallel play (the toddler plays alongside but not with other children)
• To promote the development of autonomy, allow the toddler to perform tasks independently

Normal findings in toddlers

• Average pulse rate: 100 beats/minute
• Average respiratory rate: 26 breaths/minute
• Average blood pressure: 99/64 mm Hg

Psychosocial developments in toddlers

• Egocentricity
• Separation anxiety
• Transitional objects
• Parallel play

Signs of cognitive development in the toddler

- Understands object permanence
- Engages in ritualistic behavior
- Exhibits magical thinking
- Uses symbols
- Shows curiosity
- Engages in imitative play and role play
- Points to mentioned body parts
- Recognizes himself in the mirror

Foods easily aspirated by the toddler

- Nuts
- Hot dogs
- Grapes
- Candy

● **Cognitive development**
- The toddler understands object permanence
- The toddler engages in ritualistic behavior to master skills and decrease anxiety
- The toddler exhibits magical thinking (believes that thoughts affect events)
- The toddler uses symbols (understands that gestures, such as waving bye-bye, have meaning)
- Memory and learning are enhanced by experiences
- The toddler shows curiosity about everything but isn't intentionally destructive; this curiosity can lead to aspiration or ingestion of dangerous items
- The toddler begins imitative play and role play to express his feelings
- The toddler lacks the concept of sharing and doesn't know the value of items
- The toddler points to mentioned body parts and recognizes himself in the mirror

● **Motor skills**
- The toddler explores the environment and is usually active
- The toddler uses his arms to balance
- The toddler plants his feet wide apart and walks by age 15 months; if this doesn't happen, seek further evaluation
    - Feet are flat with no arches
    - Provide push-pull toys to encourage walking
- The toddler climbs stairs at age 21 months, runs and jumps by age 2, and rides a tricycle by age 3
- The toddler has some difficulty coordinating the swallowing reflex and speaking

● **Dentition**
- First molars erupt (a child has 20 deciduous teeth by age 3)
- Introduce the toddler to a toothbrush but not yet to toothpaste; the toddler just swishes and swallows
- As necessary, continue fluoride use until age 12
- Prevent tooth decay by giving the toddler a cup containing water

● **Nutrition**
- The toddler feeds himself; provide finger foods in small portions
- Because the toddler has difficulty coordinating swallowing, avoid foods that can easily be aspirated, such as nuts, hot dogs, grapes, and candy (review with the parents)
- Nutritional needs decrease because of slow growth period
- Decreased appetite is apparent; because the child may appear to be a picky eater, nutritional content of foods is important

- The toddler shouldn't drink more than 24 oz (710 ml) of milk a day in order to have room for other nutritious foods

● **Language development**
  - Language aids the toddler's expression of feelings, experiences, and memory and provides a new way to manipulate the world
  - By age 2, the toddler uses 400 words as well as two- to three-word phrases and comprehends many more
  - Speech is egocentric
  - The toddler becomes frustrated at his inability to communicate, which may result in tantrums; allow more time for the toddler to ask questions and share feelings
  - At age 3, the toddler is a chatterbox, using about 11,000 words a day
  - The amount the toddler speaks is influenced by the amount spoken in his home
  - The toddler's speech should include four- to five-word sentences and be 75% intelligible by age 3; if not, seek further evaluation and assess his hearing
  - The toddler's ability to understand speech is more important than his ability to vocalize

● **Toilet training**
  - Training depends on the toddler's emotional readiness
    - The toddler acts to please others, trusts enough to give up his body products, and begins autonomous behavior
    - The parents must be committed to establishing a toileting pattern and must communicate well with the toddler, offering praise for success but no punishment for failure
  - Training also depends on the toddler's physical readiness
    - The toddler's bladder should reach adult functioning by age 2, with mature sphincter control
    - The toddler feels the discomfort of wet or messy pants, identifies elimination as the cause of this discomfort, and recognizes sensations before excretion
    - The toddler removes his own clothes, walks unaided, stoops and sits, talks, and imitates others
  - Toilet sitting should begin when the toddler demonstrates readiness (as described above) and shows interest
    - Provide a pleasant mood during this time
    - The toddler should use a potty seat or potty chair
    - The toddler may fear being sucked into the toilet
    - The toddler is curious about excretion products
    - Don't refer to bowel movements as being "dirty" or "yucky"
      - Excrement is the toddler's first creation

Language milestones in the toddler

- By age 2, the toddler uses 400 words as well as two- to three-word phrases.
- By age 3, the toddler uses about 11,000 words a day and should speak in four-to five-word sentences that are intelligible 75% of the time.

Toilet training tips for parents

- Begin training when the toddler demonstrates readiness.
- Provide a pleasant mood.
- Use a potty seat or potty chair.
- Be aware that the child is curious about excretion products.
- Don't refer to bowel movements as being "dirty" or "yucky."
- Teach hand washing.
- Teach front-to-back wiping.

Tips for handling a tantrum

- Don't reason, threaten, promise, hit, or give in to the toddler.
- Don't tell the toddler to wait.
- Respond calmly and consistently.

How the toddler responds to discipline

- Uses "no" excessively
- Shows assertiveness
- Is curious about how parents will react to "no"
- Becomes frustrated
- Wants immediate gratification
- May have tantrums

TOP 6

Safety guidelines for toddlers

1. Lock cabinets.
2. Don't leave the toddler unattended near bath tubs, pools, or buckets of water.
3. Check the size of toy parts and food particles.
4. Use safety plugs in electrical outlets.
5. Use safety gates on stairs.
6. Use child safety seats.

TIME-OUT FOR TEACHING

Handling tantrums

To prevent tantrums, the parents should:
- keep routines simple and consistent
- tell the toddler what behaviors are expected
- set reasonable limits and give rationales
- avoid head-on clashes
- provide limited, acceptable choices.
Instruct the parents that, during a tantrum, they should provide a safe environment for the toddler, identify the tantrum's cause, and help the toddler regain control. Also offer these tips:
- Don't reason, threaten, promise, hit, or give in to the toddler
- Don't tell the toddler to wait
- Respond calmly and consistently; follow through on discipline free of anger.

- Provide alternative toys, such as clay and water
  - Teach the toddler hand washing and front-to-back wiping
- With increased stress (such as a new baby in the family, a divorce, a vacation, a move), the toddler may regress; toileting may have to be delayed or retaught
- Introduce underpants as a badge of success and maturity
- Most toddlers achieve day dryness by age 18 months to 3 years and night dryness by ages 2 to 5
- If the toddler isn't trained by age 5, seek further evaluation

● **Discipline**
- The toddler uses "no" excessively and shows assertiveness
- The toddler is curious about how his parents will react to "no"
- The toddler becomes frustrated, wants immediate gratification, and acts out of anger; the toddler may lose control (see *Handling tantrums*)
- Overcriticizing and restricting the toddler may dampen his enthusiasm and increase shame and doubt

● **Sleep and rest guidelines**
- Total sleep required is about 12 to 14 hours
- Most toddlers continue to take a nap until age 3
- Sleep problems are common and related to fears of separation and the dark
  - Bedtime rituals help to decrease insecurity
  - Security objects, such as a blanket or favorite toy, are helpful

● **Safety guidelines (review with the parents)**
- When the toddler starts climbing over crib rails, switch to a bed
- Use locks or latches on cabinets; keep dangerous products in their original containers
- Keep the toddler away from toxic plants
- Keep pot and cup handles away from the edges of tables or stoves

- Don't leave the toddler unattended near bath tubs, pools, or buckets filled with water
- Check the size of toy parts and food particles to prevent choking
- Avoid beanbag toys; dried beans can cause instant death on aspiration
- Use safety plugs in electrical outlets
- Use safety gates at the top and bottom of stairs
- Continue to use child safety seats

PRESCHOOL CHILD (AGES 3 TO 5)

● **Introduction**
  - Slow growth continues during this period; birth length doubles by age 4
  - Average pulse rate ranges from 90 to 100 beats/minute
  - Average respiratory rate is 20 to 25 breaths/minute
  - Normal blood pressure ranges from 85/60 to 90/70 mm Hg
  - Attendance at day care or nursery school increases the child's contact with peers and the incidence of infection

● **Psychosocial development**
  - Language is egocentric and used to boast, brag, and shock others
  - The child identifies with the same-sex parent or primary caregiver; the child enjoys role playing, role modeling, and playing with dolls
  - The child shows anxiety about health care treatments and life events (use doll play to help the child prepare for or adjust to treatments)
  - The child shows fear concerning body integrity
    - Provide adhesive bandages for cuts because the child fears losing blood
    - Anticipate the child's fear of animal noises, new experiences, and the dark
  - Egocentricity decreases and awareness of others' needs increases
    - The child begins to share and take turns but continues to have difficulty with these concepts
    - The child attempts to please others
  - The child begins to develop a conscience and a superego
  - The child begins to function socially
    - The child learns rules
    - Nursery school enhances the child's social development
  - The child may exhibit sibling rivalry (reinforce the fact that each child is special)
  - The child may create an imaginary playmate to help deal with fears and loneliness; this is prevalent and normal in bright, creative children
  - Disciplinary actions should be consistent; using a time-out (no longer than 1 minute per year of age) is an effective disciplinary action (be-

---

What to expect in a toddler

- Gains 4 to 6 lb (1.8 to 2.7 kg) per year
- Exhibits egocentric behavior
- Demonstrates separation anxiety
- Climbs stairs at age 21 months, runs and jumps by age 2, and rides a tricycle by age 3
- Has first molars
- Says four- to five-word sentences and is 75% intelligible by age 3
- Begins toilet training

Normal findings in preschoolers

- Pulse rate: 90 to 100 beats/minute
- Respiratory rate: 20 to 25 breaths/minute
- Blood pressure: 85/60 to 90/70 mm Hg

Tips for disciplining a preschooler

- Use consistent disciplinary actions.
- Try using time-outs.
- Let the child know when a time-out is over.

cause the child has a poor concept of time, let the child know when a time-out is over)
- Don't compare children in terms of their psychosocial traits or abilities
- The child exhibits parallel play, associative play, group play in activities with few or no rules, and independent play accompanied by sharing or talking

● Cognitive development
- The child uses four- to five-word sentences but has difficulty with pronouns
- The child has limited perspective and focuses on one idea at a time
- The child becomes aware of racial and sexual differences
  - Boys may begin to masturbate
  - Begin sex education
- The child develops a body image
  - The parents should promote awareness of the positive aspects of both sexes
  - The parents should use appropriate names for body parts
  - The child can draw a person
- The child begins to have a concept of causality but still exhibits magical thinking
- The child begins to have a concept of time
  - The parents can explain time by referring to events
  - The child begins to have a concept of "today" and "tomorrow"
- The child begins to have a concept of numbers, letters, and colors
  - The child may count but may not understand what the numbers mean
  - The child may recognize some letters of the alphabet

● Motor skills
- The child dresses without help (but may be unable to tie his shoes until age 5)
- The child builds towers of blocks, copies circles and lines, uses scissors, strings large beads, and throws a ball overhead
- The child alternates feet on steps and hops on one foot; skips at age 5
- The child develops hand dominance
- The child enjoys the sandbox, water play, blocks, crayons, clay, and finger paints

● Nutrition
- The child may have strong food preferences
- Provide small, frequent meals with nutritious content; don't mix foods together
- The U.S. Department of Agriculture has developed the Food Guide Pyramid for Young Children, which is specifically targeted for children ages 2 to 6

Cognitive concepts developing in the preschooler

- Body image and differences
- Causality
- Time
- Letters
- Numbers
- Colors

Motor skill milestones for preschoolers

- Dresses without help
- Builds towers of blocks
- Copies circles and lines
- Uses scissors
- Strings large beads
- Throws a ball overhead
- Alternates feet on steps
- Hops on one foot
- Skips (at age 5)
- Develops hand dominance
- Enjoys the sand box, water play, blocks, crayons, clay, and finger paints

TIME-OUT FOR TEACHING

Tips for ensuring childhood health

To help ensure that a child takes in a balanced diet and maintains a healthy lifestyle, recommend these tips to parents and caregivers:

- Schedule regular mealtimes, and allow the child to participate in planning, preparing, and serving as well as cleaning up.
- Maintain variety because the child may prefer certain foods for a while and then suddenly refuse to eat them. This is normal.
- Have nutritional snacks readily available, especially when the child arrives home from school. Carrot and celery sticks and yogurt in cups or squeeze tubes are good possibilities.

- Prepare mildly flavored single-food dishes, which children tend to prefer. Many children don't like casseroles.
- Have the child get up early enough to be able to eat breakfast unhurriedly. Breakfast is an important meal.
- Encourage physical activity. Sports are increasingly an important and beneficial part of young children's lives. Also, keep in mind that physical activity other than sports is valuable as well and should be encouraged. Walks, bike rides, and other forms of loosely organized activities can be beneficial for children.

   – This guide attempts to make learning about nutrition fun and encourages the consumption of various foods
 • The child establishes eating behaviors (manners, sitting while eating, family meals, snacking) (see *Tips for ensuring childhood health*)

● **Readiness for kindergarten (age 5)**
 • The child picks up after himself
 • The child gets along without either parent for short periods
 • The child is less afraid
 • The child listens and follows directions
 • The child speaks in correct, complete sentences

SCHOOL-AGE CHILD (AGES 5 TO 12)

● **Introduction**
 • School shapes the child's cognitive and social development
 • Accidents are a major cause of death and disability during this period

● **Psychosocial development**
 • The teacher, perhaps the first important adult in the child's life besides the parents, may be a major influence
 • The child plays with peers
   – The child develops a first true friendship
   – The child develops a sense of belonging, cooperation, and compromise

Tips for ensuring childhood health

- Schedule regular mealtimes; allow the child to participate in planning, preparing, serving and cleaning up.
- Maintain variety in the diet.
- Have nutritional snacks readily available.
- Prepare mildly flavored single-food dishes.
- Make sure the child eats breakfast.
- Encourage physical activity.

Signs of kindergarten readiness

- Picks up after himself
- Gets along without either parent for short periods
- Is less afraid
- Listens and follows directions
- Speaks in correct, complete sentences

Psychosocial developments in the school-age child

- May be influenced by teacher
- Plays with peers
- Develops sense of morality
- Compares body to others
- Participates in family activities
- Becomes aware of social roles
- Engages in fantasy play and daydreaming
- May exhibit fear of death and school

– Groups offer a testing ground for the child's interpersonal interactions, development of self-concept, and sex-role behaviors
  · Groups encourage competition through fair play
  · Groups relieve the child of having to make decisions
• The child develops a sense of morality
  – The early school-age child sees actions as either right or wrong
  – After age 9, the child understands intent and differing points of view; the child's superego matures
• The child compares his own body to others and may become modest
• The child participates in family activities
• The child becomes aware of social roles
• The child engages in fantasy play and daydreaming
• The child may exhibit a fear of death and school phobias; these fears may cause psychosomatic illness

Cognitive development
• The child develops concepts of time and space, cause and effect, nesting (building blocks, puzzle pieces), reversibility, conservation (permanence of mass and volume), and numbers
• The child understands the relation of parts to the whole (fractions)
• The child learns to classify objects in more than one way
• The child learns to read and spell
• The child becomes interested in board games, cards, and collections

Physical development
• Slow growth continues during this period; height increases about 2″ (5 cm) per year, and weight doubles between ages 6 and 12
• The first primary tooth is displaced by a permanent tooth at age 6, and permanent teeth erupt by age 12, except for the final molars; the jaw grows to accommodate permanent teeth
  – This is a prime time for the development of dental caries
  – Nutrition and dental education should be reinforced in the home and school
• Vision matures by age 6
• Both sexes are about the same size until about age 9, when some females begin puberty and grow faster
• Bones grow faster than muscles and ligaments; therefore, the child is limber and prone to bone fractures
• Large and small muscle groups are refined
• Lymphoid tissue hypertrophies to maximum size
• Language development is perfected
• The child participates in group activities
  – The child likes to accomplish tasks
  – The child engages in cooperative play
  – The child's play involves group goals with interaction
  – The child plays by the rules but often cheats

Cognitive developments in the school-age child

• Time and space
• Cause and effect
• Nesting
• Reversibility
• Numbers
• Conservation (permanence of mass and volume)

Growth during the school-age years

• Period of slow growth
• Height increases about 2″ (5 cm) per year
• Weight doubles between ages 6 and 12

ADOLESCENT (AGES 12 TO 18)

● **Introduction**
- Adolescence is a rapid growth period characterized by puberty-related changes in body structure and psychosocial adjustment; nutritional needs increase significantly
- Vital signs approach adult values

● **Psychosocial and cultural development**
- Early adolescence is spent coping with changes in the physical self and becoming aware of the bodies of others
  - Fantasy thoughts and daydreams allow the adolescent to role-play different social situations
  - The adolescent may find that keeping a diary to express feelings helps
  - The adolescent may diet excessively to attempt to attain a desirable body image
- Middle adolescence involves exploring and identifying one's values and defining oneself
  - Peers may influence fad behavior, values, or conformity
  - Interest in the opposite sex increases; some adolescents may experience same-sex attractions
  - Eating is a social event and influenced by peers
- Late adolescence involves maturation, expressed by independence from parents and participation in society
  - Self-identity and personal morality develop
  - The adolescent begins to plan for the future
  - Concerns at this stage may range from acne and obesity to sexual identity and major social issues

● **Cognitive development**
- The adolescent develops abstract thinking and an increased ability to analyze, synthesize, and use logic
- The late adolescent reaches the cognitive level of an adult

● **Development of secondary sex characteristics**
- Development in the female
  - The hypothalamus signals the pituitary to release gonadotropins
    - This increases secretion of luteinizing hormone (LH) and follicle-stimulating hormone (FSH), which stimulate ovarian development and estrogen production
    - Estrogen produces all secondary sex characteristics except axillary and pubic hair, which are controlled by adrenal androgens
  - Breast development, or thelarche, is the first sign of puberty and begins at about age 9 with the bud stage
    - Breast development takes about 3 years to complete

Normal findings in adolescents

- Rapid growth
- Puberty-related changes
- Increased nutritional needs
- Vital signs approach adult values

Cognitive developments in the adolescent

- Abstract thinking
- Increased ability to analyze, synthesize, and use logic

Secondary sex characteristics in the female adolescent

- Breast development
- Increase in fatty tissue in the thighs, hips, and breasts
- Broadening of the hips
- Onset of menses
- Pubic hair growth
- Increase in sweat gland and sebaceous gland activity
- Increase in body odor
- Increase in acne

Secondary sex characteristics in the male adolescent

- Testicular enlargement
- Increase in muscle mass
- Broadening of the chest
- Increase in facial and body hair
- Voice deepens
- Pubic hair growth
- Increase in sweat gland and sebaceous gland activity
- Increase in body odor
- Increase in acne
- Nocturnal emissions
- Masturbation with ejaculation

Topics to include in sex education for adolescents

- Anatomy and physiology
- Values clarification
- Communication skills
- Role play and role modeling
- Alternatives
- Personal responsibility
- Respect for others

Common high-risk behaviors of adolescents

- Driving
- Sexual intercourse
- Smoking
- Drug abuse
- Alcohol abuse

- Breast development ends shortly after the first menses
  – Fatty tissue in the thighs, hips, and breasts increases; the hips broaden
  – The onset of menses occurs between ages 8 and 16; menses initially may be irregular
  – Pubic hair growth increases continuously for several years after menses begins
  – The female grows up to 3" (7.6 cm) a year and stops growing at about age 16
  – The sweat glands and sebaceous glands become more active; body odor and acne increase
- Development in the male
  – The hypothalamus signals the pituitary gonadotropins to release LH and FSH
    - LH results in testicular enlargement and the development of Leydig's cells in the testes, which produce testosterone
    - FSH stimulates the development of the seminiferous tubules of the testes, leading to spermatogenesis and fertility
  – Testicular enlargement signals the start of puberty
    - The scrotum enlarges, and the penis elongates and widens
    - The penis reaches adult size at about age 17
  – Muscle mass increases, the chest broadens, facial and body hair proliferates, and laryngeal cartilage growth deepens the voice
  – Pubic hair growth continues until age 20
  – The male grows up to 3½" (8.9 cm) per year and stops growing at about age 20
  – Sweat glands and sebaceous glands become more active; body odor and acne increase
  – Nocturnal emissions are common; many males who ejaculate for the first time in a nocturnal emission think that they have wet the bed
  – Masturbation with ejaculation is common

● **High-risk behaviors**
- Motor vehicle accidents are the primary cause of mortality and morbidity; car safety information is essential at this age
- One-half of all adolescents have had sexual intercourse by high school graduation
  – Sex education must be provided for both adolescents and their parents; communication between them should be encouraged
  – Sex education must include anatomy and physiology as well as values clarification, communication skills, role play and role modeling, alternatives, and the concepts of personal responsibility and respect for others

Danger signs of adolescent suicide

More than likely, you've read or heard about an adolescent committing suicide. Sometimes, young lovers or friends even commit suicide together. Do these adolescents give warning signs of their intentions? They commonly do. You should be aware of these warning signs and teach parents how to recognize them. The adolescent may:

- talk frequently about death or the futility of life
- exhibit dramatic mood changes
- appear sad or downcast or express feelings of hopelessness
- show loss of interest in friends or previous activities
- become increasingly withdrawn or spend more and more time alone
- begin having trouble at school or receiving poorer grades than usual
- exhibit behavioral changes that support alcohol or drug abuse
- start giving away favorite possessions
- seem unusually apathetic about the future.

Teach parents to never take any behavior for granted. Encourage them to follow their instincts. If they think that something is wrong with their son or daughter, they're probably right. They shouldn't try to rationalize or deny any behavior. If they suspect a problem, tell them to seek professional help. You should always stress to them the need to maintain communication with their child.

- – Discuss safe sex to prevent pregnancy and sexually transmitted diseases
- Smoking and drug and alcohol abuse are common risk-taking behaviors of adolescents
  - – Cognitive and affective information is needed
  - – Seeing the effects of drunk driving, hearing the stories of addicts, and visiting prison facilities can be effective in decreasing these behaviors
- Suicide is the third leading cause of death among adolescents
  - – Most teenagers who successfully commit suicide have made previous attempts
  - – A suicidal adolescent typically gives warning signs of his intentions (see *Danger signs of adolescent suicide*)
  - – Teach parents about such signs, and advise them to seek counseling immediately if their adolescent demonstrates these signs
  - – Suggest that parents keep guns and potentially lethal drugs properly secured

COMMUNICATING WITH A CHILD

- ● **Level of understanding**
  - Assess the child's level of understanding; use words the child can understand
  - Explain the reasons behind actions or events

Hospitalized child guidelines

- Tell the child when something will hurt.
- Avoid performing treatments in the playroom or the child's bed, if possible.
- Be aware that an adolescent requires independence; respect his privacy, allow autonomy, and anticipate concerns about the future.

Pain perception in the child

- Pain has physiologic and psychological components.
- The child may associate pain with punishment.
- Culture and child-rearing practices influence the expression of pain.
- Pain thresholds vary.

● **Self-esteem**
- Discipline is most effective if paired with praise and support for appropriate behaviors
- Allow the child to express feelings fully, and respect them
- Don't ask yes or no questions unless you'll accept either answer

● **Hospitalization guidelines**
- Prepare the child for hospitalization or treatment
  - Explain the purpose of equipment to be used
  - For young patients, demonstrate procedures on a doll first
  - Teach the child skills that will be needed after the procedure
  - Describe sensations that the child may experience
- Assess the hospitalized child's home routines, and attempt to implement them where possible
  - Develop a family-oriented environment in the hospital
  - Encourage the parents to participate; involve parents and child in the decision-making process
- Tell the child when something will hurt
- Provide play appropriate to the child's mental age and physical condition
- Provide choices
- Perform no treatments in the playroom or, if possible, the child's bed, which should be a safe place where no painful treatments are performed; take the child to the treatment room if possible
- Remember that a hospitalized adolescent faces special difficulties
  - The adolescent is in a dependent setting at a time when building independence is important
  - Encourage the family to respect the adolescent's privacy, recognize strengths, give as much autonomy as possible, and anticipate concerns about body image and how the illness will affect the future

PAIN PERCEPTION IN THE CHILD

● **Introduction**
- Pain has physiologic and psychological components
- Pain thresholds vary
- Expression of pain is influenced by culture and by child-rearing practices
- The infant consciously withdraws from pain or pulls on the affected part
- The child may associate pain with punishment

● **Assessment**
- Determine the intensity, type, location, duration, and circumstances of the pain; assess whether the child can be distracted from the pain

- Assess for crying, facial grimaces, restlessness, irritability, insomnia, anger, diaphoresis, increased pulse and respiratory rates, decreased interactions and withdrawal, diminished appetite, fatigue, and behavioral changes
- Assess the child's body language
- Use available pediatric pain assessment scales; ask the child to describe his pain, or give the child a scale to grade his pain's severity

● **Pain management interventions**
- Administer pain medication without delay to relieve the child's discomfort
- Apply comfort measures
- Apply kinesthetic comfort measures and offer tender care; give the child an adhesive bandage for minor pain
- Offer distraction, such as reading a story or playing a game
- Stay with the child; let the child assist in painful procedures (such as helping to remove a bandage) to gain a sense of control
- Reinforce the fact that pain isn't a punishment for misbehavior
- For adolescents, behavioral contracting may be useful in chronic pain experiences
- Several medications are commonly used for pain relief in children
  - Morphine is the standard for severe pain; meperidine (Demerol) is no longer the drug of choice
  - Moderate pain can be managed by nonsteroidal anti-inflammatory drugs (ibuprofen [Motrin]) and opioid analgesics (codeine)
  - Mild pain can be managed by acetaminophen (Tylenol) or ibuprofen
  - For children who require invasive procedures (lumbar punctures, multiple blood sticks or injections) or who have an intense fear of these procedures, topical EMLA cream (lidocaine and prilocaine) provides numbness to the area 1 hour after it's applied
- Patient-controlled analgesia can be used by children age 5 and older; parent-controlled analgesia can be used with younger children
- After the pain resolves, provide play that lets the child express feelings

MEDICATION ADMINISTRATION

● **Dosage calculation**
- Dosage is individualized for each child
- Dosage is commonly determined by an assessment of body surface area (BSA) or kilograms of body weight
  - The BSA method is used to calculate safe pediatric doses for a limited number of drugs, such as chemotherapeutic agents
    - BSA is measured in meters squared (m^2)

Common pain medications

- Morphine (for severe pain)
- Nonsteroidal anti-inflammatory drugs, such as ibuprofen and opioid analgesics (for moderate pain)
- Acetaminophen or ibuprofen (for mild pain)

Body surface area basics

- Used to calculate safe pediatric doses for a limited amount of drugs
- Measured in m^2
- May provide most accurate calculation because the child's BSA closely parallels his metabolic rate and organ growth and maturation

Medication administration conversions

- 1 teaspoon = 5 ml
- 1 tablespoon = 15 ml
- 1 oz = 30 ml

Administering medications

- Dosage is commonly based on BSA or kilograms of body weight.
- Don't use the dorsogluteal muscle for I.M. or S.C. injections until age 3.
- When giving I.M. or S.C. injections, use the vastus lateralis site for a child younger than age 3 and the deltoid site after toddlerhood.
- Use an infusion pump with infants and young children.
- Inspect I.V. sites frequently for infiltration and inflammation.

• This method, although not the most common, may provide the most accurate calculation because the child's BSA probably parallels his metabolic rate and organ growth and maturation
– Pediatric dosages based on body weight are usually expressed as milligrams per kilogram per day (mg/kg/day) or per dose (mg/kg/dose)
• For home medication administration: 1 teaspoon = 5 ml; 1 tablespoon = 15 ml; 1 oz = 30 ml

Oral medications
• Allow the child as much choice as possible (for instance, which pill to take first or which beverage to drink)
• Hold the infant with his head elevated to prevent aspiration
• For the infant, slowly instill liquid medication by dropper along the side of his tongue or offer it through a nipple
• For the infant and the young child, crush pills and mix them with ½ teaspoon of baby food or any sweet-tasting substance; never crush timed-release capsules or tablets or enteric-coated drugs; crushing destroys the coating that prevents stomach irritation and causes drugs to release at the right time
• For medications delivered through a gastrostomy or nasogastric tube, flush after administration

Intramuscular (I.M.) or subcutaneous (subQ) injections
• Select the needle length according to the patient's muscle size
• Don't inject into the dorsogluteal muscle until age 3
– Because the muscle isn't well developed until the child walks, the sciatic nerve occupies a larger portion of the area than it will later on and could become permanently damaged by gluteal injections
– Use the vastus lateralis site for children younger than age 3; the deltoid site can be used after toddlerhood (see *I.M. injection sites in children*)
• Don't give an infant more than 0.5 ml in any site or a child more than 1 ml in any site
• Use the Z-track method for iron dextran administration to prevent tracking the drug through the tissues

Intravenous medications
• I.V. site placement may be in a peripheral or central vein
• Because pediatric patients can tolerate only a limited amount of fluid, dilute I.V. drugs and administer I.V. fluids cautiously
• Always use an infusion pump with infants and young children
• Inspect I.V. sites frequently for signs of infiltration (cool, blanched, and puffy skin) or inflammation (warm and reddened skin)
– Do this before, during, and after the infusion because children's vessels are immature and easily damaged by drugs

I.M. injection sites in children

When selecting the best site for a child's I.M. injection, consider the child's age, weight, and muscle development; the amount of subcutaneous fat over the injection site; the type of drug you're administering; and the drug's absorption rate.

VASTUS LATERALIS AND RECTUS FEMORIS

For a child younger than age 3, you'll typically use the vastus lateralis or rectus femoris muscle for an I.M. injection. Constituting the largest muscle mass in this age-group, the vastus lateralis and rectus femoris have fewer major blood vessels and nerves.

VENTROGLUTEAL AND DORSOGLUTEAL

For a child who can walk and is older than age 3, use the ventrogluteal and dorsogluteal muscles. Like the vastus lateralis, the ventrogluteal site is relatively free of major blood vessels and nerves. Before you select either site, make sure that the child has been walking for at least 1 year to ensure sufficient muscle development.

DELTOID

For a child older than 18 months who needs rapid medication results, consider using the deltoid muscle. Because blood flows faster in the deltoid muscle than in other muscles, drug absorption should be faster. Be careful if you use this site because the deltoid doesn't develop fully until adolescence. In a younger child, it's small and close to the radial nerve, which may be injured during needle insertion.

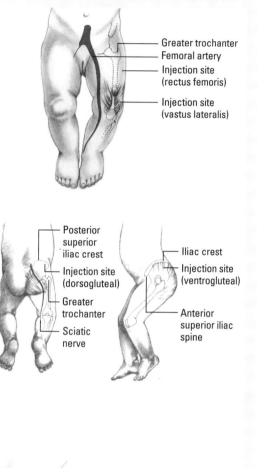

Greater trochanter
Femoral artery
Injection site (rectus femoris)
Injection site (vastus lateralis)

Posterior superior iliac crest
Injection site (dorsogluteal)
Greater trochanter
Sciatic nerve

Iliac crest
Injection site (ventrogluteal)
Anterior superior iliac spine

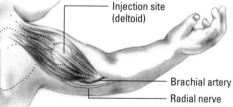

Injection site (deltoid)
Brachial artery
Radial nerve

Pediatric I.M. injection sites

- Vastus lateralis and rectus femoris muscles
- Ventrogluteal and dorsogluteal muscles
- Deltoid muscle

Factors to consider when selecting I.M. injection sites

- Age
- Weight
- Muscle development
- Amount of subcutaneous fat
- Type of drug
- Drug's absorption rate

Understanding intraosseous administration

In an emergency, intraosseous drug administration may be used for a critically ill child younger than age 6. A bone marrow needle (or spinal needle with stylette, trephin, or standard 16G to 18G hypodermic needle) inserted into the anteromedial surface of the proximal tibia ⅜″ to 1¼″ (1 to 3 cm) below the tibial tuberosity. To avoid the epiphyseal plate, the needle is directed at a perpendicular or slightly inferior angle.

After the bony cortex is penetrated and the needle is inserted in the marrow cavity, the bone marrow can be aspirated. The needle will remain upright without support, and the infusion will flow freely without subcutaneous infiltration.

When the needle is properly inserted, it's stabilized and secured with gauze dressing and tape. It will be discontinued when a secure I.V. line is established.

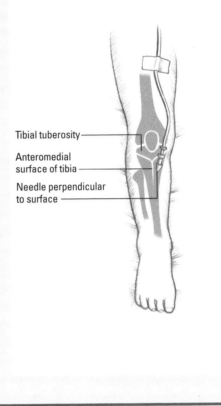

Tibial tuberosity

Anteromedial surface of tibia

Needle perpendicular to surface

● **Intraosseous administration**
- This emergency route is used to administer fluids, blood, and medication when I.V. access is unavailable (see *Understanding intraosseous administration*)
- It allows drug infusion through a needle in the medullary cavity of a long bone; from there, the medication drains through marrow sinusoids into large medullary venous channels and into the systemic circulation

● **Nose drops**
- Instill in one naris at a time in infants because they're obligate nose breathers

● **Ear medications**
- Pull the ear down and back to instill eardrops in infants; pull the ear up and out to instill eardrops in older children
- Have medication at room temperature

● **Rectal medication**
- Insert the suppository past the anal sphincter

Tips for instilling ear medications

- In infants, pull the ear down and back.
- In older children, pull the ear up and out.

- Hold buttocks together for a few seconds after insertion to prevent expulsion of the medication

● **Inhalers**

- Shake the inhaler for 2 to 5 seconds
- Position the inhaler with the canister above the mouthpiece
- After a normal exhale, have the child inhale slowly as the canister is pressed down
- Have the child hold his breath for a few seconds after the medication is released
- Inhalers without spacers aren't placed in the mouth; inhalers with spacers require the child to make a seal around the mouthpiece before inhaling; masks with spacers can be used for infants

NCLEX CHECKS

It's never too soon to begin your NCLEX preparation. Now that you've reviewed this chapter, carefully read each of the following questions and choose the best answer. Then compare your responses to the correct answers.

1. A bottle-fed infant, age 3 months, is brought to the pediatrician's office for a well-child visit. During the previous visit, the nurse taught the mother about infant nutritional needs. Which statement by the mother during the current visit indicates effective teaching?

☐ **1.** "I started the baby on cereals and fruits because he wasn't sleeping through the night."

☐ **2.** "I started putting cereal in the bottle with formula because the baby kept spitting it out."

☐ **3.** "I'm giving the baby iron-fortified formula and a fluoride supplement because our water isn't fluoridated."

☐ **4.** "I'm giving the baby skim milk because he was getting so chubby."

2. A nurse is teaching new parents about normal infant development. Voluntary grasp is usually present at what age?

☐ **1.** 2 weeks
☐ **2.** 1 month
☐ **3.** 3 months
☐ **4.** 5 months

3. A parent whose family drinks low-fat milk asks if her child can begin to drink low-fat milk. The AAP recommends that children can begin to drink low-fat milk at what age?

☐ **1.** 1 year
☐ **2.** 2 years
☐ **3.** 6 years
☐ **4.** 12 years

TOP 9

Items to study for your next test on nursing care during growth and development

1. Four developmental stages
2. Theories of growth and development
3. Nutrition guidelines for infants
4. Psychosocial characteristics of toddlers
5. Motor skill milestones for preschoolers
6. Normal growth during the school-age years
7. Cognitive development in adolescents
8. Pain assessment in children
9. Administration of oral, I.M., and subcutaneous injections

4. A nurse is teaching new parents before discharge to home. She explains that the anterior fontanel normally closes between ages:

☐ **1.** 2 and 3 months.
☐ **2.** 12 and 18 months.
☐ **3.** 3 and 6 months.
☐ **4.** 1 and 9 months.

5. A nurse is caring for children in a day-care center. According to the theorist Jean Piaget, an infant who learns about objects by placing them in his mouth is in which stage of development?

☐ **1.** Preoperational
☐ **2.** Sensorimotor
☐ **3.** Concrete operational
☐ **4.** Formal operational

6. While preparing to teach a class on child development, a nurse reviews the works of a theorist who postulated that the personality is a structure with three parts, called the id, the ego, and the superego. This theorist is:

☐ **1.** Sigmund Freud.
☐ **2.** Erik Erikson.
☐ **3.** Jean Piaget.
☐ **4.** Lawrence Kohlberg.

7. While evaluating nursing care in a community clinic, a nurse finds that toddlers are at high risk for injuries because of their increasing curiosity, advancement in cognition, and improved motor skills. All these hazards are a concern for this age-group except:

☐ **1.** burns.
☐ **2.** poisoning.
☐ **3.** sports injury.
☐ **4.** falls.

8. A nurse is preparing to administer an I.M. injection to a child who's age 2. Identify the correct area for this injection.

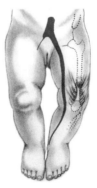

9. In a clinic, the mother of an 8-month-old asks the nurse what to feed her infant because she wants to stop breast-feeding. The nurse recommends:

☐ **1.** formula.

☐ **2.** 2% milk.

☐ **3.** whole milk.

☐ **4.** orange juice.

10. Directional trends in growth and development are easily seen in the neonate. Which term describes development in the head-to-tail direction?

☐ **1.** Sequential trend

☐ **2.** Proximodistal pattern

☐ **3.** Cephalocaudal trend

☐ **4.** Mass to specific pattern

ANSWERS AND RATIONALES

1. CORRECT ANSWER: 3

Iron-fortified formula supplies all the nutrients an infant needs during the first 6 months; however, fluoride supplementation is necessary if the local water supply isn't fluoridated. Before age 6 months, solid foods, such as cereals, aren't recommended because the GI tract tolerates them poorly. Also, a strong extrusion reflex causes the infant to push food out of his mouth. Mixing solid foods in a bottle with liquids deprives the infant of experiencing new tastes and textures and may interfere with development of proper chewing. Skim milk doesn't provide sufficient fat for an infant's neural growth.

2. CORRECT ANSWER: 4

At age 5 months, or 20 weeks, an infant can grasp an object voluntarily. At ages 2 to 6 weeks, the hands are mainly closed. At age 3 months, the hands are mostly open. At age 16 weeks, the infant begins to put his hands together.

3. CORRECT ANSWER: 2

Whole milk is recommended until a child is 2 years old to provide enough fat for the rapidly growing child. By age 2, low-fat dairy products, such as 2% milk, can be introduced.

4. CORRECT ANSWER: 2

The anterior fontanel stays open to allow for the rapid growth of brain tissue over the first year of life. It normally closes between ages 12 and 18 months. The smaller posterior fontanel closes between ages 6 and 8 weeks.

5. CORRECT ANSWER: 2

In the sensorimotor stage, from birth through age 2 years, the infant is exploring the world by gaining input through the senses and through motor activity. During the preoperational stage, a 2- to 7-year-old child uses words as symbols but hasn't yet developed a sense of logic. During the concrete operational stage, a 7- to 10-year-old child learns that matter doesn't change when its form is altered. (A ball of clay that's flattened is still clay.) The stage of formal operations is achieved when an adolescent can think abstractly about objects or concepts and consider different alternatives or outcomes.

6. CORRECT ANSWER: 1

Freud developed a theory that sexual energy is centered in specific parts of the body at certain ages: oral, anal, and genital. He also viewed the personality as a structure with three parts: the id, ego, and superego. Erikson developed a theory of psychosocial development that stresses the importance of culture and society in personality development. Piaget focused his theory on cognitive development. Kohlberg focused on a theory of moral development.

7. CORRECT ANSWER: 3

Toddlers are at risk for falls, burns, and poisoning because of their curiosity and developing motor skills. Adolescents are at high risk for sports injuries because of their increased independence.

8. CORRECT ANSWER:

For a child younger than age 3, the vastus lateralis muscle should be used to administer an intramuscular injection.

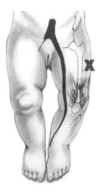

9. CORRECT ANSWER: 1

Formula is most appropriate for an 8-month-old infant when the mother decides to stop breast-feeding. Whole milk shouldn't be offered until the infant is age 12 months. Two-percent milk isn't recommended until the child is 2 years old. Orange juice is added only after the first year because of a high incidence of allergies.

10. CORRECT ANSWER: 3

A cephalocaudal trend describes development from head to tail. Sequential trends describe growth and development as a definite, predictable sequence, with each child normally passing through every stage. Proximodistal refers to the midline-to-peripheral growth pattern. Mass to specific pattern describes development from simple operations to more complex activities.

2

Conditions interfering with pediatric health

PRETEST

1. The chromosomal pattern of a cell is also known by what term?

☐ 1. Karyotype
☐ 2. Congenital
☐ 3. Genetic
☐ 4. Phenotype

CORRECT ANSWER: 1

2. Which disorder is transmitted as an autosomal recessive trait?

☐ 1. Hemophilia
☐ 2. Neurofibromatosis
☐ 3. Marfan syndrome
☐ 4. Cystic fibrosis

CORRECT ANSWER: 4

3. What type of disorders are abnormalities that result from at least two inherited abnormal genes and environmental factors?

☐ 1. Autosomal dominant
☐ 2. Multifactorial
☐ 3. Autosomal recessive
☐ 4. X-linked

CORRECT ANSWER: 2

4. What term is used to describe when a chromosome breaks and the parts connect to another chromosome?

☐ 1. Mosaicism
☐ 2. Mutation
☐ 3. Translocation
☐ 4. Deletion

CORRECT ANSWER: 3

5. Within what time frame after ingestion of a large dose of acetaminophen (Tylenol) does hepatic involvement occur?

☐ 1. 1 to 2 hours
☐ 2. 2 to 4 hours
☐ 3. 1 to 2 days
☐ 4. 3 to 4 days

CORRECT ANSWER: 4

LEARNING OBJECTIVES

After studying this chapter, you should be able to:

● Identify the physical, genetic, psychosocial, and environmental factors that can alter growth and development.

● Plan nursing interventions to prevent deficits in growth and development and to promote safety.

● Describe the impact of a chronic condition on the child and his family.

● Discuss appropriate nursing interventions for pediatric rehabilitation.

CHAPTER OVERVIEW

Conditions that interfere with pediatric health can affect the nurse's role in helping to promote the birth, growth, and development of a healthy child. Thorough assessment and prompt interventions for these conditions are essential to the practice of pediatric nursing. For children with chronic illnesses or disabilities, rehabilitation and habilitation address the special concerns of the pediatric patient to promote the child's optimal growth and development.

GENETIC ALTERATIONS

● Introduction
- Human cells contain 46 chromosomes in each nucleus (23 pairs)
  - Each chromosome contains thousands of genes
  - Chromosomes are shaped like an X (except the male Y chromosome, which is shaped like an X without a leg)
- Genes are the structures responsible for hereditary characteristics; they may or may not be expressed or passed to the next generation
- Genotype refers to the sequence and combination of genes on a chromosome
- Alleles are pairs of genes located on the same site on paired chromosomes
  - Homozygous alleles are identical (DD or dd)
  - Heterozygous alleles are two different alleles for the same trait (Dd)
- Mendel's law states that one gene for each hereditary property is received from each parent; one is dominant (expressed) and one is recessive
- A karyotype is the chromosomal pattern of a cell, including genotype, number of chromosomes, and normality or abnormality of the chromosomes
- A phenotype is the observable expression of the genes (for example, hair and eye color, body build, allergies)
- Congenital and genetic aren't synonymous
  - Congenital means present at birth because of abnormal development in utero (teratology)
  - Genetic pertains to the genes or chromosomes; some genetic disorders may be noticeable at birth and others may not appear for decades

● Types of genetic disorders
(see *Patterns of transmission in genetic disorders,* page 36)
- Mendelian or single-gene disorders are inherited in clearly identifiable patterns; they may be:
  - Autosomal, resulting from a single altered gene or a pair of altered genes on one of the first 22 pairs of autosomes

Role of genes
- Genes are responsible for hereditary characteristics.
- Genes may or may not be expressed or passed to the next generation.
- According to Mendel's law, one gene for each hereditary property is received from each parent.

Quick guide to genetic terms
- **Alleles** – pairs of genes located on the same site on paired chromosomes
- **Congenital** – present at birth because of abnormal development in utero
- **Genetic** – pertaining to genes or chromosomes
- **Genotype** – the sequence and combination of genes on a chromosome
- **Karyotype** – chromosomal pattern of a cell
- **Phenotype** – the observable expression of the genes

Types of genetic disorders
- Mendelian or single-gene disorders (includes autosomal and X-linked disorders)
- Chromosomal aberrations or abnormalities
- Multifactorial disorders

Autosomal dominant disorders

- Huntingdon's disease
- Osteogenesis imperfecta
- Neurofibromatosis
- Night blindness

Autosomal recessive disorders

- Cystic fibrosis
- Sickle cell anemia
- Phenylketonuria
- Tay-Sachs disease
- Albinism

Patterns of transmission in genetic disorders

These genetic disorders are grouped according to their pattern of transmission.

AUTOSOMAL DOMINANT
Achondroplasia (dwarfism)
Colorectal polyposis
Hereditary hemorrhagic telangiectasia
Huntington's disease
Hyperlipidemias (some types)
Marfan syndrome
Neurofibromatosis (most cases)
Night blindness
Osteogenesis imperfecta (most cases)
Pituitary diabetes insipidus
Retinoblastoma
Spherocytosis

AUTOSOMAL RECESSIVE
Albinism (some cases)
Congenital adrenal hyperplasia
Cretinism
Cystic fibrosis
Cystinuria
Fabry's disease
Fanconi's anemia
Galactosemia
Niemann-Pick disease
Osteogenesis imperfecta (some cases)
Phenylketonuria
Retinitis pigmentosa (some cases)
Sickle cell anemia

Tay-Sachs disease
Thalassemia (alpha and beta)
Xeroderma pigmentosum (most cases)

X-LINKED
Duchenne-type muscular dystrophy
Fragile X mental retardation
Glucose-6-phosphate dehydrogenase
  deficiency
Hemophilia (most types)
Pseudohypoparathyroidism
Some immunodeficiencies

CHROMOSOMAL
Cri du chat syndrome
Down syndrome (trisomy 21)
Edwards' syndrome (trisomy 18)
Klinefelter's syndrome (XXY)
Patau's syndrome (trisomy 13)
Turner's syndrome (XO)

MULTIFACTORIAL
Cleft lip or palate (some cases)
Congenital heart defects (some cases)
Diabetes mellitus (some cases)
Mental retardation (some cases)
Neural tube defects

- Autosomal dominant—a dominant allele produces its effect in heterozygotes (people who also carry a normal gene for the same trait) because the dominant allele masks the effects of the normal gene
  - Examples include Huntington's disease, osteogenesis imperfecta, neurofibromatosis, and night blindness
  - Offer genetic counseling; with each pregnancy in which only one parent is a heterozygotic carrier comes a 50% chance of having a child with the disease or disorder and a 50% chance of having a normal child
- Autosomal recessive—a recessive allele can produce a disorder only when paired with another disease-causing allele; offspring must receive one copy of the disease-causing allele from each parent to inherit the recessive trait (see *Inheritance patterns*)
  - Almost all carriers are free from symptoms
  - Examples include cystic fibrosis, sickle cell anemia, phenylketonuria, Tay-Sachs disease, and albinism

Inheritance patterns

Single-gene inheritance patterns are depicted below.

AUTOSOMAL DOMINANT DISORDERS

One heterozygous affected parent

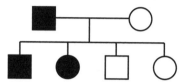

50% recurrence risk, regardless of sex

Both heterozygous affected parents

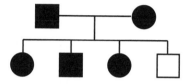

75% recurrence risk, regardless of sex

AUTOSOMAL RECESSIVE DISORDERS

One parent affected

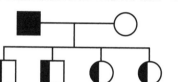

0% offspring affected; 100% carriers

Both parents carriers

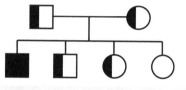

25% risk for being affected; 50% risk for being a carrier, regardless of sex

SEX-LINKED RECESSIVE DISORDERS

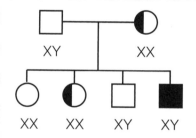

50% risk with every pregnancy with a male fetus
50% carrier risk with every pregnancy with a female fetus

100% sons normal
100% daughters carriers

KEY

☐ Male   ◻◐ Carrier
○ Female   ●■ Persons affected by disease

Sex-linked disorders

- These disorders result from an altered gene on the X chromosome.
- A father with an X-linked disorder will pass the trait on to his daughters but not his sons; none of his children will have the disease.
- Daughters with the trait have a 50% chance with each pregnancy of passing the disease or disorder to their sons.

Chromosomal aberrations and abnormalities

- Mutation: a spontaneous alteration in genes or chromosomes not present in the previous generation
- Nondisjunction: the failure of one pair of chromosomes from either parent to separate during meiosis, usually resulting in 45 or 47 chromosomes in the offspring
- Deletion: the loss of a chromosome during cell division, producing varying effects in the offspring, depending on the type and amount of genetic material lost
- Translocation: when a chromosome breaks and the parts connect to another chromosome, or when the genes switch their order or spacing
- Mosaicism: abnormal chromosomal division in the zygote resulting in two or more cell lines with different chromosomes

  - Offer genetic counseling; with each pregnancy in which each parent is a heterozygous carrier comes a 25% chance of having a child with the disease or disorder, a 50% chance of having a child who's a carrier, and a 25% chance of having a normal child
  – Sex-linked, resulting from an altered gene on the sex chromosome; almost all appear on the "X" and are recessive; they're sometimes referred to as *sex-linked* or *x-linked*
    · X-linked recessive inheritance — nearly all affected people are males because females have two X chromosomes and males have an X and a Y chromosome; recessive alleles on a male's X chromosome are expressed
    · X-linked dominant inheritance — females are affected to varying degrees; these disorders tend to be lethal in males
    · Examples include hemophilia A and B, color blindness, Duchenne-type muscular dystrophy, and glucose-6-phosphate dehydrogenase deficiency
    · Offer genetic counseling; the father with a sex-linked disorder will pass the trait to all his daughters but to none of his sons; however, none of his children will have the disease; his daughters will have a 50% chance with each pregnancy of passing the disease or disorder to their sons
- Chromosomal aberrations or abnormalities include structural defects within a chromosome, such as deletion and translocation, plus absence or addition of complete chromosomes
  – Mitosis is normal cell division, resulting in an exact copy of the parent cell
  – Meiosis is normal cell division of the ova and spermatozoon for procreation, resulting in 23 chromosomes (one chromosome from each of the 23 pairs); this is called *reduction division*
  – Mutation is a spontaneous alteration in genes or chromosomes not present in the previous generation
  – Nondisjunction is the failure of one pair of chromosomes from either parent to separate during meiosis, usually resulting in 45 or 47 chromosomes in the offspring
    · Monosomy indicates 45 chromosomes; most monosomies are incompatible with life
    · Trisomy indicates 47 chromosomes
  – Deletion is the loss of a chromosome during cell division, producing varying effects in the offspring, depending on the type and amount of genetic material lost
  – Translocation occurs when the chromosome breaks; the parts may connect to another chromosome, or the genes may switch their order or spacing

– Mosaicism refers to abnormal chromosomal division in the zygote, resulting in two or more cell lines with different chromosomes
- Multifactorial disorders are abnormalities that result from the interaction of at least two inherited abnormal genes and environmental factors
  – Such disorders don't follow the Mendelian patterns of inheritance
  – The increased incidence of specific birth defects within families suggests familial transmission

CHILD ABUSE

● **Introduction**
- Child abuse involves intentional acts of physical, emotional, psychological, or sexual abuse of a child or neglect of a child
- Infants and toddlers are the most common victims of physical abuse; school-age children and adolescents are at a higher risk for emotional and sexual abuse
- Child abuse usually indicates a serious family dysfunction in communicating and coping; the child, the focal point of stress, usually becomes a scapegoat
- Child abuse may result from the parents' unrealistic expectations of the child's physical and psychosocial abilities
- Child abusers come from all social classes and educational backgrounds; about 10% have serious psychological disturbances (see *Child abuse: Seeing the reality*)
  – Many child abusers were abused as children and may not know healthier ways to discipline a child or to show love

Types of child abuse

- Physical abuse
- Emotional and psychological abuse
- Sexual abuse
- Neglect

Child abuse: Seeing the reality

Many people believe that child abuse occurs only in poorly educated, disadvantaged families. Don't be blinded by this stereotype. Child abuse exists at every socioeconomic level and among seemingly well-adjusted parents and children.

The abusive parent may:
- feel intensely anxious about the child's behavior
- feel guilty and angry about the inability to provide for the child
- have also been a victim of child abuse
- believe that physical punishment is the best discipline
- lack a strong emotional attachment to the child
- misuse alcohol or other drugs.

Characteristics of an abused child include:
- a history of behavior problems
- unusual bruises, welts, burns, fractures, and bite marks
- long sleeves and other concealing clothing, worn to hide injuries
- frequent injuries, explained by parents as accidents
- unusual shyness toward adults and children
- a tendency to avoid physical contact with adults
- a fearful attitude around parents.

Signs of abuse

- History of behavior problems
- Unusual bruises, welts, burns, fractures, and bite marks
- Concealing clothing
- Frequent injuries (explained as accidents)
- Unusual shyness
- Tendency to avoid physical contact with adults
- Fearful attitude around parents
- Physical findings that don't match history

Your role in reporting abuse

As a nurse, you play a crucial role in recognizing and reporting incidents of suspected abuse. While caring for patients, you can readily note evidence of apparent abuse. When you do, you must pass the information along to the appropriate authorities. In many states, failure to report actual or suspected abuse constitutes a crime.

If you've ever hesitated to file an abuse report because you fear repercussions, remember that you're protected against liability by the Child Abuse Prevention and Treatment Act. If your report is bona fide (that is, if you file it in good faith), the law protects you from any suit filed by an alleged abuser.

Assessing for child abuse

- Discover any inconsistencies in the history by interviewing the child and caregivers separately.
- Don't examine the child alone.
- Observe parent-child interactions.
- Describe each injury and its stage of healing.
- Note if the injury or symptoms fit the accident or illness.
- If there has been a delay in seeking help, ask the parents to explain why.
- Suspect abuse if the injury doesn't match the accident and X-rays show old fractures.
- Suspect abuse when signs of neglect are absent.

How to intervene when you suspect abuse

- Meet the child's needs first, regardless of suspicions.
- Protect the child and try to prevent further abuse.
- Report suspected abuse to the proper authorities.

  – Child abusers characteristically have low self-esteem, little confidence, and a low tolerance for frustration
- Sexual abuse may not be perceived by the child as wrong at first because most victims know and trust their abusers

Assessment
- Try to interview the child and the caregivers separately to note inconsistencies with histories
- Don't examine the child alone
- Observe parent-child interactions, carefully noting what the child and the parents say
- Describe each sore, bruise, or burn and its stage of healing
- Note if the injury or symptoms fit the history of the accident or illness
- Note any delay in seeking help, and ask the parents to explain why they didn't seek immediate treatment
- Suspect child abuse when a child's injury doesn't match the reported accident and when X-rays show old, unexplained fractures
- Suspect abuse even when the child shows no signs of neglect, such as undernutrition, poor hygiene, or untreated illness

Interventions
- Meet the child's immediate physical and psychological needs first, regardless of suspicions
- Protect the child, help the family begin to cope, and try to prevent further abuse
- Report suspected abuse to the proper authorities; this is mandated in all states (see *Your role in reporting abuse*)
- Reinforce what the parents do correctly and encourage their participation in the child's care
- Teach the parents relevant child development principles, give them anticipatory guidance, and serve as their role model
- Provide consistent care to gain the parents' and child's trust
- Engage the child in play that encourages the expression of feelings, especially guilt and fear

• Refer the parents to a support group

ACCIDENTS

● **Introduction**
  • Accidents are the leading cause of death among children, accounting for one-third of all fatalities
  • Most accidents occur in or near the home
  • Most accidents are preventable
  • Common accidents among children include falls, ingestions, poisonings, drownings, motor vehicle accidents, and burns
    – Falls are the leading cause of head injury in children younger than age 5
  • Safety must be part of nursing care; safety teaching must be part of family-centered care

● **Nursing interventions to promote safety (review with the parents)**
  • Follow crib guidelines
    – Crib slats should be no more than 2″ (5 cm) apart
    – A firm mattress should be used with no plastic mattress cover
    – Place the crib away from windows and curtain cords
  • Check toys for sharp edges or small pieces
  • Anticipate the child's motor abilities and curiosity
  • Advocate the use of seat belts and car seats; most states have laws mandating their use
  • Teach water safety
  • Teach bicycle safety, including the use of helmets
  • Ensure safety in sports activities
  • Ensure a childproof home environment: Remove hanging cords and dangerous plants, place all medications and cleaning agents out of reach, and block electrical outlets
  • Supervise the child's activities
  • Teach the child that medicine isn't candy
  • Keep substances in their original containers
  • Post emergency numbers, including information for the poison control center
  • Review car seat safety

● **Additional safety measures in the hospital**
  • Modify the hospital environment to ensure safety based on the child's mental age, developmental level, and physical condition
  • Keep bed side rails up at all times
  • Don't allow rubber or latex balloons at a child's bedside; if popped, the child could swallow or aspirate the fragments
  • Prohibit spark-producing toys (such as a spinning top) near oxygen

---

Common accidents among children

• Falls
• Ingestions
• Poisonings
• Drownings
• Motor vehicle accidents
• Burns

Musts for childproofing a home

• Remove hanging cords and dangerous plants.
• Place all medications and cleaning agents out of reach.
• Block electrical outlets.
• Set the hot water heater at 120° F (38.9° C).

TIME-OUT FOR TEACHING

Accident prevention

Be sure to include these points in your teaching plan for parents to help prevent accidents:
- Keep all medications in original containers and out of the reach of children.
- Childproof the home.

- Supervise the child's activities.
- Provide age-appropriate toys.
- Use protective sports equipment, such as helmets and knee pads
- Set hot water heater at 120° F (38.9° C).

- Don't leave medications or syringes at the bedside
- Apply safety restraints, such as mitts or a vest restraint, if the child is a danger to himself or others
- Instruct parents in measures to prevent accidents and childproof the home when the child is discharged (see *Accident prevention*)
- Make sure parents have a car seat at discharge

ASPIRIN POISONING

Introduction
- Aspirin (acetylsalicylic acid) is an analgesic, antipyretic, and anti-inflammatory agent that inhibits platelet aggregation
- The incidence of aspirin poisoning is decreasing because aspirin is no longer recommended as a fever reducer for children
- A single ingestion of 150 to 200 mg/kg of aspirin can cause toxicity
- Aspirin's peak effect occurs in 2 to 4 hours
  – Therapeutic blood level: 15 to 30 mg/dl
  – Toxic blood level: greater than 30 mg/dl

Assessment
- Observe for increased respiratory depth and rate from metabolic acidosis; hyperapnea (deep breathing) is a classic sign of aspirin toxicity
- Note fever from the stimulation of carbohydrate metabolism
- Note decreased serum glucose levels
- Assess for GI irritation, such as occult bleeding and dyspepsia
- Note altered clotting function; assess for petechiae and blood loss
- Check for irritability, restlessness, and tinnitus or altered hearing

Interventions
- Maintain a patent airway; encourage hyperventilation
- Perform gastric lavage or induce emesis with ipecac syrup
- Ensure adequate hydration to flush the aspirin through the kidneys
- Administer calcium and potassium supplements as needed and ordered

---

Assessing for aspirin poisoning

- Hyperapnea
- Fever
- Decreased serum glucose levels
- GI irritation
- Petechiae and blood loss
- Irritability, restlessness
- Tinnitus or altered hearing

Interventions for aspirin poisoning

- Maintain a patent airway; encourage hyperventilation.
- Perform gastric lavage or induce emesis.
- Ensure adequate hydration.
- Administer calcium and potassium supplements as needed.

ACETAMINOPHEN POISONING

● **Introduction**
- Acetaminophen (Tylenol) is an analgesic and antipyretic agent that doesn't inhibit platelet aggregation
- Hepatotoxicity occurs at plasma levels greater than 200 mcg/ml by 4 hours after ingestion and 50 mcg/ml by 12 hours after ingestion
- Toxicity occurs in three stages
  - Initial period—occurs 2 to 4 hours after ingestion; the patient may experience malaise, diaphoresis, nausea, and vomiting
  - Latent phase—occurs 1 to 2 days after ingestion; GI symptoms resolve and patient appears well
  - Hepatic involvement—occurs 3 to 4 days after ingestion; hepatotoxicity is peaking, with increasing liver enzyme levels, prolonged prothrombin time, jaundice, and hepatic encephalopathy

● **Assessment**
- Assess for GI distress, such as nausea, vomiting, diarrhea, and abdominal pain
- Monitor liver function; assist with obtaining blood samples as ordered and check results frequently
- Perform frequent neurologic checks

● **Interventions**
- Maintain a patent airway
- Perform gastric lavage or induce emesis with ipecac syrup
- Administer an antidote, such as acetylcysteine (Mucomyst)
  - Acetylcysteine binds with the breakdown product of acetaminophen so that it won't bind with liver cells, thereby preventing hepatotoxicity

LEAD POISONING

● **Introduction**
- Lead, a heavy metal, is poorly absorbed by the body and slowly excreted; lead replaces calcium in the bones and increases the permeability of central nervous system membranes
- Lead poisoning can cause learning disabilities, behavioral problems and, at very high levels, seizures, coma, and death
- The major source of lead in this country is lead-based paint and lead-contaminated dust in older buildings; children are at greater risk for lead exposure than adults because they put things into their mouths
- Lead intoxication is most common in children younger than age 6
- Lead poisoning is confirmed when the child has two successive blood lead levels greater than 10 mcg/dl

---

Three stages of acetaminophen toxicity

- Initial period—2 to 4 hours after ingestion
- Latent phase—1 to 2 days after ingestion
- Hepatic involvement—3 to 4 days after ingestion

Assessing for acetaminophen poisoning

- Assess for GI distress.
- Monitor liver function.
- Perform frequent neurologic checks.

Assessing for lead poisoning

- Check for bone pain.
- Check for lead lines along gums and on X-rays.
- Monitor for symptoms of anemia.
- Assess for neurologic symptoms.
- Check for signs of GI distress.
- Monitor for peripheral neuritis.
- Test erythrocyte protoporphyrin and perform urinalysis for coproporphyrin.

⏱ TIME-OUT FOR TEACHING

Lead poisoning prevention

Share these tips with your patient's family to prevent lead poisoning:
- Carefully wash hands with hot soapy water before eating.
- Teach children to keep hands, toys, and all other objects out of the mouth.
- Wash pacifiers and other items meant to be put in the mouth (especially if the item falls on the floor or other dirty surface).
- Stress the importance of a well-balanced diet to ensure that the child receives adequate amounts of calcium, magnesium, zinc, iron, and copper.
- Allow tap water to run for 2 minutes before using water for drinking, cooking, or making formula.
- Don't use cookware or ceramic dishes that may contain lead.
- Report stomachaches, irritability, and headaches, which may be early signs of higher-than-normal lead levels.

Chelating agents

- EDTA
- BAL

Actions of chelating agents

- Bind with lead and excrete it from the body
- Remove calcium from the body

- High lead exposure can occur in some occupations and hobbies, such as ceramics, furniture, refinishing, and stained glass work

● **Assessment**
- Check for bone pain
- Check for lead lines, seen along gums and recorded on X-rays
  - Examine X-rays to check for lead lines near the epiphyseal lines (areas of increased density) of long bones
  - The thickness of the line shows the length of time the lead ingestion has been occurring
- Monitor for symptoms of anemia from the inhibition of hemoglobin formation
- Assess for increased intracranial pressure, cortical atrophy, behavioral changes, altered cognition and motor skills (such as lethargy and clumsiness), and seizures
- Check for signs of GI distress, such as constipation, vomiting, and weight loss
- Check for peripheral neuritis from calcium release into the blood
- Test erythrocyte protoporphyrin to determine blood lead levels; perform urinalysis for coproporphyrin

● **Interventions**
- Institute measures (such as oral or I.V. fluid administration) to lower the blood lead level to prevent lead encephalopathy; monitor hydration status and kidney function
- Administer chelating agents, such as EDTA by I.V. or I.M. infusion or dimercaprol (BAL) by I.M.
  - These agents bind with lead and excrete it from the body
  - They also remove calcium

- Monitor calcium levels to prevent tetany and seizures
- Discontinue iron, which binds to chelating agents
- Encourage a low-fat diet with adequate supplies of calcium, magnesium, zinc, iron, and copper to prevent more lead from being bound and stored in the body's fat tissues
- Initiate referrals to discover and remove the source of the lead contamination (see *Lead poisoning prevention*)

THE CHILD WITH A CHRONIC ILLNESS OR DISABILITY

● Introduction

- A chronic health condition is an illness or a disability that's long term; it may be relatively permanent and may result in limitations in the activities of daily living (ADLs)
- It may result from an irreversible pathological alteration, such as the morbidity resulting from prematurity
- The condition commonly requires the child to take special measures for rehabilitation or habilitation and may require long-term supervision
- Chronic conditions can affect the child's physical, psychological, and social growth and development
- A child with a chronic condition who's in a normal state of wellness should be treated as well, healthy, and normal
- An assessment of the child's disability depends on the developmental expectations for each age-group and, therefore, changes as the child ages
- A chronic condition in the child affects all members of the family
- The need for pediatric rehabilitation and habilitation has increased with the prevalence of chronic, disabling conditions and with improved technology and higher survival rates (especially for the premature infant)
  - Rehabilitation implies restoration and relearning to accomplish that which has already been learned
  - Habilitation implies achievement of skills not previously learned, such as a child with brain damage who's learning to walk for the first time
  - Both aim for the highest level of achievement possible in all aspects of the child's life
  - Both begin as soon as the child enters the health care system
  - Both continuously address the child's physical, psychological, social, and cognitive needs
  - They're comprehensive and holistic and draw on the family's active participation
  - They can apply to any chronic condition

Characteristics of a chronic health condition

- Long term; may be relatively permanent
- May result in limitations in ADLs
- Commonly requires rehabilitation or habilitation

Rehabilitation vs. habilitation

- *Rehabilitation* implies restoration and relearning to accomplish skills that have already been learned.
- *Habilitation* implies achievement of skills not previously learned.

Rehabilitation interventions

- Develop goals with the child and his family.
- Focus on the child's strengths rather than on the disability.
- Provide normal childhood experiences.

Managing the chronically ill or disabled child

- Treat a child who's in a normal state of wellness as well, healthy, and normal.
- Allow the child to grieve over the disability or chronic condition.
- Focus on the child's strengths.
- Provide therapeutic play.

● **Assessment**
- Assess the infant for deficits in stimulation
- Assess the toddler for increasingly dependent behavior
- Assess the child for abilities and disabilities
- Be alert to a child's heightened sense of loss of body integrity and awareness of "being different"
- Be sensitive to the school-age child's sense of privacy, and note a heightened fear of death
- Identify how the adolescent is coping with the stigma associated with the disability; note feelings of inferiority or inadequacy
- Be alert to sudden rebellion against treatments that have been received for years
- Determine how the parents view the child, how they define the condition, and how they expect a sick or affected child to behave; these factors influence the child's response to illness
- Assess the siblings for guilt, anger, fear, and embarrassment; additionally, they may be overprotective of their ill or affected sibling or rejected by their parents
- Identify the family's support system
- Identify available resources

● **Interventions**
- Permit the child and his family to grieve over the disability or chronic condition
  - Grieving occurs initially and whenever the child's condition interferes with developmental tasks
  - Be aware of "chronic sorrow," which families may experience when their child doesn't meet expected developmental milestones
- Help the child and his family learn to accept the condition; reinforce their coping skills at different stages of the child's development (for instance, when the condition or their expectations change)
- Focus on the child's strengths
  - Provide as much autonomy as possible, given the child's developmental age and cognitive level
  - Don't focus on the child's disability; stress what's special in each child
- Normalize the child's environment; provide consistent limits, rules, and routines
- Promote a positive body image and self-concept for the child
- Provide therapeutic play (puppets, role playing)
- Allow a child older than age 7 to participate in decisions about treatments; the child and his family are the decision makers
- Address the child's growth and development needs; rehabilitation changes as growth and development change

- Provide normal childhood experiences, even for a child connected to high-technology equipment; respect the child's body, promote sexuality, let the child experience the outdoors, encourage the child to role play, and give the child privacy
- Engage the child in activities that are appropriate for his age and condition
- Promote family involvement, home care, and respite care
- Continue meeting the child's educational needs
- Incorporate rehabilitation or habilitation measures as a routine part of the day to promote normalcy
- Develop goals with the child and his family, such as reaching developmental milestones and establishing appropriate alternatives
- Refer the family to appropriate support groups and community resources
- Be aware that case management of the child's multidisciplinary needs is essential
- Be aware of the long-term impact of chronic pain
- Familiarize the family with relevant legislation
    - Public Law 94-142 (Education for All Handicapped Children Act) promises free and appropriate education in the least restrictive environment for children with disabilities; regular schools must provide related services to assist handicapped children with their education and must develop an Individualized Education Plan for each identified child
    - Public Law 99-457, part H, an amendment to the act described above, promotes early assessment and interventions for high-risk children up to age 3; it mandates the involvement of families in planning their children's care by way of the development of an Individual Family Service Plan
    - Public Law 101-476 (Individuals with Disabilities Education Act) combines components of the two laws described above

NCLEX CHECKS

It's never too soon to begin your NCLEX preparation. Now that you've reviewed this chapter, carefully read each of the following questions and choose the best answer. Then compare your responses to the correct answers.

1. A nurse is caring for a 2-year-old with injuries that lead her to suspect child abuse. The most correct action is to:
- ☐ **1.** admit the child to the hospital.
- ☐ **2.** notify the family physician.
- ☐ **3.** report the suspected abuse.
- ☐ **4.** keep the parents away from the child.

TOP 6

Items to study for your next test on conditions interfering with pediatric health

1. Patterns of genetic transmission
2. Characteristic signs of child abuse
3. Your role in reporting suspected child abuse
4. Key ways to prevent accidents
5. Ways to prevent lead poisoning
6. Treatments for lead poisoning

2. In which child would you suspect child abuse?
- ☐ **1.** A 2-year-old with bruises on both shins
- ☐ **2.** A 2-year-old who won't make eye contact with the nurse
- ☐ **3.** A 3-year-old who is withdrawn and has bruises on his back
- ☐ **4.** A 10-year-old who comes to the emergency department (ED) with a broken arm

3. A nurse suspects that a 3-year-old has ingested lead paint. Which signs and symptoms indicate lead poisoning? Select all that apply.
- ☐ **1.** Constipation
- ☐ **2.** Lethargy
- ☐ **3.** Diarrhea
- ☐ **4.** Clumsiness
- ☐ **5.** Oliguria
- ☐ **6.** Tachycardia

4. What's the leading cause of head injury in children younger than age 5?
- ☐ **1.** Nonaccidental trauma
- ☐ **2.** Falls at home
- ☐ **3.** Motor vehicle accidents
- ☐ **4.** Trauma caused by a sibling

5. A couple has a 2-year-old with cystic fibrosis. When planning their next pregnancy, the couple should undergo:
- ☐ **1.** genetic counseling.
- ☐ **2.** psychological counseling.
- ☐ **3.** counseling regarding transmission of sexually transmitted diseases (STDs)
- ☐ **4.** a TORCH test.

6. Which drug is used as an antidote for acetaminophen poisoning?
- ☐ **1.** Furosemide
- ☐ **2.** Ampicillin
- ☐ **3.** Acetylcysteine
- ☐ **4.** EDTA

7. A nurse is teaching a class on poison prevention to parents at a day-care center. Which statement by a parent indicates a need for further instruction?
- ☐ **1.** "I've taught my child that medicine isn't candy."
- ☐ **2.** "All the household cleaners are in a locked cabinet below the kitchen sink."
- ☐ **3.** "The only medicine that isn't locked up is my Tylenol, which I carry in my purse."
- ☐ **4.** "I've removed all my poisonous houseplants from the house."

8. A nurse is caring for a child in the ED who has upper-body bruising and, possibly, parental physical abuse. Which nursing intervention is the highest priority?

☐ **1.** Report suspicions to appropriate authorities.

☐ **2.** Establish protective measures for the child.

☐ **3.** Identify circumstances surrounding the injury.

☐ **4.** Document factual, objective data to support assessment findings.

9. A nurse is caring for a child who supposedly had an accident at home. Which statement by a parent indicates the possibility of child abuse?

☐ **1.** The mother: "My husband told me my daughter fell off the bed." The father: "I heard her crying and went to her room."

☐ **2.** The mother: "I turned my back for a minute or two, and she had pulled the pot of hot water off the stove." The father: "I was at work when it happened."

☐ **3.** The mother: "She fell off a swing." The father: "She fell off the bed."

☐ **4.** The mother: "My daughter is so clumsy; she just walks into things." The father: "You really have to keep an eye on her."

10. A nurse is planning to report a child abuse case to protective services in her city. Before making the report, she must:

☐ **1.** have a suspicion that abuse has occurred.

☐ **2.** have positive evidence that the abuse has occurred.

☐ **3.** notify the parents of the intent to report the suspicions of abuse.

☐ **4.** obtain your supervisor's permission to report the suspected abuse.

ANSWERS AND RATIONALES

1. CORRECT ANSWER: 3

As a nurse, you play a crucial role in recognizing and reporting incidents of suspected abuse. When you suspect abuse, you must pass the information along to the appropriate authorities. In many states, failure to report actual or suspected abuse constitutes a crime. You aren't responsible for admitting the child to the hospital. The physician should be notified, but your responsibility to report abuse doesn't end there. You don't have authority to keep the parents away from the child unless they're hurting the child by being in the room; and the parents may not be the abusers.

2. CORRECT ANSWER: 3

A 3-year-old who acts withdrawn and has bruises on his back may be the victim of physical abuse. Three-year-olds are typically social, not withdrawn. Additionally, bruises on a child's back should be investigated. Two-year-olds often fall and bruise their shins. It's normal for a 2-year-old to be afraid of nurses and to avoid eye contact with them. Ten-year-olds are commonly injured during play.

3. CORRECT ANSWER: 1, 2, 4

Lethargy, clumsiness, irritability, anorexia, vomiting, abdominal pain, and constipation are common signs of lead poisoning. Mental retardation and seizures may also occur with high levels of lead ingestion. Oliguria, diarrhea, and tachycardia aren't symptoms of this condition.

4. CORRECT ANSWER: 2

Falls are the leading cause of head injury, and almost 70% of children younger than age 5 killed by a fall are injured at home. Head injury related to motor vehicle accidents occurs more often in adolescents. Nonaccidental trauma and trauma caused by a sibling occur less commonly than trauma caused by a fall.

5. CORRECT ANSWER: 1

Cystic fibrosis is an autosomal recessive disorder that's inherited. Genetic counseling should be offered to the couple regarding the probable outcomes of a future pregnancy. Psychological counseling could be offered at any time to the couple who have a child with this disorder, but genetic counseling is most important if the couple plans another pregnancy. Because the disease isn't sexually transmitted, STD counseling isn't appropriate. TORCH is an acronym for toxoplasmosis, rubella, cytomegalovirus, and herpes simplex antibodies. This test helps to detect exposure to pathogens that cause congenital and neonatal infections. It isn't a screening tool for cystic fibrosis.

6. CORRECT ANSWER: 3

Acetylcysteine prevents hepatotoxicity associated with acetaminophen and is used for acetaminophen poisoning. Furosemide is a diuretic, ampicillin is an antibiotic, and EDTA is a chelating agent used for lead poisoning.

7. CORRECT ANSWER: 3

All medicines should be in a locked cabinet. Medicine in a purse is easily accessible to a child, and acetaminophen (Tylenol) is the drug most commonly involved in poisoning in children. It's important for parents to teach children that medicine isn't candy. Locking up household cleaners and removing poisonous plants from the house are also important preventive measures.

8. CORRECT ANSWER: 2

Your first priority is to provide a protective environment for the child. When abuse or neglect is suspected, you're also legally required to report suspicions of abuse to child protective services. It's also important for you to determine the circumstances surrounding the injury. Assessment findings must be factual and objective and accurately describe the physical findings.

9. CORRECT ANSWER: 3

Differing reports of how an "accident" occurred is a possible indication of child abuse. When the parents relate conflicting stories or the child tells a different story than the parents, you should investigate for possible abuse. All the other statements should be investigated as well, but they may be innocent statements.

10. CORRECT ANSWER: 1

As a nurse, you have a responsibility to report cases of suspected child abuse. You don't need a supervisor's permission nor do you need to notify the parents of your intent. If your report is bona fide (that is, if you file it in good faith), the law will protect you against any suit filed by an alleged abuser. Only a court of law can give positive affirmation that abuse has taken place.

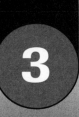

3

Pediatric assessment

---

1. What's the recommended method for testing visual acuity in a 4-year-old child?

☐ 1. Snellen chart

☐ 2. Allen cards

☐ 3. E chart

☐ 4. Hirschberg's test

CORRECT ANSWER: 3

2. At what age do children usually reach the adult respiratory rate?

☐ 1. 7

☐ 2. 11

☐ 3. 15

☐ 4. 20

CORRECT ANSWER: 3

3. A finding of pigeon chest in a child might indicate which disease?

☐ 1. Cystic fibrosis

☐ 2. Turner's syndrome

☐ 3. Rickets

☐ 4. Marfan syndrome

CORRECT ANSWER: 4.

4. At what age would you expect the Babinski reflex to disappear in a child?

☐ 1. 4 months

☐ 2. 6 months

☐ 3. 2 years

☐ 4. 8 years

CORRECT ANSWER: 3

5. The condition commonly known as bowlegs is more formally referred to by what term?

☐ 1. Genu varum

☐ 2. Genu valgum

☐ 3. Kyphosis

☐ 4. Scoliosis

CORRECT ANSWER: 1

LEARNING OBJECTIVES

After studying this chapter, you should be able to:

● Use growth grids to assess growth pattern.

● Obtain a diet history.

● Ask appropriate history questions for each body system.

● Perform a physical assessment of each body system.

CHAPTER OVERVIEW

Your health assessment may include a discussion of growth patterns and nutrition as well as an examination of body systems. Your first task is to establish rapport with the child and his parents. When you talk to the child, show empathy and understanding and use age-appropriate language. Many children are frightened at first, but by turning some of the examination into a game, you can calm a fearful child. Consider using puppets or other playthings to communicate with the child. Talk to him about toys, hobbies, pets, or other subjects he's interested in, and encourage his friendship with compliments.

GROWTH PATTERNS AND NUTRITION

● **Reasons for assessment**
- Monitor changes in a child's growth patterns
  - Failure to thrive
  - Obesity
- Assess a child's nutritional status

● **Approaches**
- Plot the child's height, weight, head circumference, and BMI (Body Mass Index) on growth grids; this allows you to screen the child's growth patterns
- The National Center for Heath Statistics has developed growth grids for children up to the age of 20
  - Plot a child's height and weight on gender-appropriate growth grids at each well visit
  - Plot an infant's head circumference until the age of 2
  - Calculate the child's BMI and plot on a gender-appropriate grid from the age of 2 to 20
- Grids use percentiles to evaluate the child's growth
  - The 50th percentile indicates an average height, weight, or head circumference for a child
  - A child usually remains in the same percentile throughout his growth periods; consider a large deviation (such as decrease from 50th to 5th percentile) abnormal
  - A BMI between 85th and 95th percentile for age and sex is considered a risk for the child to be overweight; a BMI over 95th percentile is considered overweight or obese

● **Diet history**
- Obtain a child's diet history from the parents or the child depending on age (see *Obtaining a diet history*)
  - Ask if the child was breast-fed and for length and frequency of breast-feeding

Talking with children

- Show empathy and understanding.
- Use simple language.

Growth grids

- They enable screening for early signs of nutritional deficiencies.
- They have been developed for children up to age 18.
- Findings below the 5th percentile or above the 95th percentile are considered abnormal.
- A child usually remains in the same percentile throughout his growth period.

Obtaining a diet history

For all pediatric age-groups, assess:
- daily nutritional plan (number and types of meals and snacks)
- special or modified diet
- behavioral peculiarities associated with mealtimes
- feeding problems.
 Also assess for:
- sugar intake — sugar is an empty-calorie food substance related to dental caries and obesity

- iron intake — iron deficiency anemia is a major childhood problem
- protein intake — protein is essential for growth
- fat intake — a balanced diet should allow sufficient fat to promote growth while avoiding high-cholesterol foods
- calcium intake.

Components of a diet history

- Daily nutritional plan
- Special or modified diet
- Behavioral peculiarities associated with mealtimes
- Feeding problems
- Sugar intake
- Iron intake
- Protein intake
- Fat intake

– Ask how much water, milk, juice, and soda the child drinks

– Ask if the child takes vitamins; ascertain the type and dosage

– Ask how many fruits and vegetables the child eats daily

– Find out what type of snacks the child eats

EXAMINATION OF BODY SYSTEMS

Birth history and early development
- Were there any complications during the pregnancy
- Were there any complications with the delivery, such as prematurity or birth trauma
- Did the child arrive at developmental milestones—such as sitting up, walking, and talking—at the usual ages
- Ask about childhood diseases and injuries and known congenital abnormalities
- More specific questions depend on which body system is being assessed

Skin
- Neonates and infants
    – Jaundice occurs in approximately 50% of all babies
    – Birthmarks
    – Bacterial and candidal infections may occur with diaper rash; check for papules, pustules, or vesicles (candidal rashes are severely erythematous and pustular with vesicular satellite lesions)
    – The scaling and crusting of cradle cap may entirely cover an infant's scalp
- Preschool and school-age children
    – Younger children are susceptible to common disorders, such as allergic contact dermatitis (from poison ivy, oak, or sumac or from rubber in shoes or clothing), atopic dermatitis, warts (especially on

TOP 4

Questions about birth history and development

1. Did the mother have any diseases or other problems during pregnancy?
2. Was there birth trauma or a difficult delivery?
3. Did the child arrive at developmental milestones at the usual ages?
4. Does the child have any diseases, current or previous injuries, or known congenital abnormalities?

the hands), viral exanthema, impetigo, ringworm, scabies, and skin reactions to food allergies
  – They typically have bruises on their lower extremities resulting from active play
- Adolescents
  – At puberty, hormonal changes affect the child's skin and hair
    • Androgen levels increase, causing sebaceous glands to secrete large amounts of sebum, which can clog hair follicle openings
    • Coarse hair appears on the face, axillae, and pubic area in boys, and on the axillae and pubic area in girls
  – Common dermatoses that occur during adolescence include acne, warts, sunburn, scabies, atopic dermatitis, pityriasis rosea, contact dermatitis, and fungal infections
  – For all age-groups, be aware of skin deviations that may indicate abuse

Eyes and vision

- Behavior problems or poor performance in school may relate to difficulty seeing the chalkboard
- History questions
  – Look for clues to familial eye disorders, such as refractive errors and retinoblastoma
    • Refer a child with a family history of glaucoma to an ophthalmologist, even if there are no obvious symptoms
  – Ask the parents if the child has difficulty reading the black board in school or squints, which may be a sign of myopia, or nearsightedness (the ability to see objects at close range but not at a distance); children usually don't have difficulty with reading or other close work
- Physical examination includes tests for visual acuity and inspection for strabismus (see *Characteristics of an infant's eye*)
  – Visual acuity
    • Because 20/20 visual acuity and depth perception develop fully by age 7, you can test vision in a school-age child as you would in an adult
    • Test a child age 4 or older with the E chart
      - This chart is made up entirely of capital Es, their legs pointing up, down, right, or left
      - The child identifies what he sees by indicating with his hands or fingers the position of each E
    • No method accurately measures visual acuity in children younger than age 4, but testing with Allen cards may provide useful data
      - Each card contains an illustration of a familiar object, such as a Christmas tree, birthday cake, or horse

Methods for testing visual acuity

- Test vision in school-age children as you would in adults.
- Test vision in a child age 4 or older with an E chart.
- Test vision in a child younger than age 4 with Allen cards.

Characteristics of an infant's eye

When examining an infant's eye, you'll notice several distinguishing characteristics.

- *Cornea* — thinner with a greater curvature
- *Eye structure* — larger in relation to the body than an adult's eye structure
- *Foveal light reflection* — not present for the first 3 to 4 months
- *Fundus* — gray; may also have a mottled appearance, which is normal
- *Iris* — blue from the posterior pigment layer showing through a light or transparent anterior layer (pigment, deposited in the anterior layer within the first 2 years, determines the adult iris color; small deposits of pigment make the iris appear blue or green; large deposits, brown)
- *Lens* — more refractive, compensating for the eye's shortness
- *Macula* — appears bright white and elevated
- *Pupil* — situated slightly on the nasal side of the cornea, appears larger on examination because of the high refractive power of the cornea; hard to dilate and small (the pupils widen at age 1, reaching the greatest diameter during adolescence)
- *Sclera* — blue tinge because of its thinness and translucence (it turns white as it thickens and become hydrated)

- The child is asked to identify each card with his right eye covered and then with his left eye covered
- The examiner can also back away from the child and determine the maximum distance at which the child can identify at least three pictures

– Strabismus
  • This is one of the most common abnormalities in preschool children
  • The misalignment of each eye's optic axis causes one or both of the child's eyes to turn in (crossed eyes), up, down, or out
  • A child with a deviating eye usually develops double vision (diplopia); if the child isn't treated, this can lead to amblyopia, an irreversible loss of visual acuity in the suppressed eye
  • Refer an infant or a toddler who appears to have a deviating eye to an ophthalmologist for further evaluation
  • In older children, perform the cover-uncover test
    - Ask the child to fixate on an attractive distant target, such as a stuffed animal or a cartoon figure
    - Cover his left eye with an occluder and observe his right eye; it shouldn't move or change position to view the object
    - Cover the right eye and repeat the test
  • The light reflection test (Hirschberg's test) also helps to detect strabismus
    - Shine a penlight into the child's eye

Key facts about strabismus

- One of the most common abnormalities in preschool children
- One or both eyes turn in (crossed eyes), up, down, or out
- May cause diplopia
- If left untreated, can cause an irreversible loss of visual acuity

Performing the cover-uncover test

- Ask the child to fixate on an attractive distant target.
- Cover his left eye with an occluder and observe his right eye; it shouldn't move or change position to view the object.
- Cover the right eye and repeat the test.

Performing Hirschberg's test

- Shine a penlight into the child's eye.
- The light reflection should appear in the same position on each pupil; a slight variation indicates strabismus.

- The light reflection should appear in the same position on each pupil; a slight variation indicates strabismus

● **Ears and hearing**
- Some states have mandated auditory brainstem response (ABR) test as part of newborn screening
- An infant younger than age 6 months should respond to a spoken voice; by age 6 months, an infant can localize the direction of sound; and by age 5, a child's hearing is fully developed
- Investigate the child's speech development by listening to him carefully; speech development sometimes reflects hearing acuity during childhood
- Observe behavior for possible signs of ear disorders
  - Does the child rub his ear as though it hurts
  - Does he tilt his head when listening (see *Characteristics of a child's ear*)
- The patient's birth history may provide clues to possible hearing disorders
  - Prenatal causes of congenital hearing defects include maternal infection, especially rubella during the first trimester, and maternal use of ototoxic drugs
  - Events at birth that may cause hearing loss include hypoxia, jaundice, and trauma
  - If the patient has a craniofacial deformity, such as cleft palate, he has an increased risk of developing otitis media, which can lead to hearing loss
- When asked about daily activities, parents may relate observations that indicate possible hearing loss
  - The child doesn't startle or wake up in response to a loud stimulus
  - The child has to be told several times to do something, even though he's old enough to understand
- Evaluating hearing in an infant
  - Acoustic blink reflex
  - Make a sudden loud noise, such as clapping your hands or snapping your fingers, about 12" (30.5 cm) from his ear
  - The infant should respond with the startle reflex or by blinking
- Screening hearing in a child between ages 2 and 5
  - Use play techniques, such as asking him to put a peg in a board when he hears a sound transmitted through earphones
  - Routine screening with an audiometer usually begins at age 3
- Screening hearing in an older child
  - Use the whisper test, making sure to use words he knows and taking care to prevent him from lip reading
  - The child should hear a whispered question or simple command at 8' (2.4 m)

Clues to possible hearing disorders

- Maternal infection during pregnancy
- Maternal use of ototoxic drugs during pregnancy
- Hypoxia, jaundice, or trauma at birth
- Craniofacial deformities that increase the risk of developing otitis media

Methods for evaluating hearing

1. In an older child, use the whisper test.
2. In a child between ages 2 and 5, use play techniques.
3. In an infant, use the acoustic blink reflex.

Characteristics of a child's ear

You'll recognize three major differences between an infant's or a young child's ear and an adult's ear. A child's *tympanic membrane slants horizontally,* rather than vertically, and his *external canal slants upward.* These differences require that during the otoscopic examination, you hold the child's pinna down and out instead of up and back as you would with an adult. Also, a child's *eustachian tube slants horizontally.* This causes fluid to stagnate and act as a medium for bacteria.

These anatomic differences make the infant and young child more susceptible to ear infection.

CHILD'S EAR

Tympanic membrane

External canal

Eustachian tube

ADULT'S EAR

Tympanic membrane

External canal

Eustachian tube

Anatomic characteristics of a child's ear

- Tympanic membrane slants horizontally.
- External canal slants upward.
- Eustachian tube slants horizontally.

● **Respiratory system**
  - Upper respiratory tract infections commonly occur in children because a child's respiratory tract is immature, and the mucous membranes can't produce enough mucus to warm and humidify inhaled air
  - History questions
    – Ask parents how often the child has upper respiratory tract infections
    – Find out if the child has had other respiratory signs and symptoms, such as a cough, dyspnea, wheezing, rhinorrhea, or a stuffy nose; ask if they appear related to the child's activities or to seasonal changes
  - Normal respiratory rates
    – Infants: 30 to 80 breaths/minute; apneic periods are normal in neonates as long as they last less than 15 seconds

Pediatric chest abnormalities

- Barrel chest
- Funnel chest
- Localized bulges
- Café-au-lait spots (more than five)
- Pigeon chest
- Rachitic beads
- Wide space between nipples

Normal respiratory rates in children

- Infants: 30 to 80 breaths/minute
- Toddlers: 20 to 40 breaths/minute
- Preschoolers: 20 to 30 breaths/minute
- School-age children and older: 15 to 25 breaths/minute
- Adolescents (about age 15): 12 to 20 breaths/minute (same as adult rate)

Identifying pediatric chest abnormalities

When examining a child, note these structural abnormalities of the chest:

- Barrel chest may indicate chronic respiratory disease, such as cystic fibrosis or asthma.
- Funnel chest may indicate rickets or Marfan syndrome.
- Localized bulges may indicate underlying pressures, such as cardiac enlargement or an aneurysm.
- More than five café-au-lait spots may indicate neurofibromatosis. Note that these spots may occur elsewhere on the body.
- Pigeon chest may indicate Marfan or Morquio's syndrome or a chronic upper respiratory tract condition.
- Rachitic beads (bumps at the costochondral junction of the ribs) may indicate rickets.
- An unusually wide space between the nipples may indicate Turner's syndrome (the distance between the outside areolar edges shouldn't be more than one-fourth of the child's chest circumference).

- Toddlers: 20 to 40 breaths/minute
- Preschool children: 20 to 30 breaths/minute
- Children of school age and older: 15 to 25 breaths/minute
- Children usually reach the adult rate (12 to 20 breaths/minute) at about age 15
- The best time to obtain a child's respiratory rate is when he's awake and sitting quietly or when he's sleeping
- A child's respiratory rate may double in response to exercise, illness, or emotion
- Physical assessment
  - The sitting position allows you the easiest access to the child's thorax
  - If the child is quiet, auscultate the lungs first
  - Use a flashlight and tongue blade to examine the child's mouth and throat
    - You can also use the tongue blade to elicit the gag reflex in infants
    - Never test the gag reflex or examine the pharynx in a child suspected of having epiglottiditis; these procedures can cause complete laryngeal obstruction
  - While examining the posterior thorax of the older child, make sure you check for scoliosis (see *Identifying pediatric chest abnormalities*)
  - Intracostal, subcostal, and suprasternal retractions and expiratory grunts are always serious signs in children
    - Refer an infant or a child with these signs for further evaluation and treatment immediately
    - He may have pneumonia, respiratory distress syndrome, or left-sided heart failure

● Cardiovascular system

- The two primary cardiac conditions of childhood are congenital heart defects and rheumatic fever
- History questions
  - Does the child experience dyspnea, cyanosis on exertion, orthopnea, or assume a knee-chest position (squatting position); this sign may indicate tetralogy of Fallot
  - Does the child have difficulty keeping up physically with other children his age
- Physical assessment
  - Inspection
    - Inspect the child's skin
      - Pallor can indicate a serious cardiac problem in an infant or anemia in an older child
      - Cyanosis may be an early sign of a cardiac condition in an infant or a child
      - Cyanosis of the extremities (acrocyanosis) is a common and usually normal finding in neonates less than 48 hours old, but evaluate it when present
    - Assess for clubbed fingers, a sign of cardiac dysfunction (clubbing doesn't ordinarily occur before age 2)
    - Assess for dependent edema, a late sign of heart failure in children
      - In infants, it appears in the eyelids
      - It appears in the legs only if the child can walk
    - Blood pressure can help confirm coarctation of the aorta
      - For children younger than age 1, the systolic thigh reading should equal the systolic arm reading
      - For older children, it may be 10 to 40 mm Hg higher, but the diastolic thigh value should equal the diastolic arm value
      - If thigh readings are below normal, suspect coarctation (see *Guide to pediatric pulse rate and blood pressure,* page 62)
  - Palpation, percussion, and auscultation
    - In judging cardiac enlargement, remember that in children younger than age 7, the heart is proportionately smaller and the apical impulse is at the fourth interspace
    - Palpate or percuss the liver for enlargement, which occurs with right-sided heart failure, and for systolic pulsations, which occur with tricuspid insufficiency
    - Auscultate for heart murmurs
      - Innocent murmurs are defined as benign or functional
      - Organic murmurs (noninnocent) are caused by congenital or acquired heart disease, for example, rheumatic heart disease

Guide to pediatric pulse rate and blood pressure

PULSE RATE

Age	Normal range (beats/minute)	Average (beats/minute)
Neonate	70 to 170	120
1 to 11 months	80 to 160	120
2 years	80 to 130	110
4 years	80 to 120	100
6 years	75 to 115	100
8 years	70 to 110	90
10 years	70 to 110	90
12 years (female)	70 to 110	90
12 years (male)	65 to 105	85
14 years (female)	65 to 105	85
14 years (male)	60 to 100	80
16 years (female)	60 to 100	80
16 years (male)	55 to 95	75
18 years (female)	55 to 95	75
18 years (male)	50 to 90	70

BLOOD PRESSURE

Age	Female (mm Hg)	Male (mm Hg)
4 years	98/60	98/55
6 years	105/65	105/60
8 years	108/67	105/60
10 years	112/64	110/65
12 years	115/65	110/65
14 years	112/65	114/65

Assessing the GI system

- Ease abdominal tenseness in an infant by flexing the knees and hips.
- The umbilical cord stump in a neonate should have two arteries and one vein.
- Palpate the painful quadrant last.
- Palpation in a quadrant other than the painful one should reveal a soft, nontender abdomen.
- Tenderness in the right lower quadrant may indicate an inflamed appendix.

● **GI system**
  - Abdominal pain is a common childhood complaint (see *Causes of acute abdominal pain in children*)
  - History questions
    - If the child has abdominal pain, ask him questions to help determine the pain's nature and severity
    - Determine the frequency and consistency of bowel movements and if the child suffers from constipation or diarrhea
    - Determine the characteristics of nausea and vomiting, especially projectile vomiting
  - Physical assessment
    - When examining a young child's abdomen, have a parent hold him, if possible; otherwise, position the child so that he can see his parent

Causes of acute abdominal pain in children

Acute abdominal pain (acute abdomen) commonly occurs during infancy and childhood. This table details the most common causes of this problem.

DISORDER	ASSESSMENT FINDINGS
Appendicitis Obstruction of the lumen of the appendix, leading to inflammation and, possibly, perforation with peritonitis	Vomiting common in children younger than age 8; midabdominal crampy pain, possibly progressing to right lower quadrant pain; slight fever; request to cough produces pain over site of peritoneal inflammation; bowel sounds may be depressed; rebound tenderness on palpation (performed by doctor)
Incarcerated inguinal hernia A hernia in which the bowel can't be returned to the abdominal cavity, causing complete bowel obstruction	Cramping abdominal pain; vomiting; abdominal distention; lump in inguinal area; palpable, irreducible, tender swelling or lump in inguinal area
Intussusception Telescoping of one intestinal segment into another (usually ileum into cecum), leading to acute intestinal obstruction	Colicky abdominal pain with restlessness and intense crying; passage of bloody, mucoid "currant jelly" stools; palpable sausage-shaped tender mass in right upper or right lower quadrant

– Palpation may cause distortion of normal abdominal sounds therefore, auscultate before palpation
– Abdominal tenseness can impede your examination; to ease tenseness, flex an infant's knees and hips
– Inspection
  • The contour of a child's belly may confirm a GI disorder
    - In a child younger than age 4, a mild potbelly is normal when the child stands or sits
    - From ages 4 to 13, a mild potbelly is usually noticeable only when the child stands
    - An extreme potbelly may result from organomegaly, ascites, neoplasm, defects in the abdominal wall, or starvation
    - A depressed or concave abdomen may indicate a diaphragmatic hernia
  • Look for areas of localized swelling
  • When inspecting an infant, stand at the foot of the table and direct a light across the abdomen from the right side; observe for peristaltic waves (these waves normally progress unseen across an infant's abdomen from left to right during feeding)
  • Because peristaltic waves aren't normally visible in a full-term infant, their appearance can indicate obstruction
    - Reverse peristalsis generally indicates pyloric stenosis
    - Other possible causes of visible peristaltic waves include bowel malrotation, duodenal ulcer or stenosis, and GI allergy

Causes of acute abdominal pain

- Appendicitis
- Incarcerated inguinal hernia
- Intussusception

Infant inspection instructions

- Stand at the foot of the table.
- Direct light across the abdomen from the right side.
- Observe for peristaltic waves.
- Inspect umbilical cord stump for two arteries and one vein.
- Inspect for umbilical hernia.

Significant findings of GI system auscultation

- Abdominal murmur — may indicate coarctation of the aorta
- High-pitched abdominal sounds — may indicate intestinal obstruction or gastroenteritis
- Venous hum — may indicate portal hypertension
- Splenic or hepatic friction rub — may indicate inflammation
- Double sound in the femoral artery — may indicate aortic insufficiency
- Absence of bowel sounds — may indicate paralytic ileus and peritonitis

Clues to pediatric abdominal pain

- Guarding
- Grimacing
- Change in pitch of cry

• Inspect the umbilical cord stump in a neonate; the cord should have two arteries and one vein
• Inspect for umbilical hernia; the best time to perform this inspection is when the child cries
– Auscultation
  • Auscultate a child's abdomen as you would an adult's
  • Significant findings
    - Abdominal murmur, a possible indication of coarctation of the aorta
    - High-pitched abdominal sounds, a possible indication of impending intestinal obstruction or gastroenteritis
    - Venous hum, a possible indication of portal hypertension
    - Splenic or hepatic friction rub, a possible sign of inflammation
    - Double sound, or so-called "pistol shot," in the femoral artery, a possible indication of aortic insufficiency
    - Absence of bowel sounds, a possible indication of paralytic ileus and peritonitis (no sounds within 5 minutes of continual auscultation)
– Palpation
  • Children guard their abdomens when pain is present; palpate the painful quadrant last
    - Clues to a child's pain include facial grimacing and a change in the pitch of the child's cry
    - Sudden protective movement with an arm or a leg is also a clue
  • Palpation in a quadrant other than the painful quadrant should reveal a soft, nontender abdomen
  • Tenderness in the right lower quadrant may indicate an inflamed appendix
  • Ask the child to cough; a reduced or withheld cough may confirm peritoneal irritation, contraindicating checking for rebound tenderness — a potentially painful procedure
  • Check for a hernia as you would in an adult
    - Umbilical hernias are commonly present at birth but may not always be visible
    - Press down on the child's umbilicus; if you can insert one fingertip, the child has a small hernia
– Percussion
  • Because a child swallows air when he eats and cries, you may hear louder tympanic tones when you percuss the abdomen
  • Minimal tympany with abdominal distention may result from fluid accumulation or solid masses
  • In a neonate, ascites usually results from GI or urinary perforation; in an older child, the cause may be heart failure, cirrhosis, or nephrosis

Urinary system

- History questions
  - Ask the patient's mother about problems during pregnancy and delivery that may be associated with urinary tract malformations
  - Explore a history of colic associated with voiding and persistent enuresis after age 5
    - Bladder or urethral irritation can cause bed-wetting
    - Bed-wetting can also be caused by emotional difficulties
    - Immaturity
- Physical assessment
  - Inspect the patient's skin for anemic pallor, which may indicate a congenital renal disorder such as medullary cystic disease
  - Inspect for undescended testes and inguinal hernia, anomalies associated with congenital urinary tract malformations
  - Palpate the child's abdomen carefully for bladder distention and kidney enlargement
    - Bladder distention in an older child may indicate urethral dysfunction
    - In a preschool child, a palpable, firm, smooth, and nontender mass adjacent to the vertebral column — but not crossing the midline — suggests Wilms' tumor
  - Inspect the patient's external genitalia closely for abnormalities associated with congenital anomalies of the urinary tract
    - A child may be bashful about allowing you to examine his genitalia, so take time to explain the procedures and their purpose
    - Note the location and size of a boy's urethral meatus, the size of his testes, and local irritation, inflammation, or swelling
      - The meatus should be in the center of the shaft
      - You may notice epispadias (urethral opening on the dorsum of the shaft) or hypospadias (urethral opening on the underside of the penis or on the perineum)
    - Note the location of a girl's clitoris, urethral meatus, and vaginal orifice; check for irritation, swelling, and abnormal discharge — possible signs of urethritis

Nervous system

- History questions
  - Ask if the child has experienced head or neck injuries, headaches, tremors, seizures, dizziness, fainting spells, or muscle weakness
  - Determine if the child has ever seen spots before his eyes, and if so, at what age this occurred
- Physical assessment
  - Head and neck
    - Watch a young child as he plays or interacts with his parents
      - Check for head and facial symmetry

Assessing the urinary system

- Inspect the skin for anemic pallor.
- Inspect for undescended testes and inguinal hernia.
- Palpate for bladder distention and kidney enlargement.
- Inspect the external genitalia.

Causes of bed-wetting

- Bladder irritation
- Urethral irritation
- Emotional difficulties
- Immaturity

Items to ask about when taking a history of the nervous system

- Head or neck injuries
- Headaches
- Tremors
- Seizures
- Dizziness or fainting spells
- Muscle weakness
- Spots
- Overactivity

Head and neck checklist

- Head and facial symmetry
- Cranial bones, including sutures and fontanels
- Shape and symmetry of head
- Head and neck muscles

Assessing cerebral function

- Assess LOC by using motor cues.
- Test attention span and concentration by asking the child to repeat a series of numbers after you.
- Test the child's recent memory by showing him a familiar object, waiting 5 minutes, then asking him to recall the object.

Assessing CN function

- Olfactory: Ask the child to identify familiar odors.
- Optic: Test an older child's visual acuity as you would an adult. Use Allen cards for a preschooler.
- Trigeminal: Test sensory division; make a game of the test.
- Facial: Have the child mimic your expressions.
- Acoustic: Check acuity and conduction.
- Glossopharyngeal, vagus, spinal accessory, and hypoglossal: Use games as necessary.

- Observe how he cries, laughs, turns his head, and wrinkles his forehead
- To examine an infant's cranial bones, gently run your fingers over his head, checking the sutures and fontanel; look for fullness, bulging, or swelling, which may indicate an intracranial mass or hydrocephalus
- Note the shape and symmetry of his head; abnormal shape accompanied by prominent bony ridges and poor head growth may indicate craniosynostosis (premature suture closure)
- Assess the child's head and neck muscles
  - Decreased neck mobility is an important indicator of neurologic disorders such as meningitis
  - With the child in a supine position, test for nuchal rigidity by cradling his head in your hands; supporting the weight of his head, move his neck in all directions to assess ease of movement

– Cerebral function
- To assess level of consciousness (LOC) in a young child, use motor cues
  - Observe for lethargy, drowsiness, and stupor
  - Observe for hyperactivity
  - Assess orientation to person and place
- To test attention span and concentration, ask the child to repeat a series of numbers after you
- To test a child's recent memory, show him a familiar object and tell him that you'll ask him later what it was; wait 5 minutes and then ask him to recall the object

– Cranial nerves (CNs)
- CN assessment can be difficult in a child younger than age 2, but by simple observation, you can check for symmetry of muscle movement, gaze, sucking strength, and hearing
- In a child older than age 2, assess the cranial nerves as you would in an adult, making these alterations:
  - CN I (olfactory): ask the child to identify familiar odors, such as chocolate or peppermint candy; for a very young child who may not be able to identify a smell, try a same-different game to determine whether he can distinguish one smell from another
  - CN II (optic): test a child's visual acuity as you would for an adult, but use Allen cards for a very young child or preschooler; for visual field testing, also follow the procedure for an adult but hold a bright object near the tip of your nose to help the young child keep his eyes focused

- CN V (trigeminal): test the sensory division of this nerve as you would for an adult, but make a game out of it by telling the child that a gremlin is going to brush his cheeks, pinch his forehead, and so on; test the motor division by having the child bite down hard on a tongue blade as you try to pull it away and at the same time palpate his jaw muscles for symmetry and contraction strength
- CN VII (facial): test the muscles that this nerve controls as you would for an adult, but instead of asking the child to perform certain movements, have him mimic your facial expressions; test the sensory division of the facial nerve with salt and sugar as for an adult
- CN VIII (acoustic): test the cochlear division of the acoustic nerve in a child by checking his hearing acuity and sound conduction
- CN IX, X, XI, and XII (glossopharyngeal, vagus, spinal accessory, and hypoglossal): test these nerves as you would for an adult, using games to facilitate the examination when necessary

– Motor function
  • Assess balance and coordination in a child by watching motor skills, such as dressing and undressing; you can also have the child stack blocks, put a bead in a bottle, or draw a cross
  • A child may demonstrate a preference for one-hand dominance between ages 12 and 24 months; handedness is well established by the school-age years
  • A child age 4 should be able to stand on one foot for about 5 seconds; a child age 6, along with his arms folded across his chest, for 5 seconds; and a child age 7, along with his eyes closed, for 5 seconds

– Sensory function
  • Test the sensations of pain, touch, vibration, and temperature in an older child as you would in an adult
  • Most of these tests aren't applicable to an infant or a very young child; younger children may respond to pain or touch, but their responses may be unreliable

– Reflexes
  • Many children and some adults tighten their muscles, making reflex testing almost impossible
  - Make a special effort to relax a child when assessing his reflexes; ask him to interlock the fingers of both hands and pull them tight or clench his teeth on the count of three; meanwhile, you tap the tendon
  - Keep in mind that these actions may artificially magnify the reflex

Normal infant reflexes

- Sucking
- Moro
- Rooting
- Tonic neck
- Babinski's
- Grasping
- Stepping
- Trunk incurvature

Infant reflexes

This table displays normal infant reflexes, how to elicit them, and the age at which they disappear.

REFLEX	HOW TO ELICIT	AGE AT DISAPPEARANCE
Sucking	Sucking motion begins when a nipple is placed in the neonate's mouth	6 months
Moro (startle reflex)	When lifted above the crib and suddenly lowered or in response to a loud noise, the arms and legs symmetrically extend and then abduct while the fingers spread to form a "C"	4 to 6 months
Rooting	When the cheek is stroked, the neonate turns his head in the direction of the stroke	3 to 4 months
Tonic neck (fencing position)	When the neonate's head is turned while the neonate is lying supine, the extremities on the same side straighten while those on the opposite side flex	2 to 3 months
Babinski's	When the sole on the side of the small toe is stroked, the neonate's toes fan upward	2 years
Grasping	When a finger is placed in each of the neonate's hands, the neonate's fingers grasp tightly enough to be pulled to a sitting position	3 to 4 months
Stepping	When held upright with the feet touching a flat surface, the neonate exhibits dancing or stepping movements	Variable
Trunk incurvature	When a finger is run laterally down the neonate's spine, the trunk flexes and the pelvis swings toward the stimulated side	2 months

- A positive Babinski's sign may normally be present up to age 2 (see *Infant reflexes*)

● **Musculoskeletal system**
- Between birth and adulthood, the skeleton triples in size, with normal growth spurts during infancy and adolescence
- Because a child's bones grow, osteogenic activity is greater than in an adult
- A child's bones are more porous and flexible than an adult's
    - Greenstick fractures are more common in children than in adults
    - A child's bones heal more rapidly than an adult's
- History questions

– Determine the ages at which the child reached major motor development milestones
  • For an infant, these include the age at which he held up his head, rolled over, sat unassisted, and walked alone
  • For an older child, these include the age at which he first ran, jumped, walked up stairs, and pedaled a tricycle
– Ask about a history of repeated fractures, muscle strains or sprains, painful joints, clumsiness, lack of coordination, abnormal gait, or restricted movement, any of which may indicate a musculoskeletal problem
• Physical assessment
  – Range of motion (ROM) and muscle strength
    • For infants and toddlers, assess only passive movements for ROM testing
    • For children who can follow instructions and do active ROM movements, demonstrate what you want the child to do and ask him to mimic you
    • Observe the child's muscles for size, symmetry, strength, tone, and abnormal movements
    • Test muscle strength in a preschool- or school-age child by having the child push against your hands or arms
    • To test muscle strength in an infant or a toddler who can't understand directions, observe his sucking as well as general motor activity
  – Spine and gait
    • Check the spine for scoliosis, kyphosis, and lordosis
      - Scoliosis is more common in girls than in boys; ask the child to bend over and touch her toes without bending her knees and observe for lateral curves and differences in the height of the shoulders and the illiac crests
      - Kyphosis and lordosis usually result from poor posture (see *Identifying common spine abnormalities,* page 70)
    • To check a child's gait, balance, and stance, ask him to walk, run, and skip away from you and then return
  – Hips and legs
    • Neonates should be screened for developmental dysplasia of the hip using the Ortolani and Burlow tests (should be performed only by an experienced clinician)
    • Observe the child's legs for shape, length, symmetry, and alignment
      - Genu varum (bowlegs) is common in children between ages 1½ and 2½ — to test for bowlegs, have the child stand straight with his ankles touching; in this position, the knees shouldn't be more than 1" (2.5 cm) apart

Motor development milestones

- Infant: holds up head, rolls over, sits unassisted, walks alone
- Older child: runs for the first time, walks up stairs, pedals a tricycle

Checking the musculoskeletal system

- Observe the child's muscles for size, symmetry, strength, tone, and abnormal movements.
- Test muscle strength.
- Check for scoliosis by asking the child to bend over and touch her toes without bending her knees.
- Ask the child to walk, run, and skip away from you and then return to check gait, balance, and stance.
- Observe the child's legs for shape, length, symmetry, and alignment.
- Inspect the child's feet for clubfoot, outward-turned toes, and pigeon toes.
- Test the child for tibial torsion.

Common alterations in leg alignment

- Genu varum (bowlegs): common in children between ages 1½ and 2½
- Genu valgum (knock-knees): common in preschoolers

Identifying common spine abnormalities

When examining the spine of the pediatric or adolescent patient, look for kyphosis and scoliosis. With kyphosis, the patient develops rounded shoulders and exaggerated posterior chest convexity. With scoliosis, the thoracic or lumbar spine curves laterally to the left or right in an S shape. This abnormality is particularly evident when the patient bends over.

KYPHOSIS　　　　　　　　　　**SCOLIOSIS**

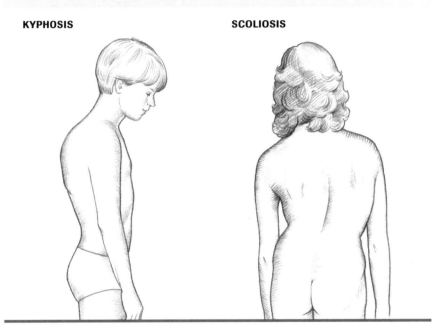

- Genu valgum (knock-knees) is common in preschoolers—to test for knock-knees, have the child stand straight with his knees touching; the ankles shouldn't be more than 1" apart in this position
- Look at the pattern of wear on the child's shoes—wear on the outside of the heel suggests bowlegs; on the inside, knock-knees
- Observe the child's feet for clubfoot (talipes equinovarus), outward-turned toes (toeing out, or pes valgus), and pigeon toes (toeing in, or pes varus)
- Test the child for tibial torsion
  - In external tibial torsion, the foot points out and the knee remains straight (toeing out)
  - In internal tibial torsion, the foot points in and the knee remains straight (toeing in or pigeon toeing)

● **Hematologic and immune systems**
- The most common hematologic disorder in children as well as the most common form of anemia is iron deficiency anemia

Most common hematologic and immune disorders

- Iron deficiency anemia
- Allergies, especially respiratory allergies

- The most common immune disorders in children are allergies, especially such respiratory allergies as rhinitis and asthma
  - Approximately one in every five children suffers from some form of allergy
  - Asthma is the leading cause of chronic illness in children, particularly those of school age
- History questions
  - Check for anemia
    - Ask the parents if the child has exhibited the common signs and symptoms: pallor, fatigue, failure to gain weight, malaise, and lethargy
    - Note a history of rhesus factor incompatibility
    - Ask if the child had jaundice that required phototherapy
    - Ask the mother who's bottle-feeding if she uses an iron-fortified formula
  - Ask about the patient's history of infections
    - For an infant, 5 to 6 viral infections a year are normal; 8 to 12 are average for school-age children
    - Continual severe infections may suggest thymic deficiency or bone marrow dysfunction
  - Obtain a thorough history of allergic conditions
  - Ask about the family's history of infections and allergic or autoimmune disorders
- Physical assessment
  - Physical examination is the same as for an adult, but normal findings are different
    - In a child younger than age 12, it's common for normal lymph nodes to be palpable
      - You may feel normal cervical and inguinal nodes ranging in size from about ⅛" (0.3 cm) to ⅜" (1 cm) across
      - Moderate numbers of nodes that are cool, firm, movable, and painless indicate prior infection
    - You may be able to palpate a normal liver and spleen in a child
      - In some children, the liver won't be palpable because it doesn't extend below the costal margin
      - If you're able to palpate a child's spleen, you should just feel the tip — anything more than that's abnormal
      - Use percussion to determine liver size
      - The liver and spleen shouldn't be tender
  - Assess the patient for signs and symptoms of inflammation around the joints, a possible sign of juvenile rheumatoid arthritis
- **Endocrine system**
  - In a neonate or an infant, endocrine disorders can cause feeding problems, constipation, jaundice, hypothermia, or somnolence

- In a child, these disorders usually cause growth and developmental abnormalities
    - Poor weight gain with little or no increase in height may indicate a lack of growth hormone
    - Hyperthyroidism can cause weight loss
- History questions
    - Obtain a thorough family history from one or both parents
        - Many endocrine disorders, such as diabetes mellitus and thyroid problems, can be hereditary
        - Others, such as delayed or precocious puberty, sometimes show a familial tendency
    - Remember that an older child or adolescent can probably give a more accurate history of his physical growth and sexual development than his parents, so interview the child when possible
- Physical assessment
    - Determine if the child's facial appearance correlates with his age; in cretinism, a child retains his infantile facial appearance
    - When inspecting the mouth, check if the number of teeth corresponds with normal expectations for the child's age; delayed eruption of teeth occurs with hypothyroidism and hypopituitarism
    - Examine the child's thyroid gland; a goiter, or swelling of the anterior neck, is caused by an enlarged thyroid gland and is often a sign of hyperthyroidism
    - When you're examining the child's breasts, abdomen, and genitalia, inspect for the developmental signs of delayed puberty or precocious puberty
        - Suspect delayed puberty if a child who has reached midadolescence has none of the physical changes associated with puberty
        - Suspect precocious puberty in females with onset of breast development, pubic and axillary hair development, and menarche before age 9

NCLEX CHECKS

It's never too soon to begin your NCLEX preparation. Now that you've reviewed this chapter, carefully read each of the following questions and choose the best answer. Then compare your responses to the correct answers.

1. What's the best time to assess the respiratory rate of a young child?
  ☐ **1.** While the child is sleeping
  ☐ **2.** While the child is playing in the playroom
  ☐ **3.** Immediately after taking the child's blood pressure
  ☐ **4.** While the child is sitting on his mother's lap

TOP 6

Items to study for your next test on pediatric assessment

1. Methods for testing visual acuity
2. Differences between a child's ear and an adult's ear
3. Common abnormal findings in cardiovascular assessment
4. Techniques for assessing motor function
5. Normal infant reflexes
6. Way to assess for scoliosis

2. A nurse observes a respiratory rate of 40 breaths/minute in a 12-hour-old neonate. The respirations are shallow with 5-second periods of apnea. What action should the nurse take?

- ☐ **1.** Notify the physician immediately.
- ☐ **2.** Request an order for supplemental oxygen.
- ☐ **3.** Continue routine monitoring.
- ☐ **4.** Bring the crash cart to the room.

3. A nurse observes that a neonate has cyanotic feet and hands 12 hours after birth. What action should the nurse take?

- ☐ **1.** Notify the physician.
- ☐ **2.** Prepare to administer supplemental oxygen.
- ☐ **3.** Make sure the neonate is warm enough, and continue observing him.
- ☐ **4.** Apply warm compresses to the feet and hands.

4. A nurse is assessing neonates in the nursery. Which of these observations would indicate respiratory problems? Select all that apply.

- ☐ **1.** Cyanosis of feet and hands
- ☐ **2.** Grunting respirations
- ☐ **3.** Respirations of 30 breaths/minute
- ☐ **4.** Respirations of 40 breaths/minute
- ☐ **5.** Intracostal, subcostal, and suprasternal retractions

5. A nurse is performing the inspection of a neonate's abdomen. Which finding of the umbilical cord is normal?

- ☐ **1.** Two arteries and one vein
- ☐ **2.** One artery and one vein
- ☐ **3.** One artery and two veins
- ☐ **4.** Two arteries and two veins

6. Which factor places an infant at greater risk than an adult for developing otitis media?

- ☐ **1.** Introduction of solid foods
- ☐ **2.** Flat, wide eustachian tubes
- ☐ **3.** Immature cardiac sphincter
- ☐ **4.** Feeding in semi-Fowler's position

7. During assessment of a child's visual acuity, which finding indicates that the child has myopia?

- ☐ **1.** The child squints all the time.
- ☐ **2.** The child closes one eye to see.
- ☐ **3.** The child has rapid eyeball movements.
- ☐ **4.** The child squints to see the blackboard.

8. Which assessment finding suggests that a 5-month-old infant has a hearing deficit?

☐ **1.** Absence of babbling
☐ **2.** Failure to localize a source of sound by age 4 months
☐ **3.** Failure to respond to spoken words
☐ **4.** Pronounced startle reflex

9. A nurse is assessing an infant during a well-child checkup. What's an easy way to determine whether an infant has strabismus?

☐ **1.** Observe for the red reflex.
☐ **2.** Observe for the reflection of a penlight in the infant's eyes.
☐ **3.** Measure the epicanthal fold of the nose.
☐ **4.** Determine whether the pupils are the same size in both eyes.

10. When performing a physical assessment on a school-age child during a well-child checkup, a nurse palpates a goiter. She suspects which condition?

☐ **1.** Diabetes insipidus
☐ **2.** Hypopituitarism
☐ **3.** Hyperpituitarism
☐ **4.** Hyperthyroidism

ANSWERS AND RATIONALES

1. CORRECT ANSWER: 1
Respirations are best determined while the child is sleeping or quietly awake. When a child is playing, respirations may increase because of activity. Respirations shouldn't be taken after the child has had his blood pressure checked because the blood pressure assessment may have upset the child. Sitting on the mother's lap doesn't guarantee that the child is quiet.

2. CORRECT ANSWER: 3
An acceptable respiratory rate for a 12-hour-old neonate is 40 breaths/minute. The normal respiratory rate is 30 to 60 breaths/minute. Periods of apnea are normal as long as they last less than 15 seconds. There isn't a need for intervention other than routine monitoring.

3. CORRECT ANSWER: 3
If the neonate's head, trunk, and mucous membranes are pink, then cyanosis of the feet and hands is probably a normal finding. Feet and hands may remain cyanotic for 48 hours, especially if they're cold. Make sure the neonate is warm enough and continue to observe him.

4. CORRECT ANSWER: 2, 5
Grunting respirations are a chief sign of respiratory distress in infants and children. These respirations are characterized by a deep, low-pitched grunting sound at the end of each breath. Intracostal, subcostal, and suprasternal retractions are another sign of respiratory distress. Cyanosis of the feet and

hands commonly occurs within the first 48 hours after birth. Respirations of 30 to 60 breaths/minute are within the normal range for a neonate.

5. CORRECT ANSWER: 1
A normal umbilical cord contains two arteries and one vein. A single artery could indicate the presence of a congenital anomaly.

6. CORRECT ANSWER: 2
Infants have flat, wide eustachian tubes that provide a relatively straight and direct route for pathogens to enter the middle ear. This makes infants more prone than older children to develop otitis media. Introducing solid foods doesn't lead to an increased incidence of otitis media. An immature cardiac sphincter would lead to reflux and vomiting, not otitis media. Feeding infants in semi-Fowler's position decreases the risk of otitis media because this position helps to prevent fluid from backing up into the respiratory tract.

7. CORRECT ANSWER: 1
Myopia is nearsightedness, or the ability to see objects clearly at close range but not at a distance. A common sign of myopia is squinting to see the blackboard. A child with strabismus (deviation of the eye) closes one eye to see more clearly. A child with a cataract might have nystagmus (involuntary movements of the eyes).

8. CORRECT ANSWER: 3
Failure to respond to spoken words indicates a possible hearing deficit. Babbling doesn't usually begin until the infant is around age 7 months. Localizing a source of sound doesn't usually begin until age 6 months. A pronounced startle reflex indicates that the infant has intact hearing.

9. CORRECT ANSWER: 2
Shining a penlight in the infant's eyes and observing for a reflection on the pupils is an easy way to check for strabismus (crossed eyes). In an infant without strabismus, the reflection of light should appear in exactly the same spot on both eyes. If the light falls off center in one eye, the infant has strabismus. The red reflex is normal and should always be seen when the eye is examined. Sometimes the epicanthal fold of the nose makes the eyes appear crossed, but this isn't an accurate measurement. Pupils should be about the same size.

10. CORRECT ANSWER: 4
A goiter, or swelling of the anterior neck, is caused by an enlarged thyroid gland and is often a sign of hyperthyroidism, or excessive production of thyroid hormone. Diabetes insipidus is hyposecretion of antidiuretic hormone, which causes polyuria and polydipsia. Hypopituitarism causes growth retardation and delayed puberty. Hyperpituitarism is an increase in growth hormones secreted by the pituitary that results in acromegaly (enlarged distal parts of the skeleton, such as nose, ears, fingers, and toes).

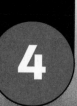

Communicable diseases and infections

PRETEST

1. Which term is used to describe the path of entry by which an infectious agent invades a susceptible host?

☐ 1. Causative agent
☐ 2. Portal of entry
☐ 3. Mode of transmission
☐ 4. Incubation period

CORRECT ANSWER: 2

2. Which method of immune protection occurs because the immune system produces antibodies after exposure to a disease?

☐ 1. Naturally acquired active
☐ 2. Naturally acquired passive
☐ 3. Artificially acquired active
☐ 4. Artificially acquired passive

CORRECT ANSWER: 1

3. Which infectious disease is transmitted through puncture wounds, burns, or open wounds?

☐ 1. Rubeola

☐ 2. Rubella

☐ 3. Pertussis

☐ 4. Tetanus

CORRECT ANSWER: 4

4. Which infectious disease is accompanied by Koplik's spots that appear on the oral mucosa?

☐ 1. Haemophilus influenza

☐ 2. Poliomyelitis

☐ 3. Rubeola

☐ 4. Erythema infectiosum

CORRECT ANSWER: 3

5. Which disease is caused by the paramyxovirus?

☐ 1. Fifth disease

☐ 2. Mumps

☐ 3. Varicella

☐ 4. Roseola infantum

CORRECT ANSWER: 2

LEARNING OBJECTIVES

After studying this chapter, you should be able to:

● Describe the five methods of obtaining immune protection against communicable diseases.

● Discuss vaccine types and their major adverse effects.

● Identify the most common communicable childhood diseases that immunization can prevent.

CHAPTER OVERVIEW

Communicable diseases and infections are common in children. Children receive protection from communicable diseases either naturally or artificially. Various immunizations are given at specific times to protect them from certain diseases.

Ways microorganisms cause cell damage

- Self-produced toxins
- Intracellular multiplication
- Competition with the host metabolism

Chain of infection

- Causative agent
- Reservoir
- Portal of exit
- Mode of transmission
- Portal of entry
- Susceptible host

Stages of infection

- Incubation
- Prodromal stage
- Acute illness
- Convalescent stage

INFECTION

- **Definition**
  - Invasion and multiplication of microorganisms in or on body tissue that produce signs and symptoms as well as an immune response
  - Such reproduction injures the host by causing cell damage from microorganism-produced toxins or intracellular multiplication or by competing with the host metabolism

- **Chain of infection**
  - Causative agent — Any microbe that can produce disease
  - Reservoir — Environment or object in or on which a microbe can survive and, in some cases, multiply; can be an inanimate object, a human being, an animal, or an insect
  - Portal of exit — Path by which an infectious agent leaves its reservoir; usually it's the site where the organisms grow; portals of exit associated with human reservoirs include the respiratory, genitourinary, and GI tracts; the skin and mucous membranes; and the placenta
  - Mode of transmission — Means by which the infectious agent passes from the portal of exit in the reservoir to the susceptible host; infections may be transmitted through one of four modes:
    - Contact
    - Airborne
    - Enteric (oral-fecal)
    - Vector-borne
  - Portal of entry — Path by which an infectious agent invades a susceptible host
  - Susceptible host — Required for the transmission of infection to occur; an infectious agent is more likely to invade the body of a weakened host rather than a healthy one and launch an infectious disease

- **Stages of infection**
  - Incubation
    - The disease may develop almost instantaneously, or this period may last for years
    - During this time, the pathogen is replicating, and the infected person is contagious and can transmit the disease
  - Prodromal stage
    - This stage occurs after incubation

– The still-contagious host complains of feeling unwell; complaints are vague
- Acute illness
  – Microbes are actively destroying host cells and affecting specific host systems
  – The patient recognizes which area of the body is affected; complaints become more specific
- Convalescent stage
  – The body's defense mechanisms have begun to confine the microbes, and damaged tissue is healing

METHODS OF OBTAINING IMMUNE PROTECTION

● Natural (innate)
- This protection, present at birth, isn't learned and doesn't depend on previous contact
- Natural immunity includes barriers against disease, such as skin and mucous membranes, and bactericidal substances of body fluids, such as intestinal flora and gastric acid
- Some species are naturally immune to some diseases

● Naturally acquired active
- The immune system produces antibodies after exposure to disease (requires contact with the disease)
- This protection lasts for life
- The risk of the child developing adverse effects is high because he contracts the disease

● Naturally acquired passive
- No active immune process is involved; the antibodies are passively received
- The antibodies are acquired through placental transfer by way of immunoglobulin (Ig) G (the smallest Ig) and through breast-feeding by way of colostrum

● Artificially acquired active
- Medically engineered substances are injected to stimulate the immune response against a specific disease
- All immunizations are included

● Artificially acquired passive
- Antibodies are injected without stimulating the immune response
- The antibodies are used either as antitoxins or for prophylaxis
- The antibodies provide immediate protection that lasts for weeks or months
- Examples include gamma globulin (a mixture of antibodies against diseases that are prevalent in the community, pooled from 1,000

Methods of obtaining immune protection
- Natural immunity
- Naturally acquired active
- Naturally acquired passive
- Artificially acquired active
- Artificially acquired passive

Means of natural immunity
- Skin
- Mucous membranes
- Intestinal flora
- Gastric acid

Examples of hyperimmune or convalescent globulin
- Tetanus antitoxin
- Hepatitis B immune globulin
- Varicella zoster immune globulin

donors of human plasma) and hyperimmune or convalescent serum globulin (such as tetanus antitoxin, hepatitis B immune globulin, and varicella zoster immune globulin)

TYPES OF IMMUNIZATIONS

Types of immunizations

- Live, attenuated
- Inactivated

● **Live, attenuated**
  - A live organism, grown under suboptimal conditions, results in a live vaccine with reduced virulence
  - The vaccine confers 90% to 95% protection for 20+ years with a single dose
  - It promotes a full range of immunologic responses
  - The vaccine is inactivated by heat
  - Examples include measles, mumps, and rubella (MMR) vaccine and varicella vaccine
  - Influenza intranasal spray (LAIV) (Live)
    - Given to children older than age 5 without a history of chronic lung disease (asthma)

● **Inactivated**
  - An inactivated vaccine offers a weaker response than a live vaccine, necessitating frequent boosters
  - A toxoid is treated with formalin or heat and rendered nontoxic but still antigenic; it provides 90% to 100% protection
  - A killed vaccine doesn't promote replication; it provides 40% to 70% protection
  - The diffusible fraction of a virus is the part of the microorganism capable of inducing immunity
  - Examples of inactivated vaccines include the diphtheria and tetanus toxoids, the Salk polio vaccine, the pertussis vaccine, the hepatitis B vaccine, the hepatitis A vaccine, and HPV
  - Influenza I.M. injection (TIV)
    - Given annually to children ages 6 to 59 months
    - Vaccinate children age 5 or older if they are high risk (heart disease, lung disease, diabetes, renal dysfunction, immunosuppression, long-term aspirin therapy, asthma, or any other chronic illness)

Live, attenuated vaccines

- Measles, mumps, and rubella vaccine
- Varicella vaccine
- Influenza intranasal (LAIV)

Inactivated vaccines

- Diphtheria and tetanus toxoids
- Salk polio vaccine
- Pertussis vaccine
- Hepatitis B vaccine
- Hepatitis A vaccine
- Influenza injection (TIV)
- HPV

IMMUNIZATION SCHEDULE

● **Doses**
  - Childhood immunizations are usually given according to a predetermined schedule (see *Recommended schedule for immunization of healthy infants and children*)
  - Hepatitis A vaccine

Recommended schedule for immunization of healthy infants and children

Before immunization, ask the parents if the child is receiving corticosteroids or other drugs that suppress the immune response or if he had a recent febrile illness. Obtain a history of allergic responses, especially to antibiotics, eggs, feathers, and past immunizations. Keep in mind that a child who's at risk for acquired immunodeficiency syndrome or who tests positive for human immunodeficiency virus infection may need special consideration.

After immunization, tell the parents to watch for and report reactions other than local swelling and pain and mild temperature elevation. Give them the child's immunization record. The following are the 2007 general vaccine recommendations approved by the Advisory Committee on Immunization Practices, the American Academy of Pediatrics, and the American Academy of Family Physicians.

AGE	IMMUNIZATION
Birth	HepB
1 to 4 months	HepB
2 months	DTaP, HIB, IPV, PCV, Rota
4 months	DTaP, HIB, IPV, PCV, Rota
6 months	DTaP, HIB, PCV, Rota
6 to 18 months	HepB, IPV
6 to 59 months	Influenza (yearly)
12 to 15 months	HIB, MMR, PCV, HepA, varicella
12 to 23 months	HepA
15 to 18 months	DTaP HepA
4 to 6 years	DTaP, IPV, MMR, varicella
11 to 12 years	HPV, Tdap, MCV4
15 years	DTaP, MCV4

Common immunizations

- Hepatitis B (HepB)
- Diphtheria and tetanus toxoids and acellular pertussis vaccine (DTaP)
- *Haemophilus influenzae* type b conjugated vaccine (Hib)
- Inactivated poliovirus (IPV)
- Pneumococcal (PCV)
- Rotavirus (Rota)
- Influenza
- Varicella
- Hepatitis A (HepA)
- Meningococcal (MCV4)
- Measles, mumps, and rubella (MMR)
- Human papillomavirus (HPV)
- Tetanus, diphtheria, and pertussis (Tdap)

- Recommended for all children; given in two doses; one at 12 months then a second given 6 months later
- Also recommended for children older than age 2 with chronic liver disease, clotting factors disorder, homosexual and bisexual adolescent males, and recreational drug users
- Hepatitis B vaccine
  - Complete series requires three doses: at birth (or before hospital discharge), 1 to 2 months, and 6 to 18 months
  - Infants born to hepatitis B surface antigen (HBsAg)-positive mothers should receive the first dose of hepatitis B vaccine and a

Adverse effects of diphtheria and tetanus toxoids

- Drowsiness
- Vomiting
- Anorexia
- Soreness and redness at injection site
- Fever

Adverse effects of MMR vaccine

- Faint, transient rash
- Arthralgia
- Low-grade fever

dose of hepatitis B immune globulin (HBIG) within 12 hours of birth at different injection sites
  – Infants born to mothers with unknown HBsAg status should receive the first dose of hepatitis B vaccine within 12 hours of birth
  – Common adverse effects include swelling or redness at the injection site
- Diphtheria and tetanus toxoids and acellular pertussis vaccine (DTaP)
  – Five doses are given: at 2 months, 4 months, 6 months, 15 to 18 months, and 4 to 6 years
  – Tetanus and diphtheria toxoids and acellular pertussis (Tdap) (adolescent preparation) is recommended at age 11 to 12 for those who have completed the recommended childhood diphtheria and tetanus toxoids and pertussis/diphtheria and tetanus toxoids and acellular pertussis (DTP/DTaP) vaccination series and haven't received the tetanus and diphtheria toxoids (Td) booster
  – Subsequent Td boosters are recommended every 10 years
  – Common adverse effects include drowsiness, vomiting, anorexia, soreness and redness at the injection site, and fever
- *Haemophilus influenzae* type B (HIB) vaccine
  – Four doses are given: at 2 months, 4 months, 6 months, and 12 to 15 months
  – Common adverse effects are redness and pain at the injection site
- Human papillomavirus vaccine (Gardasil)
  – Three doses are given to females ages 11 to 12 (no younger than age 9); the second dose 2 months after the first dose and the third dose 6 months after the first dose
  – Common adverse reactions include fever, nausea, dizziness, and injection site reactions, including pain, swelling, itching, and redness
- Inactivated poliovirus vaccine (IPV)
  – Four doses are given: at 2 months, 4 months, 6 to 18 months, and 4 to 6 years
  – Oral polio vaccine is no longer used
  – Common adverse effects are pain at the injection site and fever
- Influenza
  – The first time a child age 8 or younger receives the influenza vaccine, he should receive two doses, separated by 4 weeks for TIV and at least 6 weeks for LAIV
- MMR vaccine
  – Two doses are given: at 12 to 15 months and 4 to 6 years
  – Common adverse effects include faint, transient rash; arthralgia; and low-grade fever
  – Postpubertal females shouldn't become pregnant within 3 months of immunization

- Varicella virus vaccine
  - Two doses are given: at 12 to 15 months and at 4 to 6 years
  - Two-dose series is given to all susceptible adolescents age 13 and older
  - Common adverse effects include faint rash, fever, and varicella-like rash at the injection site
- Pneumococcal vaccine
  - Four doses are given: at 2 months, 4 months, 6 months, and 12 to 15 months
  - Common adverse effects are drowsiness, irritability, restless sleep, diarrhea, vomiting, decreased appetite, and injection site reactions, including edema, erythema, induration, inflammation, skin discoloration, and tenderness
  - Pneumoconjugate isn't given to children age 5 or older
- Rotavirus vaccine (Rotateq)
  - Three-dose series given: at 2 months, 4 months, and 6 months
  - Given orally
  - May give first dose as early as 6 weeks and third dose no later than 32 weeks
  - Common adverse reactions are mild diarrhea and vomiting

- **Principles of vaccine administration**
  - Divided doses don't decrease the risk of adverse effects
  - If the child has one severe reaction, don't administer a booster without further evaluation; ask which adverse effects (if any) the child had from the previous immunization
  - Withhold the DTaP vaccine if the child has a progressive and active central nervous system (CNS) problem; a child with cerebral palsy can receive immunizations
  - Don't vaccinate if the child's temperature is elevated; a vaccine's adverse effect would be difficult to differentiate from an exacerbation of the original disease
  - Don't vaccinate with a live virus vaccine if the child's immune system is suppressed or if he has received gamma globulin within the past 6 weeks, is allergic to the contents of the immunization, or has been on chemotherapy
  - Don't give the tuberculin purified protein derivative test and the measles vaccine at the same time; the measles vaccine may make a tuberculosis (TB)-positive person appear to be TB-negative
  - The rubella vaccine can cause transient arthritis, arthralgia, and joint pain 1 month after vaccination; rare in young children but occurs more commonly in postpubertal females
  - The risk of adverse effects from a vaccine is significantly less than the risk of adverse effects caused by the disease

Adverse effects of varicella virus vaccine

- Faint rash
- Fever
- Varicella-like rash at injection site

Adverse effects of pneumococcal vaccine

- Drowsiness
- Irritability
- Restless sleep
- Diarrhea
- Vomiting
- Decreased appetite
- Injection site reactions

Key facts about immunizations

- Divided doses don't increase the risk of adverse effects.
- The risk of adverse effects from a vaccine is significantly less than the risk of adverse effects caused by the disease.
- All routinely recommended pediatric vaccines contain no, or only trace amounts of, mercury.

- Assess for pregnancy in teenagers; some vaccines shouldn't be given during pregnancy
- Teach parents about the complications of communicable diseases and the potential adverse effects of vaccines (see *Communicable diseases*)
- All routinely recommended pediatric vaccines contain no, or only trace amounts of, mercury (thimerosal)
- Meningococcal vaccine should be offered to all older adolescents going to college or joining the military
- Foreign-born adopted children should have their immunization status checked carefully; immunizations should be started as soon as possible

BACTERIAL INFECTIONS

● Diphtheria
- General information
  - Acute, highly contagious toxin-mediated infection
  - Caused by *Corynebacterium diphtheriae*, a gram-positive rod that usually infects the respiratory tract, primarily the tonsils, nasopharynx, and larynx
  - More serious in infants because of their smaller airways
  - Rare in many parts of the world, including the United States
- Assessment findings
  - Thick, patchy, grayish green membrane over the mucous membranes of the pharynx, larynx, tonsils, soft palate, and nose
  - Fever
  - Sore throat, rasping cough, hoarseness
  - Airway obstruction (tachypnea, stridor, possibly cyanosis, suprasternal retractions, and suffocation, if untreated)
  - Positive throat culture for bacilli
- Complications
  - Thrombocytopenia
  - Myocarditis

Key facts about diphtheria

- Highly contagious
- Toxin-mediated
- Caused by *Corynebacterium diphtheriae*
- Usually infects respiratory tract
- Rare

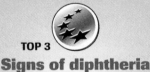

TOP 3

Signs of diphtheria

1. Thick, patchy, grayish green membrane over pharynx, larynx, tonsils, soft palate, and nose
2. Sore throat, rasping cough, hoarseness
3. Airway obstruction

– Severe neuritis with paralysis of the soft palate, eye muscles, and diaphragm

– Renal, cardiac, and peripheral CNS damage

• Nursing interventions

– Maintain infection precautions until after two consecutive negative nasopharyngeal cultures to prevent spread of the disease

– Rule out the child's sensitivity to horse serum because antitoxin is derived from it

– Administer antitoxin in large doses as ordered

– Administer penicillin or erythromycin, as ordered

– Maintain bed rest during the acute stage

● Pertussis (whooping cough)

• General information

– Highly contagious respiratory tract infection; characteristically produces an irritating cough that becomes paroxysmal and commonly ends in a high-pitched inspiratory whoop

– Usually caused by the nonmotile, gram-negative coccobacillus *Bordetella pertussis* and, occasionally, by the related, similar bacteria *B. parapertussis* and *B. bronchiseptica*

– Typically transmitted by direct inhalation of contaminated droplets from a person in the acute stage

– Spreads indirectly through soiled linen and other articles contaminated by respiratory secretions

• Assessment findings

– Spasmodic, recurrent coughing with tenacious mucus; cough typically ends in a loud, crowing inspiratory whoop

– Infants can have symptoms of choking and gasping for air

– Vomiting, if the patient chokes on mucus

– Epistaxis during paroxysmal coughing

– Exhaustion and cyanosis after coughing spell

– Sneezing, lacrimation, and rhinorrhea

– Diminished breath sounds, upper airway wheezing

• Complications

– Increased venous pressure

– Anterior eye chamber hemorrhage; detached retina and blindness

– Rectal prolapse

– Inguinal or umbilical hernia

– Encephalopathy, seizures

– Atelectasis, pneumonitis, or pneumonia

– In infants: apnea, anoxia

– Rib fractures

• Nursing interventions

– Maintain a patent airway; keep suctioning equipment readily available

– Create a quiet environment to decrease coughing stimulation
– Anticipate using a mist tent to help loosen secretions
– Maintain respiratory isolation (mask only) for 5 to 7 days after antibiotic therapy begins

● **Tetanus (lockjaw)**
  • General information
    – An acute exotoxin-mediated infection that's usually systemic but possibly localized
    – Caused by *Clostridium tetani*, an anaerobic, spore-forming bacteria
    – Transmitted through puncture wounds, burns, or open wounds contaminated by soil, dust, or animal excreta that contains *C. tetani*
    – Reaches the axons of the nerves, causing involuntary muscle contraction, muscle rigidity, and painful paroxysmal seizures
    – No transplacental immunity; attacks equally dangerous to adults and children
  • Assessment findings
    – Rigid neck and facial muscles, resulting in lockjaw (trismus) and a grotesque, grinning expression (risus sardonicus)
    – Rigid somatic muscles, causing arched-back rigidity (opisthotonos)
    – Spasm and increased muscle tone near the wound (local infection)
    – Irregular heartbeat and tachycardia
    – Hyperactive deep tendon reflexes
    – Profuse sweating, low-grade fever
  • Complications
    – Pneumonia
    – Airway obstruction
    – Respiratory arrest
    – Heart failure, cardiac arrhythmias
    – Fractures
    – Severe pain
    – Death
  • Nursing interventions
    – If the child has a clean wound that's less than 6 hours old and has been immunized less than 5 years ago, no treatment is needed
    – If the child has a clean wound and was immunized less than 10 years ago, administer a toxoid
    – If the child has a dirty wound and didn't complete the initial series of immunizations, or if the child's immunizations are more than 10 years old, give the toxoid and Ig
    – Maintain an adequate airway and ventilation; keep emergency airway equipment readily available

● *Haemophilus influenzae* type B (HIB) infection

- General information
  - Bacterial disease that's a common cause of epiglottiditis, laryngo-tracheobronchitis, pneumonia, bronchiolitis, otitis media, and meningitis
  - Caused by *H. influenzae*, a gram-negative, pleomorphic aerobic bacillus
  - Transmitted by direct contact with secretions or airborne droplets
- Assessment findings
  - Generalized malaise, high fever
  - Other signs and symptoms depend on presenting infection
- Complications
  - Permanent neurologic sequelae from meningitis
  - Complete upper airway obstruction from epiglottiditis
  - Cellulitis
  - Pericarditis, pleural effusion
  - Respiratory failure from pneumonia
- Nursing interventions
  - Maintain respiratory isolation
  - Maintain adequate respiratory function through cool humidification, oxygen as needed, and croup or face tents; suction as needed
  - Keep emergency resuscitation equipment readily available
  - Maintain adequate nutrition and elimination

VIRAL INFECTIONS

● Rubeola (measles)

- General information
  - Acute, highly contagious infection that causes a characteristic maculopapular rash
  - Can be severe or fatal in patients with impaired cell-mediated immunity; mortality highest in children younger than age 2 and in adults
  - Caused by rubeola virus
  - Spread by direct contact or by inhalation of contaminated airborne droplets; portal of entry in the upper respiratory tract
- Assessment findings
  - Fever, periorbital edema, conjunctivitis
  - Koplik's spots (tiny gray-white specks surrounded by red halo) on oral mucosa opposite the molars that may bleed
  - Red, blotchy rash that begins on the face and becomes generalized
  - Severe cough, rhinorrhea, lymphadenopathy
- Complications
  - Secondary bacterial infection

Key facts about *H. influenzae* type B infection

- Transmitted by direct contact with secretions or airborne droplets
- Signs and symptoms depend on presenting infections but may include generalized malaise and high fever

Key facts about rubeola

- Also called *measles*
- Caused by rubeola virus
- Highly contagious
- Spread by direct contact or by inhalation of contaminated airborne droplets
- Causes maculopapular rash
- Mortality is highest in children younger than age 2 and in adults

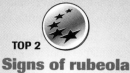

TOP 2

Signs of rubeola

1. Koplik's spots on oral mucosa
2. Red, blotchy rash that begins on the face and becomes generalized

– Autoimmune reaction
– Bronchitis, otitis media, pneumonia
– Encephalitis
- Nursing interventions
  – Institute respiratory isolation measures for 4 days after rash onset
  – Encourage bed rest during the acute period
  – Report measles cases to local public health officials
  – Administer antipyretics for fever, as ordered
  – Keep the child well-hydrated

● Rubella (German measles)

- General information
  – Acute, mildly contagious viral disease that causes a distinctive maculopapular rash (resembling that of measles or scarlet fever) and lymphadenopathy
  – Caused by rubella virus (a togavirus)
  – Virus enters the bloodstream, usually through the respiratory tract
- Assessment findings
  – Rash accompanied by a low-grade fever
  – Exanthematous, maculopapular, mildly pruritic rash; typically begins on the face and spreads rapidly, covering the trunk and extremities within hours
  – Small, red, petechial macules on the soft palate (Forschheimer spots) preceding or accompanying the rash
  – Suboccipital, postauricular, and postcervical lymph node enlargement
- Complications
  – Arthritis
  – Postinfectious encephalitis
  – Thrombocytopenic purpura
  – Congenital rubella
  – In fetal infection (rare after 20 weeks' gestation): intrauterine death, spontaneous abortion, congenital malformations of major organ systems
- Nursing interventions
  – Institute isolation precautions until 5 days after the rash disappears; keep an infant with congenital rubella in isolation for 3 months, until three throat cultures are negative
  – Keep the patient's skin clean and dry
  – Ensure that the patient receives care only from nonpregnant hospital workers who aren't at risk for rubella; as ordered, administer immune globulin to nonimmunized people who visit the patient
  – Report confirmed rubella cases to local public health officials

● Mumps (parotitis)

- General information

Key facts about rubella

- Also called *German measles*
- Acute viral disease
- Caused by rubella virus
- Transmitted via respiratory tract
- Mildly contagious

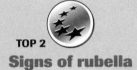

TOP 2

Signs of rubella

1. Exanthematous, maculopapular, mildly pruritic rash
2. Suboccipital, postauricular, and postcervical lymph node enlargement

Parotid inflammation in mumps

The mumps virus (paramyxovirus) attacks the parotid glands — the main salivary glands. Inflammation causes characteristic swelling and discomfort associated with eating, drinking, swallowing, and talking.

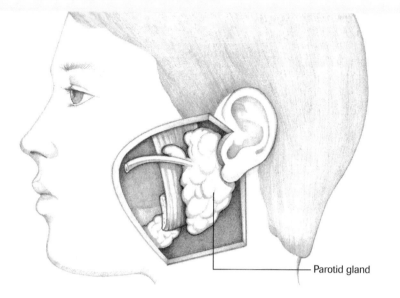

Parotid gland

- Acute inflammation of one or both parotid glands and sometimes the sublingual or submaxillary glands
- Caused by a paramyxovirus found in the saliva of an infected person
- Transmitted by droplets or by direct contact with the saliva of an infected person
- Assessment findings
  - Myalgia
  - Anorexia
  - Malaise
  - Headache, an earache aggravated by chewing, and pain when drinking sour or acidic liquids
  - Fever
  - Swelling and tenderness of the parotid glands (see *Parotid inflammation in mumps*)
  - Simultaneous or subsequent swelling of one or more other salivary glands
- Complications
  - Epididymoorchitis
  - Meningoencephalitis
  - Male infertility (rare)
  - Pancreatitis
  - Transient sensorineural hearing loss (typically unilateral)

Key facts about mumps

- Caused by a paramyxovirus
- Transmitted by droplets or direct contact with saliva of an infected person
- Causes acute inflammation of one or both parotid glands
- Sometimes causes acute inflammation of sublingual or submaxillary glands

TOP 2

Signs of mumps

1. Swelling and tenderness of parotid glands
2. Simultaneous or subsequent swelling of other salivary glands

Classifying poliomyelitis

- Inapparent (subclinical)
- Abortive (minor illness)
- Major (nonparalytic or paralytic)

Signs and symptoms of nonparalytic poliomyelitis

- Moderate fever
- Headache
- Vomiting
- Lethargy
- Irritability
- Pains in the neck, back, arms, legs, and abdomen
- Muscle tenderness, weakness, and spasms in the extensors of the neck or back

Signs and symptoms specific to paralytic poliomyelitis

- Asymmetrical weakness of various muscles
- Loss of superficial and deep reflexes
- Paresthesia
- Hypersensitivity to touch
- Urine retention
- Constipation
- Abdominal distention

– Arthritis
– Nephritis
- Nursing interventions
  – Apply warm or cool compresses to the neck area to relieve pain
  – Report all cases of mumps to local public health officials

● **Poliomyelitis (polio)**
- General information
  – Acute communicable disease that may range in severity from inapparent infection to fatal paralytic illness
  – Caused by the poliovirus
  – Transmitted by direct contact with infected oropharyngeal secretions or stool
- Assessment findings
  – Inapparent (subclinical) — no signs or symptoms
  – Abortive poliomyelitis (minor illness) — slight fever, headache, malaise, sore throat, inflamed pharynx, and vomiting
  – Major poliomyelitis — involves the CNS and may be nonparalytic or paralytic
    · Nonparalytic — moderate fever, headache, vomiting, lethargy, irritability, and pains in the neck, back, arms, legs, and abdomen; muscle tenderness, weakness, and spasms in the extensors of the neck and back
    · Paralytic — symptoms similar to those of nonparalytic poliomyelitis, with asymmetrical weakness of various muscles, loss of superficial and deep reflexes, paresthesia, hypersensitivity to touch, urine retention, constipation, and abdominal distention
- Complications
  – Hypertension
  – Urinary tract infection
  – Urolithiasis
  – Atelectasis
  – Pneumonia
  – Myocarditis
  – Skeletal and soft-tissue deformities
  – Paralytic ileus
- Nursing interventions
  – To control the spread of poliomyelitis, wash your hands thoroughly after contact with the patient, especially after contact with excretions (only facility personnel who have been vaccinated against poliomyelitis may have direct contact with the patient)
  – Observe the patient carefully for signs of paralysis and other neurologic damage, which can occur rapidly
  – Maintain a patent airway, and watch for respiratory weakness and difficulty swallowing

– Apply high-top sneakers or use a footboard to prevent footdrop

● **Varicella (chickenpox)**

• General information
  – Acute, highly contagious infection that can occur at any age
  – Caused by the varicella-zoster virus, which also causes herpes zoster (shingles)
  – Transmitted through direct contact (primarily with respiratory secretions, less common with skin lesions) and indirect contact (through airwaves)

• Assessment findings
  – Fever
  – Crops of small, erythematous macules on the trunk or scalp
  – Macules progress to papules and then clear vesicles on an erythematous base (so-called dewdrops on rose petals)
  – Vesicles become cloudy and break easy; then scabs form
  – Rash spreads to face and torso; less distribution of rash to extremities
  – Rash is a combination of red papules, vesicles, and scabs in various stages
  – Ulcers on mucous membranes of the mouth, conjunctivae, and genitalia

• Complications
  – With scratching due to severe pruritus: infection, scarring, impetigo, furuncles, and cellulitis
  – Reye's syndrome
  – Myocarditis
  – Bleeding disorders
  – Arthritis
  – Nephritis
  – Hepatitis
  – Pneumonia
  – Meningitis

• Nursing interventions
  – Institute strict isolation measures until all skin lesions have crusted
  – Observe an immunocompromised patient for manifestations of complications, such as pneumonitis and meningitis, and report them immediately
  – Provide skin care comfort measures (calamine lotion, cornstarch, oatmeal baths, sponge baths, or showers); administer oral antihistamines (preferred over topical itch medications)
  – Keep the child's fingernails short and clean
  – Don't give aspirin when a viral infection is suspected; the combination of these may result in Reye's syndrome, an acute encephalopathy with cerebral cortex swelling but without

---

Key facts about varicella

• Also called *chickenpox*
• Highly contagious
• Can occur at any age
• Caused by varicella-zoster virus
• Transmitted through direct or indirect contact

Complications of scratching chickenpox

• Infection
• Scarring
• Impetigo
• Furuncles
• Cellulitis

Comfort measures for varicella

• Calamine lotion
• Cornstarch
• Oatmeal baths
• Sponge baths
• Showers

Reye's syndrome

• What is it? Acute encephalopathy with cerebral cortex swelling but without inflammation.
• How do you prevent it? Don't give aspirin when a viral infection is suspected.

inflammation, accompanied by impaired liver function and hyperammonemia
  - Advise the parents that the child can't return to day care or school until all lesions are crusted

● **Fifth disease (erythema infectiosum)**
  - General information
    - Contagious disease characterized by rose-colored eruptions diffused over the skin, usually starting on the cheeks
    - Caused by human parvovirus B19
    - Transmitted by way of the respiratory tract
  - Assessment findings
    - Mildly erythematous pharynx and conjunctivae
    - Intensely red facial rash, forming a "slapped face" appearance 4 to 7 days after resolution of symptoms
    - Rash on extensor surfaces of extremities 1 day after facial rash appears
    - Rash on flexor surface and trunk 1 day later and lasting 1 or more weeks
  - Complications
    - Arthritis and arthralgia
    - Myocarditis, encephalitis (both rare)
  - Interventions
    - Isolation isn't necessary
    - Cut the child's fingernails to avoid injury from scratching
    - Provide lukewarm water baths with baking soda to soothe itching

● **Roseola infantum (exanthema subitum)**
  - General information
    - Common acute, benign, presumably viral illness characterized by fever with subsequent rash
    - Caused by human herpesvirus types 6 and 7
    - May be transmitted by saliva and, possibly, genital secretions
  - Assessment findings
    - High fever (102° F to 105° F [38.9° C to 40.6° C]), with rash appearing after the fever breaks
    - Maculopapular, nonpruritic rash that blanches with pressure
    - Profuse rash on the trunk, arms, and neck; mild rash on the face and legs; rash fades within 24 hours
  - Complications
    - Encephalopathy
    - Thrombocytopenic purpura
    - Febrile seizures
  - Nursing interventions
    - Give tepid sponge baths and administer antipyretics (not aspirin), as ordered

– Replace fluids and electrolytes as needed

– Institute seizure precautions

NCLEX CHECKS

It's never too soon to begin your NCLEX preparation. Now that you've reviewed this chapter, carefully read each of the following questions and choose the best answer. Then compare your responses to the correct answers.

1. A nurse is assessing a child with a rash. Which finding would lead her to conclude that the child has chickenpox?

☐ **1.** Rash that starts on the face and moves to the trunk

☐ **2.** Red, raised rash that begins on the trunk

☐ **3.** Central rash that's sparse on distal limbs

☐ **4.** Scaling of the palms and soles

2. The American Academy of Pediatrics (AAP) recommends that the first dose of the hepatitis B vaccine be given at what age?

☐ **1.** Neonate

☐ **2.** 2 months

☐ **3.** 4 months

☐ **4.** 6 months

3. Place in chronological order the correct sequence for the stages of infection.

1. Prodromal stage	
2. Convalescent stage	
3. Incubation	
4. Acute illness	

4. A child is born to a woman who tested HBsAg positive. When should this infant receive the first dose of hepatitis B vaccine?

☐ **1.** Within 12 hours of birth

☐ **2.** Within the first 2 months after birth

☐ **3.** Between ages 1 and 4 months

☐ **4.** Between ages 6 and 18 months

5. A nurse is assessing a child who may have measles. Which clinical manifestation most commonly appears in a child suffering from measles?

☐ **1.** Arthritis

☐ **2.** Parotid gland enlargement

☐ **3.** Erythematous rash

☐ **4.** Encephalitis

TOP 6

Items to study for your next test on pediatric communicable diseases and infections

1. Methods of obtaining immune protection
2. Recommended schedule for pediatric immunizations
3. Adverse reactions of frequently administered vaccines
4. Classifications of poliomyelitis
5. Prevention of Reye's syndrome
6. Nursing interventions for the child with varicella

6. The live intranasal influenza vaccine is recommended for:
- ☐ **1.** children with immunosuppression.
- ☐ **2.** preschool-age children.
- ☐ **3.** children older than age 5 years.
- ☐ **4.** adolescents only.

7. The nurse is caring for a 12-year-old child who has a laceration on his ankle and whose last immunizations were at age 5. What immunization should she expect the child to receive?
- ☐ **1.** DTaP
- ☐ **2.** DT
- ☐ **3.** Td
- ☐ **4.** Tdap

8. What route is recommended for the administration of the rotavirus vaccine?
- ☐ **1.** Subcutaneous injection
- ☐ **2.** Intramuscular injection
- ☐ **3.** Orally as a liquid
- ☐ **4.** Orally as a tablet

9. Preadolescent females should receive the human papillomavirus vaccine in order to prevent:
- ☐ **1.** cervical cancer.
- ☐ **2.** birth defects to their future children.
- ☐ **3.** genital herpes.
- ☐ **4.** menstrual irregularities.

10. A nurse is caring for a child with an infectious disease that produces a rash when the child's fever breaks. The child has:
- ☐ **1.** fifth disease.
- ☐ **2.** roseola infantum.
- ☐ **3.** poliomyelitis.
- ☐ **4.** mumps.

ANSWERS AND RATIONALES

1. CORRECT ANSWER: 3
A child with chickenpox has a centralized rash that's sparse on the distal limbs, along with lesions in different stages on one area of the body. The rash doesn't start on the face and move to the trunk, and it usually doesn't start as a red, raised rash. Scaling of the palms and soles isn't seen in chickenpox.

2. CORRECT ANSWER: 1

The AAP recommends that the first dose of hepatitis B vaccine be given in the neonatal nursery.

3. CORRECT ANSWER:

| **3.** Incubation |
| **1.** Prodromal stage |
| **4.** Acute illness |
| **2.** Convalescent stage |

Infection begins with incubation. During that time, the pathogen is replicating and the infected person is contagious. The prodromal stage occurs after incubation; the host is still contagious and has vague complaints of not feeling well. During acute illness, microbes actively destroy host cells. During the convalescent stage, the body's defense mechanisms have begun to confine the microbes and damaged tissue is healing.

4. CORRECT ANSWER: 1

An infant born to an HBsAg-positive mother should receive the hepatitis B vaccine and HBIG within 12 hours of birth at different injection sites. An infant born to an HBsAg-negative mother should receive the vaccine before discharge from the hospital after birth.

5. CORRECT ANSWER: 3

A rash is seen with measles. It usually occurs after spots develop in the prodromal stage (when early symptoms appear). Arthritis symptoms are seen with such diseases as fifth disease and the mumps. Parotid gland enlargement occurs with the mumps. Encephalitis can be a complication of measles, but it isn't a clinical manifestation.

6. CORRECT ANSWER: 3

The live intranasal influenza vaccine is given to children older than age 5 years. Children with immunosuppression shouldn't receive this live virus vaccine because it can cause them to develop influenza from the vaccine, which can be life-threatening.

7. CORRECT ANSWER: 4

Tdap should be given to this child because it has been more than 5 years since his last dose of DTaP. An adolescent who has never received Tdap before is recommended to receive it. DTaP is given to younger children (less than age 6 years).

8. CORRECT ANSWER: 3

Rotavirus is for infants. The recommended administration is at ages 2, 4, and 6 months. The vaccine is given orally, not via injection. Infants shouldn't be given medications in tablet form because they could choke on them.

9. CORRECT ANSWER: 1

HPV vaccine can prevent most cases of cervical cancer. It doesn't prevent birth defects or affect menses. There's no vaccine for genital herpes.

10. CORRECT ANSWER: 2

Roseola infantum is accompanied by a high fever of 102° F to 105° F (38.9° C to 40.6° C) with a rash that appears as soon as the fever breaks. Fifth disease is accompanied by a rash that appears 4 to 7 days after resolution of symptoms. Poliomyelitis and mumps are accompanied by a rash.

5

Altered hematologic functioning

PRETEST

1. What's the average life cycle of a red blood cell?
- [ ] 1. 24 hours
- [ ] 2. 72 hours
- [ ] 3. 130 days
- [ ] 4. 120 days

CORRECT ANSWER: 4

2. What structure or structures maintain acid-base balance?
- [ ] 1. White blood cells
- [ ] 2. Red blood cells
- [ ] 3. Plasma
- [ ] 4. Lymphocytes

CORRECT ANSWER: 2

3. Hemophilia A is caused by a deficiency in which coagulation factor?
- [ ] 1. VII
- [ ] 2. VIII
- [ ] 3. IX
- [ ] 4. X

CORRECT ANSWER: 2

4. Hemorrhage into the skin resulting in red discoloration is indicative of what disorder?

- ☐ 1. Hemophilia
- ☐ 2. Iron deficiency anemia
- ☐ 3. Idiopathic thrombocytopenic purpura
- ☐ 4. Sickle cell anemia

CORRECT ANSWER: 3

5. Which diagnostic indicator suggests sickle cell trait?

- ☐ 1. Less than 50% hemoglobin S
- ☐ 2. More than 50% hemoglobin S
- ☐ 3. Less than 50% factor
- ☐ 4. More than 50%

CORRECT ANSWER: 1

LEARNING OBJECTIVES

After studying this chapter, you should be able to:

- List at least five functions of blood.
- Describe appropriate nursing interventions for the child with hyperbilirubinemia.
- Discuss conditions associated with alterations in red blood cell and platelet functioning.
- Plan appropriate nursing care for pediatric patients with anemia and clotting deficiencies.

CHAPTER OVERVIEW

Knowledge of normal RBC and clotting function provides the foundation for understanding the conditions associated with altered hematologic function. Assessment and nursing interventions are geared to preventing and controlling the problems associated with the alteration and promoting normal function.

KEY CONCEPTS

● **Structures**
  • Blood composition
    – Cells—erythrocytes (RBCs) that carry oxygen to the tissues and remove carbon dioxide, thrombocytes (platelets) that contribute to clotting, and three types of leukocytes WBCs that participate in the immune response: lymphocytes, monocytes, and granulocytes
      · All five blood cell types are produced in the bone marrow and originate from the same stem cell (see *Human blood cell development,* page 100)
      · Early in utero, all blood cells are made by the liver and spleen; these organs retain some hematopoietic ability throughout life
      · Before birth, the bone marrow becomes the main producer of blood cells
    – Plasma—largely water; also includes plasma proteins, electrolytes and dissolved nutrients, clotting factors, anticoagulants, and antibodies

● **Functions**
  • Blood
    – Carries oxygen to tissues and removes carbon dioxide
    – Provides cellular nutrition by carrying nutrients from the GI tract to the tissues
    – Removes waste products by transporting them to the lungs, kidneys, liver, and skin for excretion
    – Maintains acid-base balance
    – Regulates body temperature by transferring heat from deep within the body to small vessels near the skin
    – Defends against foreign antigens by transporting leukocytes and antibodies to the sites of infection, injury, and inflammation
    – Transports hormones from the endocrine glands to various parts of the body
  • Plasma
    – Carries antibodies and nutrients to tissues and carries wastes away
  • RBC functioning
    – RBCs transport oxygen from the lungs to the tissues and carbon dioxide from the tissues to the lungs

Five blood cell types

- Erythrocytes (RBCs)
- Platelets
- Lymphocytes
- Monocytes
- Granulocytes

What's in plasma

- Water
- Plasma proteins
- Electrolytes
- Dissolved nutrients
- Clotting factors
- Anticoagulants
- Antibodies

Functions of blood

- Carries oxygen to tissues and removes carbon dioxide
- Provides cellular nutrition
- Removes waste products
- Maintains acid-base balance
- Regulates body temperature
- Defends against foreign antigens
- Transports hormones from the endocrine glands to various parts of the body

Human blood cell development

All five blood cell types originate from the same stem cell. The flowchart below shows how this stem cell becomes differentiated, developing into each blood cell type.

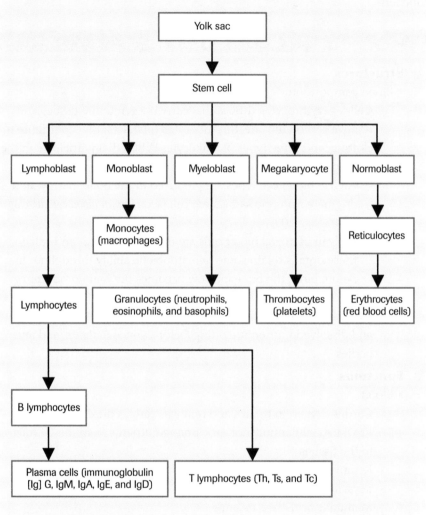

Key facts about RBCs

- RBCs transport oxygen from the lungs to the tissues and carbon dioxide from the tissues to the lungs.
- Reticulocytes are precursors of mature RBCs.
- RBCs live 120 days.
- RBC production is stimulated by erythropoietin.
- Excess RBC production is called *polycythemia*.
- Neonates normally have high RBC counts.
- Hb is the iron-containing pigment in RBCs.
- RBCs are classified by size and color.

– Reticulocytes are precursors of mature RBCs; they constitute 2% of total RBCs and predict RBC production
– RBCs live 120 days
  · At death, most of their iron is conserved
  · The remaining products produce indirect bilirubin
  · Liver enzyme converts indirect bilirubin to direct bilirubin so it can be excreted in bile
– RBC production is stimulated by erythropoietin (made in the kidneys) in response to hypoxia

– Excess RBC production is called *polycythemia;* it results in increased blood viscosity

– Neonates normally have high RBC counts (4.8 to 7.1 million/mm^3)

– Hemoglobin (Hb) is the iron-containing pigment in the RBC; it carries oxygen to the tissues

  • Normal Hb changes

    - During the first 6 months of fetal life, 90% of Hb is fetal hemoglobin (HbF), which absorbs oxygen at a lower tension; at birth, 75% of Hb is HbF

  • The production of adult hemoglobin (HbA) begins during the last 2 months in utero; it slowly replaces HbF and reaches adult levels by age 2

  • The infant's Hb level is lowest between ages 4 and 6 months, when HbF is decreasing and HbA is developing

    - This state is called physiologic anemia

    - Iron should be added to the infant's diet during this time

– RBCs are classified by size (macrocytic, microcytic, normocytic) and color (hyperchromic, hypochromic, normochromic)

• Clotting functioning

  – Normal platelet (thrombocyte) function

    • Platelets are the smallest blood element

      - They aren't nucleated

      - They live 4 to 10 days

    • Platelets cause capillary homeostasis by adhering to the inner surface of a vessel and sticking to one another

    • They produce a temporary mechanical plug

    • They repair breaks in small blood vessels and capillaries, especially in the skin, mucous membranes, and internal organs

    • Heparin, aspirin, guaifenesin (Robitussin), indomethacin (Indocin), and phenylbutazone (Butazolidin) interfere with platelet function

  – Normal clotting mechanism

    • In the intrinsic pathway, platelet factor, antihemophilic factor (factor VIII), and multiple clotting factors (including calcium) result in thromboplastin formation; generation of thromboplastin is measured by partial thromboplastin time (PTT)

    • In the extrinsic pathway, injured tissue cells release incomplete thromboplastin; this plus multiple clotting factors result in thromboplastin formation

    • Prothrombin and vitamin K (with the help of thromboplastin) result in thrombin production, which is measured by prothrombin time (PT)

    • Fibrinogen, thrombin, and factor VIII produce a fibrin clot, which is measured by thrombin time

Normal hemoglobin changes

● During the first 6 months of fetal life, 90% of Hb is HbF.
● At birth, 75% of Hb is HbF.
● Production of adult Hb begins during last 2 months in utero; reaches adult levels by age 2.
● The infant's Hb level is lowest between ages 4 and 6 months.

Key facts about platelets

● Smallest blood element
● Life span is 4 to 10 days
● Cause capillary homeostasis by adhering to inner surface of a vessel and sticking to one another
● Repair breaks in small blood vessels and capillaries

Drugs that interfere with platelet function

● Heparin
● Aspirin
● Guaifenesin
● Indomethacin
● Phenylbutazone

DIAGNOSTIC TESTS

● Blood typing
- Purpose
  - To determine the antigens present in a patient's RBCs; reaction with standardized sera indicates the presence of specific antigens
- Nursing interventions
  - Explain the procedure to the child and his family
  - Handle the sample gently to prevent hemolysis
  - Apply pressure to the venipuncture site to prevent hematoma formation and bleeding

● Coagulation study
- Purpose
  - To analyze platelet function, platelet count, PT, International Normalized Ratio, PTT, coagulation time, and bleeding time
- Nursing interventions
  - Note the child's current drug therapy before the procedure
  - Check the venipuncture site for bleeding after the procedure

NURSING DIAGNOSES

● Probable nursing diagnoses
- Activity intolerance
- Fatigue
- Imbalanced nutrition: Less than body requirements
- Impaired gas exchange
- Ineffective thermoregulation
- Ineffective tissue perfusion: Peripheral

● Possible nursing diagnoses
- Acute pain
- Risk for activity intolerance
- Risk for imbalanced body temperature
- Risk for imbalanced fluid volume
- Risk for impaired skin integrity

APLASTIC ANEMIA

● Definition
- Group of disorders characterized by pancytopenia (anemia, granulocytopenia, and thrombocytopenia) resulting from the decreased functional capacity of a hypoplastic, fatty bone marrow

● Causes
- Congenital

- Congenital hypoplastic anemia (Blackfan-Diamond anemia); develops between ages 2 and 3 months
- Fanconi syndrome (characterized by pancytopenia, hypoplasia of bone marrow, and patchy brown discoloration of the skin) develops between birth and age 10; chromosomal abnormalities usually associated with multiple congenital anomalies

• Acquired
- Drug-induced; occurs as an adverse effect from chemotherapy, chloramphenicol (Chloromycetin), phenylbutazone (Apo-Phenylbutazone), phenytoin (Dilantin), some antibiotics, and some recreational drugs
- Chemical exposure
- Idiopathic (no known cause)
- Radiation
- Viral hepatitis
- Human parvovirus
- Overwhelming infection
- Autoimmune disorders such as lupus

● **Pathophysiology**
• Aplastic anemias usually develop when damaged or destroyed stem cells inhibit RBC production
• Less commonly, they develop when damaged bone marrow microvasculature creates an unfavorable environment for cell growth and maturation

● **Complications**
• Life-threatening hemorrhage
• Immunosuppression

● **Assessment findings**
• Anorexia
• Dyspnea, tachypnea
• Epistaxis
• Fatigue, weakness
• Gingivitis
• Headache
• Melena
• Multiple infections, fever
• Palpitations, tachycardia
• Purpura, petechiae, ecchymosis, pallor

● **Diagnostic test findings**
• Bone marrow biopsy shows fatty marrow with reduction of stem cells
• Fecal occult blood test is positive
• Hematology shows decreased granulocytes, thrombocytes, and RBCs
• Peripheral blood smear shows pancytopenia
• Urine chemistry reveals hematuria

Key facts about Fanconi syndrome

● Characterized by pancytopenia, hypoplasia of bone marrow, and patchy brown discoloration of the skin
● Develops between birth and age 10
● Chromosomal abnormalities usually associated with multiple congenital anomalies

Drugs that cause acquired aplastic anemia

● Chemotherapeutic drugs
● Chloramphenicol
● Phenylbutazone
● Phenytoin

TOP 3
Findings in aplastic anemia

1. Fatigue and weakness
2. Multiple infections and fever
3. Purpura, petechiae, ecchymosis, and pallor

Managing aplastic anemia

- Implementation of a high-protein, high-calorie, high-vitamin diet
- Transfusion of platelets and packed RBCs
- Drug therapy
- Bone marrow transplantation
- Peripheral stem-cell transplants

Key nursing interventions for aplastic anemia

- Assess vital signs and respiratory and cardiovascular status.
- Monitor for infection, bleeding, and bruising.
- Encourage fluid intake.
- Administer oxygen to improve tissue oxygen supply.
- Maintain the patient's diet to promote RBC production.
- Avoid giving I.M. injections to reduce the risk of hemorrhage.
- Avoid taking rectal temperatures to reduce the risk of tissue trauma.
- Avoid contact sports and excessive exercise.

● **Medical management**
- Dietary changes, including establishing a high-protein, high-calorie, high-vitamin diet
- Transfusion of platelets and packed RBCs
- Drug therapy
  - Analgesics: ibuprofen (Motrin), acetaminophen (Tylenol)
  - Androgens: fluoxymesterone (Halotestin), oxymetholone (Anadrol-50)
  - Antibiotics (if infection present): according to the sensitivity of the infecting organism
  - Antithymocyte globulin and cyclosporin (Gengraf)
  - Hematopoietic growth factor: epoetin alfa (Procrit)
  - Human granulocyte colony-stimulating factor: filgrastim (Neulasta)
- Bone marrow transplantation
- Peripheral stem-cell transplants

● **Nursing interventions**
- Assess respiratory status to detect hypoxemia caused by low Hb levels
- Assess vital signs for signs of hemorrhage, infection, and activity intolerance
- Assess cardiovascular status to detect arrhythmias or myocardial ischemia
- Monitor and record intake and output and urine specific gravity to determine fluid balance
- Monitor laboratory values to determine effectiveness of therapy
- Assess stool, urine, and emesis for occult blood loss caused by decreased platelet levels
- Monitor for infection, bleeding, and bruising caused by decreased levels of WBCs and platelets
- Encourage fluids and administer I.V. fluids to replace fluids lost by fever and bleeding
- Administer oxygen to improve tissue oxygen because low Hb levels reduce the blood's oxygen-carrying capacity
- Administer transfusion therapy, as prescribed, to replace low levels of blood components
- Maintain the patient's diet to promote RBC production and fight infection
- Avoid giving I.M. injections to reduce the risk of hemorrhage
- Avoid taking rectal temperatures to reduce the risk of tissue trauma
- Prepare for possible bone marrow transplantation, the treatment of choice for anemia caused by severe aplasia and for the patient who needs constant RBC transfusions
- Avoid contact sports
- Avoid excessive exercise

HEMOPHILIA

Definition
- Hereditary bleeding disorder
- Caused by a deficiency in one of the coagulation factors
- Types
  - Hemophilia A (classic hemophilia): results from a deficiency of factor VIII
  - Hemophilia B (Christmas disease): results from a deficiency of factor IX

Causes
- X-linked recessive disorder
  - If the father has hemophilia and the mother doesn't, all daughters will be carriers but sons won't have the disease
  - If the mother is a carrier and the father doesn't have hemophilia, each son has a 50% chance of getting hemophilia and each daughter has a 50% chance of being a carrier

Pathophysiology
- Abnormal bleeding occurs because of a specific clotting factor deficiency
  - Factor VIII is a critical cofactor that accelerates the activation of factor X by several thousandfold
  - Factor IX is an essential factor
- After a platelet plug forms at a bleeding site, the lack of clotting factors impairs formation of a stable fibrin clot
- Immediate hemorrhage isn't prevalent; delayed bleeding is common

Complications
- Hemorrhage
- Hepatitis
- Human immunodeficiency virus (HIV) infection secondary to transfusions
- Chronic liver disease

Assessment findings
- Bleeding into the throat, mouth, and thorax
- Hemarthrosis
- Multiple bruises without petechiae
- Peripheral neuropathies from bleeding near peripheral nerves
- Prolonged bleeding after circumcision, immunizations, or other minor injuries

Diagnostic test findings
- Hemophilia A
  - Factor VIII assay 0% to 25% of normal
  - Prolonged PTT
  - Normal platelet count and function, bleeding time, and PT

Types of hemophilia
- Hemophilia A: deficiency of factor VIII
- Hemophilia B: deficiency of factor IX

Diagnostic test findings specific to hemophilia A
- Factor VIII assay 0% to 25% of normal
- Prolonged PTT
- Normal platelet count and function
- Normal bleeding time
- Normal PT

- Hemophilia B
  - Deficient factor IX assay
  - Baseline coagulation results similar to those in hemophilia A, with normal factor VIII
- Hemophilia A or B
  - Degree of factor deficiency defines severity:
    - Mild hemophilia—factor levels 5% to 25% of normal
    - Moderate hemophilia—factor levels 1% to 5% of normal
    - Severe hemophilia—factor levels less than 1% of normal

● **Medical management**

- Avoidance of aspirin, sutures, and cauterization, which may aggravate bleeding
- Avoid anti-inflammatory agents such as ibuprofen
- Blood transfusion if necessary
- Frequent assessment of HIV status (child is at increased risk for acquiring HIV through blood product transfusions)
- Administration of fresh frozen plasma to restore deficient coagulation factors
- Promotion of vasoconstriction during bleeding episodes by applying ice, pressure, and hemostatic agents
- Drug therapy
  - Fibrinolysis inhibitor: aminocaproic acid
  - For hemophilia A
    - Hemostatic: desmopressin (DDAVP) to promote release of factor VIII in patients with mild or moderate hemophilia A; factor VIII concentrate
    - Antihemophilic: cryoprecipitated antihemophilic factor (AHF), lyophilized AHF, or both
  - For hemophilia B
    - Hemostatic: factor IX concentrate

● **Nursing interventions**

- Monitor vital signs and intake and output to assess renal status, and monitor for fluid overload or dehydration
- Assess cardiovascular status and check for signs of bleeding (fever, tachycardia, or hypotension may indicate hypovolemia)
- Measure the affected joint's circumference and compare it with that of an unaffected joint to assess for bleeding into the joint, which may lead to hypovolemia
- Note swelling, pain, or limited joint mobility; changes may indicate progressive decline in function
- Assess for joint degeneration from repeated hemarthroses to detect extent of damage

- Pad toys and other objects in the child's environment to promote child safety and prevent bleeding; discourage play activities that may result in trauma or injury
- Recommend using protective head gear, softening the toothbrush under warm water, and administering stool softeners as appropriate to prevent bleeding
- Discourage abnormal weight gain, which increases the load on joints
- During bleeding episodes
  - If the patient has surface cuts or epistaxis, apply pressure; this is commonly the only treatment needed
  - With deeper cuts, pressure may stop the bleeding temporarily; cuts deep enough to require suturing may also require factor infusions to prevent further bleeding
  - Give the deficient clotting factor or plasma, as ordered
  - The body uses up AHF in 48 to 72 hours; repeat infusions as ordered, until the bleeding stops
  - Apply cold compresses or ice bags, and elevate the injured part
  - To prevent recurrence of bleeding, restrict activity for 48 hours after bleeding is under control
  - Control pain with analgesics as ordered
  - Avoid I.M. injections because of possible hematoma formation at the injection site
  - Avoid aspirin and aspirin-containing medications, which are contraindicated because they decrease platelet adherence and may increase bleeding
  - If the patient can't tolerate activities because of blood loss, provide rest periods between activities
- During bleeding in a joint
  - Immediately elevate the joint
  - To restore joint mobility, begin range-of-motion (ROM) exercises at least 48 hours after the bleeding is controlled
  - Restrict weight bearing until bleeding stops and swelling subsides
  - Administer analgesics for the pain associated with hemarthrosis
  - Apply ice packs and elastic bandages to alleviate pain

HYPERBILIRUBINEMIA

● Definition
- Also called *neonatal jaundice*
- Characteristics of bilirubin level
  - Exceeds 6 mg/dl within the first 24 hours after delivery
  - Increases greater than 5 mg/dl/day
  - Remains elevated beyond 7 days in a full-term neonate
  - Remains elevated for 10 days in a premature neonate

TOP 4

Actions to take during a bleeding episode

1. For surface cuts, apply pressure.
2. Apply cold compresses or ice bags and elevate the injured part.
3. Restrict activity for 48 hours after bleeding is under control.
4. Administer analgesics for the pain associated with hemarthrosis.

Actions to take during bleeding in a joint

- Immediately elevate the joint.
- Begin ROM exercises at least 48 hours after bleeding is controlled.
- Restrict weight bearing.
- Administer analgesics.
- Apply ice packs and elastic bandages.

Characteristics of bilirubin level in hyperbilirubinemia

- Exceeds 6 mg/dl within the first 24 hours after delivery
- Increases greater than 5 mg/dl/day
- Remains elevated beyond 7 days in a full-term neonate
- Remains elevated for 10 days in a premature neonate

Assessment findings in hyperbilirubinemia

- Decreased reflexes
- High-pitched crying
- Jaundice
- Lethargy
- Opisthotonos
- Seizures

Managing hyperbilirubinemia

- Exchange transfusion
- Increased fluid intake
- Phototherapy
- Treatment for anemia (if jaundice is caused by hemolytic disease)

Causes

- Absence of intestinal flora needed for bilirubin passage in the bowel
- Enclosed hemorrhage
- Erythroblastosis fetalis (hemolytic disease of the neonate)
- Hypoglycemia
- Hypothermia
- Impaired hepatic functioning
- Neonatal asphyxia (respiratory failure in the neonate)
- Polycythemia
- Prematurity
- Reduced bowel motility and delayed meconium passage
- Sepsis
- Cephalohematoma
- Maternal complications, such as gestational hypertension and hemolysis, elevated liver enzymes, and low platelet count (HEELP) syndrome

Pathophysiology

- The neonate's bilirubin levels rise as bilirubin production exceeds the liver's capacity to metabolize it and the bowel's ability to excrete it
- Unbound, unconjugated bilirubin can easily cross the blood-brain barrier, leading to kernicterus (an encephalopathy)

Complications

- Kernicterus

Assessment findings

- Decreased reflexes
- High-pitched crying
- Jaundice (of the skin and sclera)
- Lethargy
- Opisthotonos
- Seizures

Diagnostic test findings

- Bilirubin levels exceed 12 mg/dl in premature and full-term neonates

Medical management

- Exchange transfusion to remove maternal antibodies and sensitized RBCs if phototherapy fails
- Increased fluid intake
- Phototherapy (preferred treatment)
- Treatment for anemia if jaundice is caused by hemolytic disease

Nursing interventions

- Assess neurologic status for signs of encephalopathy, which indicates the potential for permanent damage
- Maintain a neutral thermal environment to prevent hypothermia

TIME-OUT FOR TEACHING

Home phototherapy

Be sure to include the following points in your teaching plan for the parents whose infant is receiving home phototherapy:

- pathophysiology of hyperbilirubinemia, including causes, tests, and treatments
- signs and symptoms of jaundice
- use of home phototherapy unit (fiber-optic blanket) according to protocol and use of eye patches if appropriate
- fluid needs
- stool characteristics
- skin care measures
- need for stimulation and cuddling
- monitoring parameters
  - stool color
  - skin inspection for redness and dehydration
  - temperature
- follow-up laboratory tests and physician visits.

- Encourage fluid intake at least every 2 hours to hasten the elimination of bilirubin
- Monitor serum bilirubin levels to assess for decrease in levels
- Initiate phototherapy; use bilirubin reduction lights to decompose unconjugated bilirubin beneath the skin, promoting excretion
- During phototherapy, keep the infant unclothed (except for a diaper), frequently reposition the infant, shield the infant's eyes, and maintain proper body temperature and hydration
  - If using bilirubin lights, keep them at least 12" (30.5 cm) away from the infant
  - If using a fiber-optic blanket, keep the infant wrapped in it at all times, including during feeding; eye patches aren't necessary
- Keep the neonate's anal area clean and dry; frequent, greenish stools result from bilirubin excretion and can lead to skin irritation
- Assist with an exchange transfusion if the child doesn't respond to phototherapy
- Teach parents safe use of home phototherapy equipment (see *Home phototherapy*)

IDIOPATHIC THROMBOCYTOPENIC PURPURA

● **Definition**
- Acquired hemorrhagic disorder that results in the autoimmune destruction of platelets in the spleen
- Typically preceded by an upper respiratory tract infection or other viral illness

TOP 4

Nursing interventions during phototherapy

1. Keep the infant unclothed (except for a diaper).
2. Frequently reposition the infant.
3. Shield the infant's eyes.
4. Maintain proper body temperature and hydration.

Causes of ITP

- Viral infection
- Immunization with a live virus vaccine
- Immunologic disorders
- Drug reactions

What happens in ITP

- Circulating IgG molecules react with host platelets.
- Host platelets are then destroyed in the spleen and, to a lesser extent, the liver.
- Platelets survive 1 to 3 days or less (normal life span is 7 to 10 days).

Key assessment findings in ITP

- Hemorrhage into the skin, mucous membranes, and other tissues, causing red discoloration (purpura)
- Small, purplish hemorrhagic spots on the skin (petechiae)

Medications used to treat ITP

- Glucocorticoids
- Immunoglobulin

Key nursing interventions for ITP

- Administer cortisone, chemotherapeutic drugs, and I.V. immunoglobulins as prescribed.
- Instruct the child and his parents about safety measures to prevent trauma.

Causes
- Viral infection
- Immunization with a live virus vaccine
- Immunologic disorders
- Drug reactions

Pathophysiology
- ITP occurs when circulating immunoglobulin (Ig) G molecules react with host platelets, which are then destroyed in the spleen and, to a lesser degree, the liver
- Normally, the life span of platelets in circulation is 7 to 10 days; in ITP, platelets survive 1 to 3 days or less

Complications
- Hemorrhage
- Cerebral hemorrhage
- Purpuric lesions of vital organs (such as the brain and kidneys)

Assessment findings
- Epistaxis
- Oral bleeding
- Hemorrhage into the skin, mucous membranes, and other tissues, causing red discoloration of the skin (purpura)
- Small, purplish hemorrhagic spots on the skin (petechiae)
- Excessive menstrual bleeding

Diagnostic test findings
- Coagulation tests reveal a platelet count less than 20,000/µl, prolonged bleeding time, and normal PT and PTT
- Bone marrow studies show abundant megakaryocytes (platelet precursor cells) and a circulating platelet survival time of only several hours to a few days
- Humoral tests that measure platelet-associated IgG (may help to establish the diagnosis; half the patients have elevated IgG levels)

Medical management
- In children, the disease usually runs its course without medical treatment
- In more severe cases, plasmapheresis, platelet pheresis
- Drug therapy
  - Glucocorticoids to prevent further platelet destruction
  - Immunoglobulin to prevent platelet destruction

Nursing interventions
- Instruct the child and his parents about safety measures to prevent trauma such as avoiding contact sports
- Administer cortisone or chemotherapeutic drugs to stop the autoimmune process
- Avoid using injections; if necessary, inject subcutaneously and apply pressure to the site for 5 minutes

- Don't administer aspirin, which increases bleeding
- Administer I.V. immunoglobulins, if prescribed (they may prevent platelet self-destruction)

IRON DEFICIENCY ANEMIA

● **Definition**
- Inadequate supply of iron for optimal formation of RBCs, resulting in smaller (microcytic) cells with less color on staining
- Most common nutritional anemia of childhood

● **Causes**
- Blood loss secondary to drug-induced GI bleeding (from anticoagulants, aspirin, steroids) or because of heavy menses, hemorrhage from trauma, GI ulcers, or cancer
- Inadequate dietary intake of iron, which may occur after prolonged, unsupplemented breast- or bottle-feeding or when the body is stressed such as during rapid growth periods
- Iron malabsorption, as in chronic diarrhea and malabsorption syndromes, such as celiac disease and pernicious anemia
- Intravascular hemolysis-induced hemoglobinuria or paroxysmal nocturnal hemoglobinuria
- Mechanical erythrocyte trauma caused by a prosthetic heart valve or vena cava filters
- Chronic disease (increases risk)

● **Pathophysiology**
- Most commonly, iron deficiency anemia occurs when the child experiences rapid physical growth, low iron intake, inadequate iron absorption, or loss of blood
- Insufficient body stores of iron lead to:
  - Depleted RBC mass
  - Decreased Hb concentration (hypochromia)
  - Decreased oxygen-carrying capacity of blood

● **Complications**
- Infection and pneumonia
- Pica, causing the child to eat lead-based paint, which results in lead poisoning
- Bleeding
- Hemochromatosis (excessive iron deposits in tissue) or iron poisoning caused by overreplacement of oral or I.M. iron supplements

● **Assessment findings**
- Anemia progresses gradually, and many children are initially asymptomatic, except for symptoms of an underlying condition; children with advanced anemia display these symptoms:
  - Dyspnea on exertion

Factors that contribute to iron deficiency anemia

- Rapid physical growth
- Blood loss
- Inadequate dietary intake of iron
- Inadequate iron absorption

Effects of iron deficiency anemia

- Depleted RBC mass
- Decreased Hb concentration
- Decreased oxygen-carrying capacity of blood

Complications of iron deficiency anemia

- Infection and pneumonia
- Pica
- Bleeding
- Hemochromatosis or iron poisoning

TOP 7

Assessment findings in iron deficiency anemia

1. Fatigue
2. Pallor
3. Tachycardia
4. Numbness and tingling in the extremities
5. Smooth tongue
6. Spoon-shaped, brittle nails
7. Vasomotor disturbances

Managing iron deficiency anemia

- Implementation of iron-rich diet
- Iron supplements
- Vitamin B$_{12}$ supplement

Nursing interventions for iron deficiency anemia

- Assess the child's drug history.
- Provide passive stimulation.
- Allow frequent rest.
- Give small, frequent feedings.
- Elevate the head of the bed.

– Fatigue
– Headache
– Inability to concentrate
– Irritability
– Listlessness
– Pallor
– Susceptibility to infection
– Tachycardia

- In cases of chronic iron deficiency anemia, children display the following symptoms:
  – Cracks in corners of the mouth
  – Dysphagia
  – Neuralgic pain
  – Numbness and tingling in the extremities
  – Smooth tongue
  – Spoon-shaped, brittle nails
  – Vasomotor disturbances

● Diagnostic test findings

- Bone marrow studies reveal depleted or absent iron stores and normoblastic hyperplasia
- Hematocrit (HCT) and Hb and serum ferritin levels are low
- Mean corpuscular Hb is decreased
- RBC count is low, with microcytic and hypochromic cells (in early stages, RBC count may be normal, except in infants and children)
- Serum iron levels are low with high binding capacity

● Medical management

- Increase iron intake by adding foods rich in iron to diet (for children and adolescents) or adding iron supplements (for infants)
- Drug therapy
  – Oral preparation of iron or a combination of iron and ascorbic acid (which enhances iron absorption)
  – Vitamin supplement: cyanocobalamin (vitamin B$_{12}$) if intrinsic factor is lacking
  – Iron supplement: iron dextran if additional therapy is needed

● Nursing interventions

- Carefully assess the child's drug history; certain drugs, such as pancreatic enzymes and vitamin E, may interfere with iron metabolism and absorption; other drugs, such as aspirin and steroids, may cause GI bleeding
- Provide passive stimulation; allow frequent rest; give small, frequent feedings; and elevate the head of the bed to decrease oxygen demands
- Provide foods high in iron (liver; dark, leafy vegetables; whole grains; and legumes) to replenish iron stores
- Ensure that parents are providing their infant with iron-fortified formula and cereals

- Administer iron with citrus juice before meals (iron is best absorbed in an acidic environment)
- Give liquid iron through a straw to prevent staining the skin and teeth; for infants, administer by oral syringe toward the back of the mouth
- Don't give iron with milk products because they may interfere with iron absorption
- Ensure that parents are keeping the iron safely stored out of the child's reach at home
- Brush teeth after administration of iron
- Advise parents to expect black, tarry stools

SICKLE CELL ANEMIA

- **Definition**
  - Congenital hemolytic disease resulting from a defective Hb molecule (HbS) that causes RBCs to become sickle-shaped
  - The child may experience periodic, painful attacks called sickle cell crises; a sickle cell crisis may be triggered or intensified by:
    - Dehydration
    - Deoxygenation
    - Acidosis
- **Causes**
  - Autosomal recessive inheritance (homozygous inheritance of the HbS–producing gene
- **Pathophysiology**
  - The abnormal HbS found in the patient's RBCs becomes insoluble whenever hypoxia occurs
  - The RBCs become rigid, rough, and elongated, forming a crescent or sickle shape (see *Comparing normal and sickled red blood cells,* page 114)
  - Sickling can produce hemolysis (cell destruction)
  - The altered cells accumulate in capillaries and smaller blood vessels, making the blood more viscous
  - Normal circulation is impaired, causing pain, tissue ischemia and infarctions, and swelling
- **Complications**
  - Retinopathy, nephropathy, and cerebral vessel occlusion caused by organ infarction
  - Hypovolemic shock and death caused by massive cell entrapment
  - Necrosis
  - Infection and gangrene
- **Assessment findings**
  - Infants
    - Before age 4 months, symptoms are rare because HbF prevents excessive sickling

Administration guidelines for iron preparations

- Administer before meals with citrus juice.
- Give liquid through a straw to prevent staining the skin and teeth.
- Don't give with milk products.
- Brush teeth after administration.

Sickle cell crisis triggers

- Dehydration
- Deoxygenation
- Acidosis

Effects of sickled cells

- Hemolysis
- Increased blood viscosity
- Impaired circulation

Comparing normal and sickled red blood cells

When a child with sickle cell anemia develops hypoxia, the abnormal hemoglobin S found in his red blood cells (RBCs) becomes insoluble. This causes the RBCs to become rigid, rough, and elongated, forming the characteristic sickle shape.

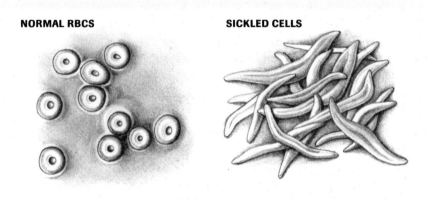

NORMAL RBCS   **SICKLED CELLS**

Assessment findings in sickle cell anemia

● Infants: colic, splenomegaly
● Toddlers and preschoolers: hypovolemia, shock, pain at site of vaso-occlusive crisis
● School-age children and adolescents: enuresis, extreme pain at site of crisis, priapism

    – Colic from pain caused by an abdominal infarction
    – Dactylitis or hand-foot syndrome from infarction of the small bones of the hands and feet
    – Splenomegaly from sequestered RBCs
● Toddlers and preschoolers
    – Hypovolemia and shock from sequestration of large amounts of blood in spleen
    – Pain at site of vaso-occlusive crisis
    – Possible functional asplenia by age 4, leading to an increased risk of infection
● School-age children and adolescents
    – Delayed growth and development and delayed sexual maturity
    – Enuresis
    – Extreme pain at site of crisis
    – History of pneumococcal pneumonia and other infections caused by atrophied spleen
    – Poor healing of leg wounds from inadequate peripheral circulation of oxygenated blood
    – Priapism
● Suspect any of the following crises in a patient with sickle cell anemia who has pale lips, tongue, palms, or nail beds; lethargy; listlessness; sleepiness; irritability; severe pain; and fever:
    – Aplastic crisis (megaloblastic crisis) due to bone marrow depression; associated with infection, usually viral, and characterized by pallor, lethargy, sleepiness, dyspnea, markedly de-

creased bone marrow activity, RBC hemolysis and, possibly, coma
  – Acute sequestration crisis due to the sudden massive entrapment of cells in the spleen and liver; affects infants ages 8 months to 2 years and may cause lethargy, pallor, and hypovolemic shock
  – Hemolytic crisis (rare), which usually affects patients who also have glucose-6-phosphate dehydrogenase deficiency; degenerative changes cause liver congestion and enlargement and chronic jaundice worsens
  – Vaso-occlusive crisis (most common non-life-threatening crisis) characterized by migratory pain, ischemia of tissue and bones, and abdominal pain from visceral hypoxia

● **Diagnostic test findings**
  • Laboratory studies show Hb level is 6 to 9 g/dl (in a toddler)
  • More than 50% HbS indicates sickle cell disease; a lower level of HbS indicates sickle cell trait
  • RBCs are crescent-shaped and prone to agglutination

● **Medical management**
  • Bed rest with crises
  • Avoidance of stress and extreme temperatures
  • Hydration with I.V. fluid (may be increased to 3 L/day during crisis)
  • Short-term oxygen therapy (long-term oxygen decreases bone marrow activity, further aggravating anemia)
  • Transfusion therapy as needed
  • Drug therapy
    – Analgesic: meperidine (Demerol)
    – Antineoplastic: hydroxyurea
    – Vaccine: pneumococcal vaccine

● **Nursing interventions**
  • Administer sufficient pain medication to promote comfort; concerns regarding addiction are clinically unfounded
  • Assess cardiovascular, respiratory, and neurologic status; tachycardia, dyspnea, or hypotension may indicate fluid volume deficit or electrolyte imbalance; change in level of consciousness may signal neurologic involvement
  • Assess for symptoms of acute chest syndrome from a pulmonary infarction to identify early complications
  • Promote fluid intake to prevent dehydration, which may result from the kidney's inability to concentrate urine
  • Assess vision to monitor for retinal infarction
  • Teach relaxation techniques to decrease the child's stress level
  • Provide proper skin care to prevent skin breakdown
  • Remove tight clothing that impedes circulation

Crises to watch for with sickle cell anemia

- Aplastic crisis
- Acute sequestration crisis
- Vaso-occlusive crisis
- Hemolytic crisis (rare)

Diagnostic indicators of sickle cell anemia

- More than 50% HbS indicates sickle cell disease.
- Less than 50% HbS indicates sickle cell trait.

Managing sickle cell anemia

- Hydration
- Transfusion as necessary
- Analgesics
- Antineoplastics

Key nursing interventions for sickle cell anemia

- Administer sufficient pain medication to promote comfort.
- Assess cardiovascular, respiratory, and neurologic status.
- Assess for symptoms of acute chest syndrome.
- Promote fluid intake.
- Assess vision.
- Teach relaxation techniques.
- Provide proper skin care.

Key facts about thalassemia

- Group of hemolytic anemias characterized by defective synthesis in the polypeptide chains necessary for Hb production
- Autosomal recessive disorder
- Most common in children of Mediterranean ancestry
- Also occurs in blacks and children from southern China, southeast Asia, and India

Forms of thalassemia

- Major (Cooley's anemia, Mediterranean disease, erythroblastic anemia)
- Intermedia
- Minor

- Reduce the child's energy expenditure to improve oxygenation
- Maintain the child's normal body temperature
- Initiate genetic counseling
- Suggest family screening for possible carriers of the disease
- Instruct the child to avoid activities that precipitate a crisis, such as excessive exercise, mountain climbing, and deep sea diving; advise the family to seek early treatment of illness to prevent dehydration

THALASSEMIA

● **Definition**
- Hereditary group of hemolytic anemias characterized by defective synthesis in the polypeptide chains necessary for Hb production; consequently, RBC synthesis is also impaired
- Most common in children of Mediterranean ancestry (especially Italian and Greek) but also occurs in blacks and children from southern China, southeast Asia, and India
- Occurs in three clinical forms: major (also known as *Cooley's anemia, Mediterranean disease,* and *erythroblastic anemia*), intermedia, and minor

● **Causes**
- Autosomal recessive disorder
- Thalassemia major and thalassemia intermedia: result from homozygous inheritance of the partially dominant autosomal gene responsible for this trait
- Thalassemia minor: results from heterozygous inheritance of the same gene

● **Pathophysiology**
- Total or partial deficiency of beta-polypeptide chain production impairs Hb synthesis and results in continual production of HbF, lasting even past the neonatal period
- Normally, immunoglobulin synthesis switches from gamma- to beta-polypeptides at birth; this conversion doesn't happen in thalassemic infants; their RBCs are hypochromic and microcytic

● **Complications**
- Iron overload from RBC transfusions
- Pathologic fractures
- Cardiac arrhythmias
- Liver failure
- Heart failure
- Death

● **Assessment findings**
- Thalassemia major

- Healthy infant at birth; severe anemia, bone abnormalities, failure to thrive, and life-threatening complications develop during second 6 months of life
- Pallor and jaundice (yellow skin and sclera) at ages 3 to 6 months
- Splenomegaly or hepatomegaly with abdominal enlargement; frequent infections; bleeding tendencies (especially nosebleeds); anorexia
- Small body and large head (characteristic features); possibly mental retardation
- Features similar to Down syndrome in infants because of thickened bone at the base of the nose from bone marrow hyperactivity
- Thalassemia intermedia
  - Some degree of anemia, jaundice, and splenomegaly
  - Possibly signs of hemosiderosis because of increased intestinal absorption of iron
- Thalassemia minor
  - Mild anemia (usually produces no symptoms and is commonly overlooked; should be differentiated from iron deficiency anemia)

● Diagnostic test findings
- Complete blood count showing decreased Hb level, HCT, and mean corpuscular volume
- Decreased reticulocyte count
- In thalassemia major, X-rays of the skull and long bones show thinning and widening of the marrow space because of overactive bone marrow; long bones may show areas of osteoporosis; the phalanges may also be deformed (rectangular or biconvex); the bones of the skull and vertebrae may appear granular (see *Skull changes in thalassemia major,* page 118)

● Medical management
- No treatment for mild or moderate forms
- Iron supplements contraindicated in all forms
- Avoidance of iron-rich foods
- Avoidance of strenuous activity
- Transfusions of packed RBCs
- Surgery: splenectomy or bone marrow transplantation
- Drug therapy: deferoxamine (Desferal) for chelation therapy

● Nursing interventions
- Prepare for and administer multiple blood transfusions (every 3 to 4 weeks throughout the child's life)
- Administer chelating agents, such as Desferal, to remove excess iron from the system
- Prepare the child for a possible splenectomy

TOP 3

Assessment findings in thalassemia major

1. Pallor and yellow skin and sclera
2. Splenomegaly or hepatomegaly
3. Small body and large head

Managing thalassemia

- No treatment for mild or moderate forms
- Iron supplements contraindicated in all forms
- Avoidance of iron-rich foods
- Avoidance of strenuous exercise
- Transfusions of packed RBCs
- Splenectomy or bone marrow transplantation
- Drug therapy

Key nursing interventions for thalassemia

- Prepare for and administer multiple blood transfusions.
- Administer chelating agents.

Skull changes in thalassemia major

This illustration of an X-ray shows a characteristic skull abnormality in thalassemia major: diploetic fibers extending from the internal lamina and resembling hair standing on end.

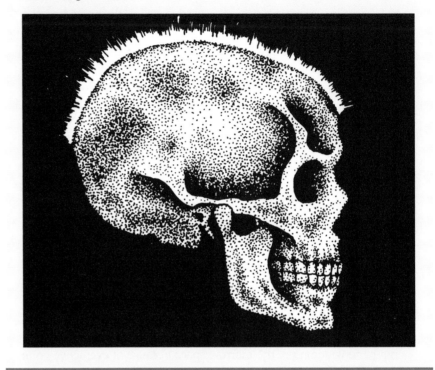

TOP 7

Items to study for your next test on the hematologic system

1. Functions of blood
2. Role of platelets in clotting
3. Types of hemophilia
4. Interventions during a bleeding episode in a patient with hemophilia
5. Interventions for an infant during phototherapy
6. Proper way to administer iron preparations
7. The three forms of thalassemia

NCLEX CHECKS

It's never too soon to begin your NCLEX preparation. Now that you've reviewed this chapter, carefully read each of the following questions and choose the best answer. Then compare your responses to the correct answers.

1. A child is admitted to the pediatric unit with ITP. Which finding should the nurse expect?

☐ **1.** Petechiae
☐ **2.** Dark-colored urine
☐ **3.** External hemorrhage
☐ **4.** Temperature more than 101° F (38.3° C)

2. A nurse is caring an 8-year-old child who has hemophilia A, a hereditary bleeding disorder. Hemophilia is:

☐ **1.** a Y-linked recessive disorder that leads to deficient factor IX production.
☐ **2.** an X-linked recessive disorder that leads to deficient factors VIII or IX production.

☐ **3.** seen only in males and is likely to produce a platelet count greater than 500,000/µl.

☐ **4.** transmitted at the time of delivery and usually isn't apparent until the child is age 2.

3. A 1-year-old boy with a history of sickle cell disease is admitted to the emergency department complaining of abdominal pain. While examining him, the nurse palpates an enlarged liver. The abdominal X-ray reveals an enlarged liver and spleen. These findings indicate which type of crisis?

☐ **1.** Aplastic
☐ **2.** Sequestration
☐ **3.** Vaso-occlusive
☐ **4.** Hemolytic

4. An 8-year-old with iron deficiency anemia is being discharged from the facility. In a nurse's discharge teaching, she includes appropriate activities to decrease oxygen demands on the body. Which activity is most appropriate?

☐ **1.** Dancing
☐ **2.** Playing video games
☐ **3.** Reading a book
☐ **4.** Riding a bicycle

5. A 2-year-old boy with iron deficiency anemia is brought to the clinic for a follow-up visit. He has been taking ferrous iron supplements to correct the iron deficiency. Which vitamin should the nurse make sure the child is taking with the iron?

☐ **1.** Folic acid
☐ **2.** Ascorbic acid
☐ **3.** Niacin
☐ **4.** Riboflavin

6. Which instruction is most important when teaching home management of a child with hemophilia?

☐ **1.** Toothbrushes should be held under warm water before use.
☐ **2.** Aspirin should be used for mild joint pain and inflammation.
☐ **3.** Bleeding extremities should be held in a dependent position to encourage stasis and clot formation.
☐ **4.** Wall-to-wall carpeting shouldn't be used anywhere in the home.

7. A nurse is caring for a client with ITP. The main cause of symptoms with this disorder is:

☐ **1.** destruction of platelets through an autoimmune process.
☐ **2.** decreased platelet production.
☐ **3.** an enlarged spleen.
☐ **4.** bleeding and petechiae.

8. An infant with jaundice is treated using phototherapy. Which precaution is used during this treatment?
- ☐ **1.** Leave the infant's clothes on.
- ☐ **2.** Check the infant's temperature once a day.
- ☐ **3.** Reposition the infant infrequently.
- ☐ **4.** Cover the infant's eyes.

9. A nurse is caring for a 5-year-old with hemophilia who's bleeding. Which intervention should she perform?
- ☐ **1.** Apply pressure.
- ☐ **2.** Apply warm packs to the site.
- ☐ **3.** Administer aspirin for pain.
- ☐ **4.** Perform ROM exercises to the injured area immediately after bleeding stops.

10. Place in chronological order the stages of human blood cell development for plasma cells.

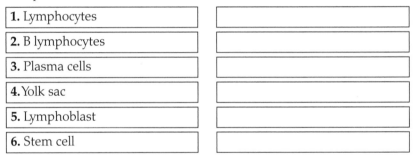

1. Lymphocytes	
2. B lymphocytes	
3. Plasma cells	
4. Yolk sac	
5. Lymphoblast	
6. Stem cell	

ANSWERS AND RATIONALES

1. CORRECT ANSWER: 1
The common symptoms of ITP include easy bruising, petechiae, and bleeding from mucous membranes. Dark-colored urine may indicate concentrated urine. Hemorrhage is a rare physical finding. Fever isn't always present with ITP.

2. CORRECT ANSWER: 2
Hemophilia is an X-linked recessive disorder that leads to deficiency in the production of factors VIII or IX. It's hereditary and transmitted genetically, not at the time of delivery. The platelet count of a child with hemophilia is usually low (normal platelet count is 150,000 to 450,000/µl).

3. CORRECT ANSWER: 2
Sequestration crisis results from pooling of large amounts of blood in the liver and spleen, which causes these organs to enlarge. Aplastic crisis occurs from decreased RBC production, resulting in profound anemia. Vaso-occlusive crisis is usually preceded by a respiratory tract or GI infection because clumps of sickled RBCs obstruct vessels and cause occlusion, ischemia, and infarction of adjacent tissues. Hemolytic crisis is a rare form in which RBCs are rapidly destroyed; it occurs in conjunction with glucose-6-phosphate dehydrogenase deficiency.

4. CORRECT ANSWER: 3

Reading a book is a restful activity and can keep the child from becoming bored and withdrawn. Dancing to music, riding a bicycle, and even playing video games requires too much energy for a child with anemia and can increase stress demands on the body.

5. CORRECT ANSWER: 2

Ascorbic acid (vitamin C) facilitates iron absorption in the body and is usually prescribed with iron supplements. Folic acid, niacin, and riboflavin are necessary for the body but don't facilitate iron absorption.

6. CORRECT ANSWER: 1

Softening the toothbrush under warm water decreases the risk of bleeding gums. Aspirin is contraindicated because it interferes with platelet function. Bleeding extremities should be kept elevated. The home should have wall-to-wall carpeting to cushion falls.

7. CORRECT ANSWER: 1

ITP involves the destruction of platelets caused by an autoimmune process. It's as if the body is fighting against itself. This can lead to an enlarged spleen, bleeding, and petechiae. Decreased platelet production doesn't occur with this disease.

8. CORRECT ANSWER: 4

Covering the infant's eyes decreases exposure to the light. Remove the infant's clothes, except for the diaper, so that as much skin surface as possible is exposed to the light. Check the infant's temperature more frequently to prevent hypothermia or hyperthermia. Change the infant's position frequently to expose his body to light.

9. CORRECT ANSWER: 1

Applying pressure is one intervention to control bleeding. Applying warm packs to the site, administering aspirin, and moving the injured area after bleeding stops prolong the bleeding.

10. CORRECT ANSWER:

4. Yolk sac
6. Stem cell
5. Lymphoblast
1. Lymphocytes
2. B Lymphocytes
3. Plasma cells

Human plasma blood cell development begins with the yolk sac and is followed by the stem cell, lymphoblast, lymphocytes, B lymphocytes and, finally, plasma cells.

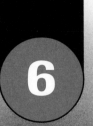

6

Altered immunologic functioning

1. Which type of immune cell is responsible for many of the symptoms of anaphylaxis?

☐ 1. Neutrophils
☐ 2. Monocytes
☐ 3. Basophils
☐ 4. Eosinophils

CORRECT ANSWER: 3

2. Which immunoglobin (Ig) prevents viruses and bacteria from adhering to mucous membranes?

☐ 1. Secretory IgA
☐ 2. IgD
☐ 3. IgE
☐ 4. IgM

CORRECT ANSWER: 1

3. What's the most common allergy that's an immunoglobin (Ig) E–mediated response against the allergen?

☐ 1. Type I
☐ 2. Type II
☐ 3. Type III
☐ 4. Type IV

CORRECT ANSWER: 1

4. In the five stages of Reye's syndrome, which stage involves coma?

☐ 1. Stage 1
☐ 2. Stage 2
☐ 3. Stage 3
☐ 4. Stage 4

CORRECT ANSWER: 3

5. Which immune disorder predisposes clients to infection from all classes of microorganisms?

☐ 1. Allergic rhinitis
☐ 2. Acquired immunodeficiency syndrome
☐ 3. Reye's syndrome
☐ 4. Severe combined immunodeficiency disease

CORRECT ANSWER: 4

LEARNING OBJECTIVES

After studying this chapter, you should be able to:

● Discuss conditions associated with alteration in immunologic function.
● Discuss different types of hypersensitivity disorders.
● Plan appropriate nursing interventions for a patient with acquired immunodeficiency syndrome.
● Describe appropriate nursing interventions for a patient with juvenile rheumatoid arthritis.

CHAPTER OVERVIEW

Knowledge of normal white blood cells (WBCs) and immune function provides the foundation for understanding the conditions associated with altered immunologic function. Assessment and interventions are geared to controlling the problems associated with the alteration and promoting normal function. Prevention plays a primary role in hypersensitivity reactions.

KEY CONCEPTS

● **Structures**
  • Immune cells and their functions
    – Neutrophil (polymorphonuclear leukocyte) — short-lived phagocyte; first immune cell at the trauma site
      · It attacks bacteria and fungi
      · A band is an immature cell; a segmented neutrophil (seg) is a mature cell
    – Eosinophil — effective in phagocytizing parasites; also inactivates histamine and increases with allergic attack
    – Basophil — releases histamine, bradykinin, serotonin, and heparin during an allergic attack
      · It's responsible for many symptoms of anaphylaxis
      · In the tissues, it's known as a mast cell
    – Monocyte — phagocytizes antigens and presents antigenic markers to lymphocytes
      · It appears later than a neutrophil but lasts longer
      · It includes Kupffer's cells of the liver
      · A macrophage is a monocyte that has left the circulation and entered the tissues
      · An increase indicates chronic inflammation
    – B lymphocyte (B cell) — produces antibodies
      · Immunoglobulin (Ig) M is the largest immunoglobulin; it stays in the blood, activates complement, and is responsible for making antibodies against the ABO blood groups
      · IgG is the smallest immunoglobulin and the only one that passes the placenta, thus offering the neonate passive protection; it activates complement and has an excellent memory
      · IgD is a lymphocyte receptor whose actions aren't well understood
      · Secretory IgA is present in all moist body secretions, including breast milk, saliva, and tears; it prevents viruses and bacteria from adhering to the mucous membranes
      · IgE governs the allergic response by stimulating basophils to release their products after contact with the allergen

Immune cells

● Neutrophils
● Eosinophils
● Basophils
● Monocytes
● B lymphocytes (B cells)
● T lymphocytes (T cells)

Facts about immunoglobulin

● IgM – largest immunoglobulin; responsible for making antibodies against ABO blood groups
● IgG – smallest immunoglobulin and the only one that passes the placenta; activates complement and has an excellent memory
● IgD – lymphocyte receptor whose actions aren't well understood
● Secretory IgA – present in all moist body secretions; prevents viruses and bacteria from adhering to mucous membranes
● IgE – governs the allergic response by stimulating basophils to release their products after contact with an allergen

- T lymphocyte (T cell)—carries out functions directly or by its cell products; releases soluble factors (lymphokines) that stimulate the immune system
  - Th (helper T or CD4+) tells the B cells when to make antibodies and how many to make
  - Ts (suppressor T or CD8) tells the B cells to stop making antibodies
  - Tc (cytotoxic T) has a direct killing effect
- Human leukocyte antigen (HLA)
  - Major histocompatibility complex normally found on the cell surface of every nucleated cell (not on red blood cells)
  - Allows the body to recognize self versus nonself
    - For organ transplants, markers are matched as closely as possible to decrease the odds of rejection
    - The cornea is avascular and thus doesn't need HLA matching
  - Genetically transmitted on chromosome 6, so the child gets markers from both parents
  - Contains a genetic predisposition or susceptibility to a disorder; doesn't pass the disorder itself
  - Consists of four main loci: HLA-A, HLA-B, HLA-C, HLA-D/DR
  - Carries a 1-in-30,000 chance that two nonrelated persons have the same HLA
- Natural first line of defense against disease invasion
  - Skin
  - Body secretions (tears, saliva, sebum, mucus, acidic environments, normal body flora, and salt in sweat)
  - Nasal hairs and cilia
  - Controlled body temperature
  - Adequate renal function

● **Functions**
- Immune system functions
  - Defense against nonself antigens
    - Hyperfunctioning results in an allergy
    - Hypofunctioning results in an immunodeficiency
  - Homeostasis
    - Homeostasis is the phagocytosis of debris from cellular warfare or of dead cells
    - Hyperfunctioning results in an autoimmune disease
  - Surveillance against any antigenic invasion; hypofunctioning results in cancer
- Function of immune cells in the inflammatory reaction
  - Histamine causes vasodilation, and granulocytes and monocytes are attracted to the site

Types of T cells

- Th – tells B cells when to make antibodies and how many to make
- Ts – tells B cells to stop making antibodies
- Tc – has a direct killing effect

Natural defenses against disease invasion

- Skin
- Body secretions
- Nasal hairs and cilia
- Controlled body temperature
- Adequate renal function

Immune system functions

- Defense against nonself antigens
- Homeostasis
- Surveillance against antigenic invasion

Types of hypersensitivity disorders

- Type I – atopy or anaphylaxis
- Type II – cytotoxic reaction
- Type III – immune complex disease
- Type IV – delayed hypersensitivity

Type I hypersensitivity disorders

- Anaphylaxis
- Allergic rhinitis
- Asthma (in some cases)

Type II hypersensitivity disorders

- Transfusion reactions
- Rh incompatibility
- Idiopathic thrombocytopenic purpura
- Autoimmune hemolytic anemia

Type III hypersensitivity disorders

- Systemic lupus erythematosus
- Rheumatic fever
- Glomerulonephritis
- Rheumatoid arthritis

Type IV hypersensitivity disorders

- Contact dermatitis
- Poison ivy
- Tuberculin reactions
- Graft rejection

– Cells leave the blood and enter the damaged site, resulting in redness, warmth, swelling, pain, and altered function

● **Hypersensitivity disorders**
- Exaggerated or inappropriate immune response may lead to various hypersensitivity disorders
- Type I (atopy or anaphylaxis) is an IgE-mediated response against the allergen; it's the most common type of allergy
  – IgE attaches to the mast cell, causing it to release histamine, leukotrienes, and chemotaxic substances
  – Anaphylaxis can result
  – Examples include anaphylaxis, allergic rhinitis and, in some cases, asthma
- In type II (cytolytic-cytotoxic), antibody is directed against cell surface antigens
  – Binding of antigen and antibody activates complement, which ultimately disrupts cellular membranes
  – Examples include transfusion reactions, Rh incompatibility, idiopathic thrombocytopenic purpura, and autoimmune hemolytic anemia
- In type III (immune complex disease), excessive circulating antigen-antibody complexes (immune complexes) result in the deposition of these complexes in tissue, most commonly in the kidneys, joints, skin, and blood vessels
  – Deposited immune complexes activate the complement cascade, resulting in local inflammation; they also trigger platelet release of vasoactive amines that increase vascular permeability
  – Examples include systemic lupus erythematosus, rheumatic fever, glomerulonephritis, and rheumatoid arthritis (RA)
- In type IV (delayed hypersensitivity), antigen is processed by macrophages and presented to T cells
  – The sensitized T cells then release lymphokines, which recruit and activate other lymphocytes, monocytes, macrophages, and polymorphonuclear leukocytes; coagulation, kinin, and complement pathways contribute to tissue damage in this type of reaction
  – Examples include contact dermatitis, poison ivy, tuberculin reactions, and graft rejection

DIAGNOSTIC TESTS

● **Laboratory studies**
- Purpose
  – Laboratory studies such as CD4+ T-cell count and enzyme-linked immunosorbent assay (ELISA) are used to assess immunosuppression

- Nursing considerations
  - Explain the procedure to the child and family
  - Handle the sample gently to prevent hemolysis
  - Apply pressure to the venipuncture site to prevent hematoma or bleeding

● **Liver function studies**
- Purpose
  - Liver function studies measure levels of hepatic enzymes, such as aspartate aminotransferase (AST) and alanine aminotransferase (ALT)
- Nursing considerations
  - Before the test, prepare the child for venipuncture
  - After the test, check the venipuncture site for bleeding

NURSING DIAGNOSES

● **Probable nursing diagnoses**
- Risk for infection
- Ineffective protection
- Deficient fluid volume
- Delayed growth and development
- Ineffective thermoregulation
- Deficient knowledge
- Acute pain
- Fatigue

● **Possible nursing diagnoses**
- Imbalanced nutrition: Less than body requirements
- Decreased intracranial adaptive capacity
- Risk for deficient fluid volume
- Disturbed body image
- Social isolation
- Impaired physical mobility

ACQUIRED IMMUNODEFICIENCY SYNDROME

● **Definition**
- Acquired immunodeficiency syndrome (AIDS) results from the human immunodeficiency virus (HIV) attacking helper T cells
- Three main groups of children are infected with HIV
  - Infants of HIV-infected mothers
  - Adolescents who acquire the infection through sexual contact or I.V. drug abuse
  - Infants, children, and adolescents who acquired the virus via contaminated blood products

Probable nursing diagnoses for a patient with an immune disorder

- Risk for infection
- Ineffective protection
- Deficient fluid volume
- Delayed growth and development
- Ineffective thermoregulation
- Deficient knowledge
- Acute pain
- Fatigue

Key facts about AIDS

- Results from HIV attacking helper cells
- Spreads by an exchange of body fluid, including breast milk
- HIV infection has a shorter incubation period in children than in adults

Key causes of AIDS in children

- Contaminated blood products
- Infected mother
- Sexual contact with infected partner
- I.V. drug abuse

Complications of AIDS

- Repeated opportunistic infections
- Neoplasms
- Premalignant diseases
- Organ-specific syndrome

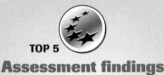

TOP 5

Assessment findings in AIDS

1. Failure to thrive
2. Mononucleosis-like prodromal symptoms
3. Night sweats
4. Recurring diarrhea
5. Weight loss

- AIDS isn't spread by casual contact with an infected child; it's spread only by an exchange of body fluids, including breast milk
- HIV infection has a much shorter incubation period in children than in adults
  - In adults, the incubation period may last 10 or more years
  - Children who acquire the virus by placental transmission are usually HIV-positive by age 6 months and develop clinical signs by age 3 years
- Because of passive antibody transmission, all infants born to HIV-infected mothers test positive for antibodies to the virus up to about age 18 months; confirmation of diagnosis during this time requires detection of the HIV antigen

Causes
- Contaminated blood products
- Infected mother
- Sexual contact with infected partner
- I.V. drug abuse

Pathophysiology
- HIV strikes helper T cells bearing the CD4 antigen
- The antigen serves as a receptor for the retrovirus and lets it enter the cell
- After invading a cell, HIV replicates, leading to cell death, or becomes latent
- HIV infection leads to profound pathology either directly, through destruction of CD4+ cells, other immune cells, and neuroglial cells, or indirectly, through the secondary effects of CD4+ T-cell dysfunction and resultant immunosuppression

Complications
- Repeated opportunistic infections
- Neoplasms
- Premalignant diseases
- Organ-specific syndrome

Assessment findings
- Failure to thrive
- Lymphadenopathy
- Mononucleosis-like prodromal symptoms
- Neurologic impairment, such as loss of motor milestones and behavioral changes
- Night sweats
- Recurrent opportunistic infections or malignancies
- Recurring diarrhea
- Weight loss
- Hepatosplenomegaly

Diagnostic test findings

- CD4+ T-cell count measures the severity of immunosuppression
- Culture and sensitivity tests reveal infection with opportunistic organisms
- ELISA and Western blot are positive for HIV antibody
- Viral culture or p24 antigen test reveals the presence of the virus in children younger than age 18 months

Medical management

- Blood administration, if necessary
- Follow-up laboratory studies
- High-calorie diet provided in small, frequent meals
- I.V. fluids to maintain hydration
- Nutritional supplements, if necessary
- Parenteral nutrition, if necessary
- Drug therapy
  - Antibiotic therapy according to the sensitivity of the infecting opportunistic organism
  - Antiviral agents: zidovudine
  - Monthly gamma globulin administration
  - Prophylactic antibiotic therapy with co-trimoxazole (Bactrim) to prevent *Pneumocystitis jiroveci* pneumonia
  - Routine immunizations (varicella vaccine isn't recommended for HIV-infected children); no live vaccinations or yearly influenza vaccine

Nursing interventions

- Monitor developmental progress at regular intervals to detect changes in level of functioning and, as appropriate, adapt activity program
- Provide appropriate play activities to promote development
- Encourage fluid intake to prevent dehydration
- Assess respiratory and neurologic status to detect early signs of compromise
- Maintain standard precautions to prevent the spread of infection
- Administer medications, as ordered, to help boost immune response and prevent opportunistic infections
- Instruct the child and parents in infection control measures in the home (see *The child with HIV infection,* page 130)
- Because an AIDS diagnosis is devastating for the child and his family, provide psychosocial support
- Assess the child's support system, and provide referrals as necessary

---

Diagnostic test findings for AIDS

- Low CD4+ T-cell count
- Positive screen for HIV antibody on ELISA and Western blot
- Viral presence on viral culture or p24 antigen test

Managing AIDS

- Blood administration, if necessary
- Follow-up laboratory studies
- High-calorie diet provided in small, frequent meals
- I.V. fluids
- Nutritional supplements, if necessary
- Parenteral nutrition, if necessary
- Drug therapy

Medications used to treat AIDS

- Antibiotic therapy according to the sensitivity of the infecting opportunistic organism
- Antiviral agents (zidovudine)
- Monthly gamma globulin administration
- Prophylactic antibiotic therapy (co-trimoxazole)

Key nursing interventions for AIDS

- Encourage fluid intake.
- Maintain standard precautions.
- Administer medications as ordered.
- Teach infection control measures to use at home.

Causes of allergic rhinitis

- Seasonal allergens — tree, grass, and weed pollens
- Perennial allergens — animal dander, dust mites, and mold spores

Complications of allergic rhinitis

- Sinusitis
- Otitis media
- Secondary infection
- Decreased pulmonary function
- Nasal polyps

TOP 5

Assessment findings in allergic rhinitis

1. Paroxysmal sneezing
2. Profuse watery rhinorrhea
3. Nasal obstruction or congestion
4. Pruritus of the nose and eyes
5. Dark circles under the eyes (allergic shiners)

TIME-OUT FOR TEACHING

The child with HIV infection

Be sure to include the following points in your teaching plan for the parents of a child with human immunodeficiency virus (HIV) infection:
- hand-washing procedures
- how and when to use protective equipment, such as gloves, gowns, and masks
- household and laundry cleaning measures
- care of the patient's eating utensils
- spill clean-up
- disposal of contaminated equipment and supplies
- trash disposal.

ALLERGIC RHINITIS

- ● **Definition**
  - Reaction to airborne (inhaled) allergens that's characterized by nasal congestion, rhinorrhea, sneezing, itchy nose, and postnasal drainage
  - Depending on the allergen, the resulting rhinitis may occur seasonally (hay fever) or year-round (perennial allergic rhinitis)
- ● **Causes**
  - Seasonal allergens: tree, grass, and weed pollens
  - Perennial allergens: animal dander, dust mites, and mold spores
- ● **Pathophysiology**
  - Allergic rhinitis reflects an IgE-mediated type I hypersensitivity response to an environmental antigen (allergen) in a genetically susceptible person (see *What happens in allergic rhinitis*)
- ● **Complications**
  - Sinusitis
  - Otitis media
  - Secondary infection
  - Decreased pulmonary function
  - Nasal polyps
- ● **Assessment findings**
  - Paroxysmal sneezing
  - Profuse watery rhinorrhea
  - Nasal obstruction or congestion
  - Pruritus of the nose (provokes the classic allergic salute, accomplished by pushing the palm up along the tip of the nose) and eyes
  - Red, edematous eyelids and conjunctivae
  - Dark circles under the eyes (allergic shiners) caused by venous congestion of the maxillary sinuses
  - Excessive lacrimation
  - Headache or sinus pain

What happens in allergic rhinitis

The nose is a highly sensitive organ. Nasal mucosa, mucus-secreting membranes that line the nasal cavity, react to various environmental factors, which may include allergens (such as pollen and mold) and irritants (such as cigarette smoke and formaldehyde). When the mucosa encounters substances that interfere with proper functioning, the turbinates swell and mucus production increases in an effort to carry away offending irritants. The result is sneezing, nasal stuffiness, itching, a runny nose, and other signs and symptoms.

LATERAL CROSS-SECTION OF THE NASAL CAVITY

- Itching in the throat
- Malaise
- Chronic nasal obstruction in perennial allergic rhinitis
- Wheezing

● **Diagnostic test findings**
  - Microscopic examination of sputum and nasal secretions reveals many eosinophils
  - Blood chemistry shows normal or elevated IgE level
  - Skin testing paired with testing responses to environmental stimuli can pinpoint the responsible allergens, given the patient's history

● **Medical management**
  - Treatment aims to control symptoms by eliminating the environmental antigen, if possible, and providing drug therapy and immunotherapy
    – Drug therapy
      · Antihistamines (first-generation): diphenhydramine (Benadryl)
      · Antihistamines (second-generation—nondrowsy): cetirizine (Zyrtec), fexofenadine (Allegra), loratadine (Alavert)
      · Corticosteroids: flunisolide (Aerobid), beclomethasone (Beclovent), triamcinolone (Azmacort)

Diagnostic test findings for allergic rhinitis

- High eosinophil level
- Elevated IgE level

Medications used to treat allergic rhinitis

- First-generation antihistamines such as diphenhydramine (Benadryl)
- Second-generation (nondrowsy) antihistamines such as cetirizine (Zyrtec), fexofenadine (Allegra), and loratadine (Alavert)
- Corticosteroids such as flunisolide, beclomethasone, and triamcinolone (Azmacort)

- Leukotriene inhibitor (Montelukast) helps control allergy symptoms such as asthma
  – Immunotherapy—desensitization with injections of extracted allergens, administered before or during allergy season or perennially

● **Nursing interventions**

- Advise the patient to use intranasal steroids as ordered by the physician for optimal effectiveness
- To reduce environmental exposure to airborne allergens, suggest that the patient sleep with the windows closed, avoid the countryside during pollination seasons, use air conditioning to filter allergens and minimize moisture and dust, and eliminate dust-collecting items, such as stuffed animals, wool blankets, deep-pile carpets, and heavy drapes, from the home

ATOPIC DERMATITIS

● **Definition**

- Also called *eczema*, atopic dermatitis is a chronic skin condition characterized by superficial skin inflammation and intense itching
- Typically, it begins during infancy or early childhood; it may then subside spontaneously, followed by exacerbations in late childhood, adolescence, or early adulthood

● **Causes**

- Exact cause unknown
- Exacerbating factors
  – Irritants
  – Infections (commonly caused by *Staphylococcus aureus*)
  – Some allergens
    - Although no reliable link exists between atopic dermatitis and exposure to inhalant allergens (such as house dust and animal dander), exposure to food allergens (such as soybeans, fish, and nuts) may coincide with flare-ups

● **Pathophysiology**

- Several theories attempt to explain the pathogenesis of atopic dermatitis
  – One theory suggests an underlying metabolically or biochemically induced skin disorder that's genetically linked to elevated serum IgE levels
  – Another theory suggests defective T-cell function

● **Complications**

- Secondary skin infection
- Psychological problems

Key nursing interventions for allergic rhinitis

- Instruct the patient on the use of intranasal steroids.
- Provide guidelines on reducing environmental exposure.

Key facts about atopic dermatitis

- Also called *eczema*
- Chronic skin condition characterized by superficial skin inflammation and intense itching
- Typically begins during infancy or early childhood
- Possibly caused by an underlying metabolically or biochemically induced skin disorder that's genetically linked to elevated serum IgE levels

Lesion patterns in pediatric atopic dermatitis

Rash and lesions in atopic dermatitis form a characteristic pattern, depending on the child's age. This chart shows the approximate progression of lesions over 4 years.

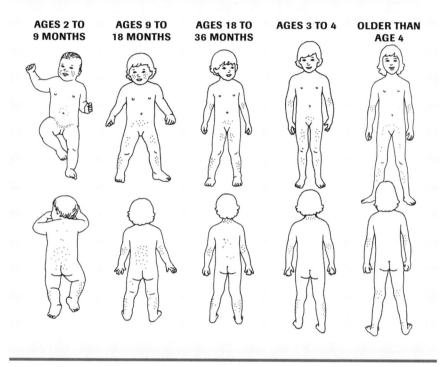

| AGES 2 TO 9 MONTHS | AGES 9 TO 18 MONTHS | AGES 18 TO 36 MONTHS | AGES 3 TO 4 | OLDER THAN AGE 4 |

Assessment findings

- Scratching the skin causes vasoconstriction and intensifies pruritus, resulting in erythematous, weeping lesions
- Eventually, the lesions become scaly and lichenified
- The rash and lesions form a characteristic pattern, depending on the child's age (see *Lesion patterns in pediatric atopic dermatitis*)
- Children with atopic dermatitis are prone to unusually severe:
  - Viral infections
  - Bacterial infections
  - Fungal skin infections
  - Ocular complications
  - Allergic contact dermatitis

Diagnostic test findings

- Laboratory tests reveal eosinophilia and elevated serum IgE levels
- Allergy skin testing or radioallergosorbent testing can help identify specific allergens that may trigger the child's reactivity

Assessment findings in atopic dermatitis

- Pruritus
- Scaly lesions
- Characteristic rash pattern

The role of scratching in atopic dermatitis

- Causes vasoconstriction
- Intensifies pruritus
- Ultimately results in erythematous, weeping lesions that become scaly and lichenified

Measures to ease atopic dermatitis

- Frequent application of topical lubricant, especially after bathing or showering
- Minimizing exposure to allergens and irritants
- Drug therapy consisting of topical corticosteroids, oral antihistamines, and topical macrolides

Personal hygiene recommendations for the child with atopic dermatitis

- Use only water and a small amount of unscented soap when bathing.
- Use lanolin-rich skin cream or emulsions after bathing to seal in moisture.

Medical management

- Measures to ease this chronic disorder include meticulous skin care, environmental control of offending allergens, and drug therapy
- Because dry skin aggravates itching, frequent application of nonirritating topical lubricants is important, especially after bathing or showering
- Minimizing exposure to allergens and irritants, such as wools and harsh detergents, helps to control symptoms
- Drug therapy
  - Topical corticosteroids
    - Fluocinolone acetonide (Synalar)
    - Flurandrenolide (Cordran)
    - Should be applied immediately after bathing for optimal penetration
  - Antipruritics and antihistamines
    - Hydroxyzine (Atarax)
    - Phenothiazine derivatives
      - Methdilazine (Tacaryl)
      - Trimeprazine (Temaril)
  - Topical immunomodulators
    - These medications are steroid free
      - Tacrolimus (Protopic)
      - Pimecrolimus (Elidel)
  - Antibiotics (for secondary infections)
- Counseling because the disorder may frustrate the patient and strain family ties

Nursing interventions

- Monitor the patient's compliance with drug therapy
- Teach the patient when and how to apply topical drug therapy during flare-ups
- Emphasize the importance of regular personal hygiene
  - Use only water and a small amount of unscented soap
  - Use lanolin-rich skin cream or emulsions after bathing to seal in moisture
- Be alert for signs and symptoms of secondary infection; teach the patient how to recognize them as well
- If the patient's diet is modified to exclude food allergens, monitor his nutritional status
- Breast-fed infants are less likely to develop eczema, especially if the mother eliminates cow's milk from her diet
- Offer support to help the patient and his family cope with this chronic disorder
- Discourage use of laundry additives
- Discourage the child from scratching to help prevent further pruritus and infection

- Cut nails short to prevent secondary infection
- Interventions to decrease dryness, inflammation, and pruritus:
  - Avoid heat and sweating; keep the child dry
  - Bathe the child only twice per week, without soap if possible
  - Apply topical emollient to the skin immediately after the bath; pat dry
  - To prevent complications from scratching, keep the child's nails short; use hand mitts if necessary, and cover affected areas with light clothing
  - Rinse laundry thoroughly, and use a mild detergent
  - Encourage parents to humidify the home during the winter
  - Avoid wool; use lightweight cotton

JUVENILE RHEUMATOID ARTHRITIS

● Definition
- Juvenile rheumatoid arthritis (JRA) refers to several conditions characterized by chronic synovitis and joint swelling, pain, and tenderness
- Major types
  - Pauciarticular JRA: asymmetrical involvement of fewer than five joints; usually affects large joints, such as the knees, ankles, and elbows, and eye complications such as iridocyclitis
  - Polyarticular JRA: symmetrical involvement of five or more joints, especially the hands and weight-bearing joints, such as the hips, knees, and feet; involvement of the temporomandibular joint may cause earache; involvement of the sternoclavicular joint may cause chest pain
  - Systemic disease with polyarthritis: involves the lining of the heart and lungs, blood cells, and abdominal organs; exacerbations may last for months; fever, rash, and lymphadenopathy may occur

● Causes
- Unknown
- Suggested link to genetic factors or an abnormal immune response
- Viral or bacterial (streptococcal) infection, trauma, and emotional stress

● Pathophysiology
- If JRA isn't arrested, the inflammatory process in the joints occurs in four stages:
  - Synovitis develops from congestion and edema of the synovial membrane and joint capsule
  - Pannus covers and invades cartilage and eventually destroys the joint capsule and bone
  - Fibrous tissue and ankylosis occludes the joint space
  - Fibrous tissue calcifies, resulting in bony ankylosis and total immobility

---

Ways to decrease dryness, inflammation, and pruritus

- Avoid heat and sweating.
- Bathe the child only twice per week.
- Apply a topical emollient immediately after the bath.
- Use a mild clothes detergent; rinse laundry thoroughly.
- Encourage parents to humidify the home during the winter.

Key facts about JRA

- Refers to several conditions characterized by chronic synovitis and joint swelling, pain, and tenderness
- Linked to genetic factors or an abnormal immune response

Major types of JRA

- Pauciarticular: asymmetrical involvement of fewer than five joints
- Polyarticular: symmetrical involvement of five or more joints
- Systemic disease with polyarthritis: involvement of the lining of the heart and lungs, blood cells, and abdominal organs

What happens in JRA

- Synovitis develops from congestion and edema of the synovial membrane and joint capsule
- Pannus covers and invades cartilage and eventually destroys the joint capsule and bone
- Fibrous tissue and ankylosis occludes the joint space
- Fibrous tissue calcifies, resulting in bony ankylosis and total immobility

● **Complications**
  • Flexion contractures
  • Ocular damage and vision loss

● **Assessment findings**
  • Inflammation around the joints
  • Stiffness, pain, and guarding of the affected joints

● **Diagnostic test findings**
  • Decreased serum hemoglobin levels and increased neutrophil (neutrophilia) and platelet (thrombocytosis) levels; other findings include elevated erythrocyte sedimentation rate and elevated C-reactive protein, serum haptoglobin, immunoglobulin, and C3 complement levels
  • Positive antinuclear antibody test in patients with polyarticular JRA and in those with pauciarticular JRA with chronic iridocyclitis
  • Rheumatoid factor (RF) appears in about 15% of patients with JRA; in contrast, about 85% of patients with RA test positive for RF; patients with polyarticular JRA may test positive for RF
  • HLA-B27 forecasts later development of ankylosing spondylitis
  • X-ray studies demonstrate early structural changes associated with JRA, including soft-tissue swelling, effusion, and periostitis in affected joints

● **Medical management**
  • Heat therapy: warm compresses, baths
  • Splint application
  • Drug therapy
    – Low-dose corticosteroids
    – Low-dose methotrexate (used as a second-line medication)
    – Nonsteroidal anti-inflammatory drugs (NSAIDs): naproxen (Aleve), ibuprofen (Advil)

● **Nursing interventions**
  • Focus nursing care on reducing pain and promoting mobility
  • During inflammatory exacerbations, administer NSAIDs or prescribed medication on a regular schedule
  • Allow the patient to rest frequently throughout the day to conserve energy for times when he must be mobile
  • Arrange the patient's environment for participation in activities of daily living so that he feels capable of accomplishing tasks
  • Instruct the patient to receive regular slit-lamp examinations to enable early diagnosis and treatment of iridocyclitis

REYE'S SYNDROME

● **Definition**
  • Acute illness that causes fatty infiltration of the liver, kidneys, brain, and myocardium

---

Medications used to treat JRA

• Low-dose corticosteroids
• Low-dose methotrexate (used as a second-line medication)
• Nonsteroidal anti-inflammatory drugs such as naproxen and ibuprofen

Key nursing interventions for JRA

• Institute measures to reduce pain and promote mobility.
• Administer NSAIDs as prescribed.
• Provide frequent rest periods.

- It can lead to hyperammonemia, encephalopathy, and increased intracranial pressure (ICP)
- Incidence commonly rises during influenza outbreaks and may be linked to aspirin use; for this reason, use of aspirin for children under age 15 should be avoided

Causes
- Acute viral infection, such as upper respiratory tract, type B influenza, or varicella (Reye's syndrome almost always follows within 1 to 3 days of infection)
- Concurrent aspirin use (high incidence)

Pathophysiology
- Damaged hepatic mitochondria disrupt the urea cycle, which normally changes ammonia to urea for its excretion from the body
  - This results in hyperammonemia, hypoglycemia, and an increase in serum short-chain fatty acids, leading to encephalopathy
- Simultaneously, fatty infiltration occurs in renal tubular cells, neuronal tissue, and muscle tissue, including the heart

Complications
- Increased ICP
- Respiratory alkalosis and subsequent impaired gas exchange, respiratory arrest, and decreased cardiac output

Assessment findings
- Reye's syndrome develops in five stages; the severity of signs and symptoms varies with the degree of encephalopathy and cerebral edema
  - Stage 1: vomiting, lethargy, hepatic dysfunction
  - Stage 2: hyperventilation, delirium, hyperactive reflexes, hepatic dysfunction
  - Stage 3: coma, hyperventilation, decorticate rigidity, hepatic dysfunction
  - Stage 4: deepening coma, decerebrate rigidity, large fixed pupils, minimal hepatic dysfunction
  - Stage 5: seizures, loss of deep tendon reflexes, flaccidity, respiratory arrest (death is usually a result of cerebral edema or cardiac arrest)

Diagnostic test findings
- Blood test results show elevated serum ammonia levels; serum fatty acid and lactate levels are also increased
- Cerebrospinal fluid (CSF) analysis shows WBCs less than 10/µl; with coma, there's increased CSF pressure
- Coagulation studies reveal prolonged prothrombin time and partial thromboplastin time
- Liver biopsy shows fatty droplets uniformly distributed throughout cells
- Liver function studies show that AST and ALT are elevated to twice normal levels

---

Key facts about Reye's syndrome
- An acute illness that causes fatty infiltration of the liver, kidneys, brain, and myocardium
- Can lead to hyperammonemia, encephalopathy, and increased intracranial pressure
- Incidence commonly rises during influenza outbreaks
- May be linked to aspirin use

Complications of Reye's syndrome
- Increased ICP
- Respiratory alkalosis and subsequent impaired gas exchange, respiratory arrest, and decreased cardiac output

Assessment findings in the five stages of Reye's syndrome
- **Stage 1** — vomiting, lethargy, hepatic dysfunction
- **Stage 2** — hyperventilation, delirium, hyperactive reflexes, hepatic dysfunction
- **Stage 3** — coma, hyperventilation, decorticate rigidity, hepatic dysfunction
- **Stage 4** — deepening coma, decerebrate rigidity, large fixed pupils, minimal hepatic dysfunction
- **Stage 5** — seizures, loss of deep tendon reflexes, flaccidity, respiratory arrest

Managing Reye's syndrome

- Ventilation support as necessary
- Fresh frozen plasma
- Osmotic diuretic
- Vitamin K

TOP 4

Nursing interventions for Reye's syndrome

1. Assess cardiac, respiratory, and neurologic status.
2. Maintain seizure precautions.
3. Elevate the head of the bed to decrease ICP and promote venous return.
4. Maintain oxygen therapy.

Key facts about SCID

- Also known as *bubble-boy disease*
- Cell-mediated and humoral immunity either deficient or absent
- Predisposes the infant to infection from all classes of microorganisms
- Transmitted as an autosomal recessive trait but may be X-linked

● **Medical management**
- Craniotomy
- Endotracheal intubation and mechanical ventilation to control partial pressure of arterial carbon dioxide levels
- Enteral or parenteral nutrition as needed
- Exchange transfusion
- Induced hypothermia
- Transfusion of fresh frozen plasma
- Drug therapy
    - Osmotic diuretic: mannitol
    - Vitamin: phytonadione (vitamin K) to treat hypoprothrombinemia
    - Barbiturate: pentobarbital
    - Neuromuscular blocking agent: pancuronium bromide

● **Nursing interventions**
- Monitor ICP with a subarachnoid screw or other invasive device to closely assess for increased ICP
- Assess cardiac, respiratory, and neurologic status
- Monitor fluid intake and output to prevent fluid overload
- Monitor serum glucose levels
- Maintain seizure precautions to prevent injury
- Keep the head of bed elevated 30 degrees to decrease ICP and promote venous return
- Maintain oxygen therapy, which may include intubation and mechanical ventilation, to promote oxygenation and maintain thermoregulation
- Administer blood products as necessary to increase oxygen-carrying capacity of blood and prevent hypovolemia
- Maintain hypothermia blanket as needed, and monitor temperature every 15 to 30 minutes while in use
- Check for loss of reflexes and signs of flaccidity
- Provide good skin and mouth care and range-of-motion exercises
- Provide postoperative craniotomy care if necessary
- Maintain a minimal stimulation environment to avoid increases in ICP
- Be supportive of the family, and keep them informed of the child's status

SEVERE COMBINED IMMUNODEFICIENCY DISEASE

● **Definition**
- Cell-mediated (T-cell) and humoral (B-cell) immunity either deficient or absent
- Predisposes the patient to infection from all classes of microorganisms during infancy
- Also known as *SCID* and *bubble-boy disease*

Causes
- Transmitted as autosomal recessive trait but may be X-linked
- Possibly, enzyme deficiency
- Thymus or bursa equivalent may fail to develop normally or possible defect in thymus and bone marrow (responsible for T- and B-cell development)

Pathophysiology
- Three types of SCID have been identified
  - reticular dysgenesis, the most severe type, in which the hematopoietic stem cell fails to differentiate into lymphocytes and granulocytes
  - Swiss-type agammaglobulinemia, in which the hematopoietic stem cell fails to differentiate into lymphocytes alone
  - Enzyme deficiency, such as adenosine deaminase deficiency, in which the buildup of toxic products in the lymphoid tissue causes damage and subsequent dysfunction

Complications
- Without treatment, death due to infection within 1 year of birth
- Pneumonia
- Oral ulcers
- Failure to thrive
- Dermatitis

Assessment findings
- Extreme susceptibility to infection within the first few months of life but probably no signs of any gram-negative infections until about age 6 months because of protection by maternal IgG
- Emaciated appearance and failure to thrive
- Assessment findings that depend on the type and site of infection
- Signs of chronic otitis media and sepsis
- Signs of the usual childhood diseases such as chickenpox

Diagnostic test findings
- Defective humoral immunity is difficult to detect before an infant reaches age 5 months
- Blood tests show a severely diminished or absent T-cell number and function
- A chest X-ray characteristically shows bilateral pulmonary infiltrates
- Lymph node biopsy that shows an absence of lymphocytes can be used to confirm a diagnosis of SCID

Medical management
- Strict protective isolation (germ-free environment)
- Gene therapy (experimental)
- Drug therapy
  - Immunoglobulin

Types of SCID
- Reticular dysgenesis
- Swiss-type agammaglobu-linemia
- Enzyme deficiency

Complications of SCID
- Without treatment, death due to infection within 1 year of birth
- Pneumonia
- Oral ulcers
- Failure to thrive
- Dermatitis

Assessment findings in SCID
- Extreme susceptibility to infection within the first few months of life
- Emaciated appearance and failure to thrive
- Signs of chronic otitis media, sepsis, and childhood diseases such as chickenpox

Managing SCID
- Strict protective isolation
- Immunoglobulin and antibiotic therapy
- Possible bone marrow transplant or fetal thymus and liver transplant

– Antibiotic therapy
- Surgical interventions
    – Histocompatible bone marrow transplantation
    – Fetal thymus and liver transplantation

● **Nursing interventions**
- Monitor for signs and symptoms of infection
- If infection develops, provide prompt and aggressive drug therapy and supportive care as ordered
- Watch for adverse effects of any medications given
- Avoid vaccinations, and give only irradiated blood products if a transfusion is ordered
- Although the infant with SCID must remain in strict protective isolation, try to provide a stimulating atmosphere to promote growth and development
- Encourage parents to visit their child often, to hold him, and to bring him toys that can be easily sterilized
- Maintain a normal day and night routine, and talk to the child as much as possible; if parents can't visit, call them often to report on the infant's condition
- Provide emotional support for the family

TOP 5

Items to study for your next test on the immune system

1. Functions of the immune system
2. Key facts about AIDS
3. Assessment findings in allergic rhinitis
4. Major types of JRA
5. Stages of Reye's syndrome

NCLEX CHECKS

It's never too soon to begin your NCLEX preparation. Now that you've reviewed this chapter, carefully read each of the following questions and choose the best answer. Then compare your responses to the correct answers.

1. A 17-year-old client with allergic rhinitis has to drive a long distance to work at night. Which medication used for allergic rhinitis doesn't cause sedation and would therefore be the best choice for this client?
- ☐ **1.** Brompheniramine and pseudoephedrine (Dimetapp)
- ☐ **2.** Diphenhydramine (Benadryl)
- ☐ **3.** Pseudoephedrine (Triaminic)
- ☐ **4.** Loratadine (Claritin)

2. A nurse is taking a history from the mother of a pediatric client suspected of having Reye's syndrome. The history reveals the use of several medications. Which medications might be implicated in the development of Reye's syndrome?
- ☐ **1.** Phenytoin (Dilantin)
- ☐ **2.** Furosemide (Lasix)
- ☐ **3.** Phytonadione (AquaMEPHYTON)
- ☐ **4.** Aspirin

3. A nurse is caring for a child with AIDS. Which precautions must the nurse maintain?

- ☐ **1.** Airborne precautions
- ☐ **2.** Standard precautions
- ☐ **3.** Protective isolation
- ☐ **4.** Strict hand washing

4. A child has JRA, an autoimmune disease of the connective tissue characterized by chronic inflammation of the synovia and, possibly, joint destruction. In planning the child's care, which goal has the highest priority?

- ☐ **1.** Preserve joint function.
- ☐ **2.** Be alert for complications such as pericarditis.
- ☐ **3.** Make the child more comfortable.
- ☐ **4.** Educate the family about the disease.

5. Which type of immune cell is the first to arrive at a site of trauma?

- ☐ **1.** Basophils
- ☐ **2.** Eosinophils
- ☐ **3.** Monocytes
- ☐ **4.** Neutrophils

6. Which type of immune cell is responsible for the body's recognition of self versus nonself?

- ☐ **1.** T lymphocyte
- ☐ **2.** HLA
- ☐ **3.** B lymphocyte
- ☐ **4.** Monocyte

7. Which T lymphocyte cell tells B cells when to make antibodies?

- ☐ **1.** Tc
- ☐ **2.** CD8
- ☐ **3.** Th
- ☐ **4.** Ts

8. Which type of hypersensitivity disorder is anaphylaxis?

- ☐ **1.** Type I
- ☐ **2.** Type II
- ☐ **3.** Type III
- ☐ **4.** Type IV

9. In which stage of Reye's syndrome would you expect to find seizures, loss of deep tendon reflexes, and flaccidity?

- ☐ **1.** Stage 2
- ☐ **2.** Stage 3
- ☐ **3.** Stage 4
- ☐ **4.** Stage 5

10. Place in chronological order the four stages of the inflammatory process of juvenile rheumatoid arthritis.

1. Fibrous tissue calcifies.	
2. Synovitis develops.	
3. Fibrous tissue occludes joint space.	
4. Pannus invades the cartilage.	

ANSWERS AND RATIONALES

1. CORRECT ANSWER: 4

Loratadine is a nonsedating antihistamine used for allergic symptoms. All the other listed oral histamine-1 blocking agents cause drowsiness in more than 50% of people who take them.

2. CORRECT ANSWER: 4

Aspirin use has been implicated in the development of Reye's syndrome in children with a history of recent acute viral infection. Phenytoin, furosemide, and phytonadione aren't associated with the development of Reye's syndrome.

3. CORRECT ANSWER: 2

The nurse caring for a child with AIDS should maintain standard precautions. Airborne precautions are instituted for clients known or suspected to be infected with microorganisms transmitted by airborne droplet nuclei such as clients with tuberculosis. Protective isolation is instituted for clients who require added protection from infection, such as those who have undergone bone marrow transplantation and those with burns. Strict hand washing should be performed when caring for all clients.

4. CORRECT ANSWER: 1

There's no specific cure for JRA. The highest priority goals of therapy are to preserve joint function, prevent physical deformities, and relieve symptoms without therapeutic harm. The next most important goals concern treating potential complications, such as pericarditis, profound anemia, and vasculitis. After these goals have been accomplished, making the child more comfortable and educating the family are important nursing interventions.

5. CORRECT ANSWER: 4

Neutrophils are the first immune cell to arrive at the site of trauma. They attack bacteria and fungi. Basophils, eosinophils, and monocytes appear later than neutrophils.

6. CORRECT ANSWER: 2

HLAs allow the body to recognize self versus nonself. T lymphocytes carry out functions directly or by its cell products. B lymphocytes produce antibodies. Monocytes phagocytize parasites. T and B lymphocytes and monocytes don't help the body recognize self versus nonself.

7. CORRECT ANSWER: 3

Th (helper T or CD4+) cells tell the B cells when to make antibodies and how to make them. Tc (cytoxic T) cells have a direct killing affect. Ts (suppressor T or CD8) cells tell B cells to stop making antibodies.

8. CORRECT ANSWER: 1

Anaphylaxis is a type I hypersensitivity disorder. A transfusion reaction is an example of a type II hypersensitivity disorder. Rheumatic fever is an example of a type III hypersensitivity disorder. Contact dermatitis is an example of a type IV hypersensitivity disorder.

9. CORRECT ANSWER: 4

In stage 5, the client experiences seizures, loss of deep tendon reflexes, flaccidity, and respiratory arrest. In stage 2, hyperventilation, delirium, hyperactive reflexes, and hepatic dysfunction occur. In stage 3, coma, hyperventilation, decorticate rigidity, and hepatic dysfunction occur. In stage 4, the client has a deepening coma, decerebrate rigidity, large fixed pupils, and minimal hepatic dysfunction.

10. CORRECT ANSWER:

2. Synovitis develops.

4. Pannus invades the cartilage.

3. Fibrous tissue occludes joint space.

1. Fibrous tissue calcifies.

Synovitis develops from congestion and edema of the synovial membrane and joint capsule. Then the pannus covers and invades cartilage and eventually destroys the joint capsule and bone. Fibrous tissue and ankylosis occludes the joint space. Finally, the fibrous tissue calcifies, resulting in bony anklyosis and total immobility.

7

Altered neurosensory functioning

1. A neonate is diagnosed with hydrocephalus. Which sign is consistent with this diagnosis?

☐ 1. Lethargy
☐ 2. Closed suture lines
☐ 3. Cephalohematoma
☐ 4. Diarrhea

CORRECT ANSWER: 1

2. Which part of the brain stem contains a respiratory and cranial nerve center?

☐ 1. Mesencephalon
☐ 2. Medulla
☐ 3. Pons
☐ 4. Cerebrum

CORRECT ANSWER: 3

3. Which type of cerebral palsy involves hyperactive stretch reflex in associated muscle groups?

☐ 1. Rigid
☐ 2. Spastic
☐ 3. Athetoid
☐ 4. Ataxic

CORRECT ANSWER: 2

4. Which term refers to the marbling and speckling of the iris in Down syndrome?

☐ 1. Koplik spots
☐ 2. Gowers' sign
☐ 3. Hill's sign
☐ 4. Brushfield's spots

CORRECT ANSWER: 4

5. Which term describes the type of blindness that involves difficulty reading newsprint with correction?

☐ 1. Low vision
☐ 2. Legal blindness
☐ 3. Visually impaired
☐ 4. Severe visual impairment

CORRECT ANSWER: 3

LEARNING OBJECTIVES

After studying this chapter, you should be able to:

- Describe alterations in sensory, integrative, and motor functions of the central nervous system.
- Discuss interventions to promote the growth, development, safety, and comfort of a child with alterations in the components of the sensory motor arc.
- Differentiate between the disorders that can increase intracranial pressure.

Key facts about the central nervous system

- Coordinates information to and from the peripheral nervous system
- Regulates and controls the entire body
- Receives sensory stimuli from the external or internal environment
- Perceives, integrates, interprets, or retains the stimulus in memory and produces a motor response
- Consists of the brain and spinal cord

The brain's structures

- Cerebrum (two hemispheres)
- Cerebellum
- Brain stem

Parts of the brain stem

- Mesencephalon – contains cranial nerve nuclei
- Pons – a respiratory and cranial nerve center
- Medulla – a respiratory control center

CHAPTER OVERVIEW

Knowing how the normal nervous system functions provides a foundation for understanding conditions associated with its altered functioning. Rapid assessment and prompt intervention are necessary to stabilize the patient, promote an optimal level of functioning, and prevent complications. In addition, continuous monitoring for signs and symptoms of increased intracranial pressure (ICP) is crucial.

KEY CONCEPTS

- **The nervous system**
  - Grows more rapidly before birth than other systems
  - At birth, the brain is 12% of the neonate's body weight
  - The brain's weight doubles in the first year and triples by age 5 or 6

- **Structures and functions**
  - Central nervous system (CNS) (see *A close look at the CNS*)
    - Coordinates information to and from the peripheral nervous system
    - Regulates and controls the entire body
    - Receives sensory stimuli from the external (exteroceptive) or internal (interoceptive or proprioceptive) environment
    - Perceives, integrates, interprets, or retains the stimulus in memory and produces a motor response
      - The five senses are vision, hearing, touch, taste, and smell
      - The infant's early responses are primarily reflexive; he learns to discriminate stimuli and bring motor responses under conscious control
    - The CNS consists of the brain and spinal cord
      - The brain, consisting of three structures, regulates and controls body functions
        - Cerebrum
          - ·· Composed of two hemispheres that are divided into the frontal, parietal, occipital, and temporal lobes
          - ·· Controls consciousness, memory, sensory input, motor activity, and thought
        - Cerebellum
          - ·· Coordinates and refines all muscle movements
          - ·· Controls muscle tone, balance, talking, and walking
        - Brain stem
          - ·· Mesencephalon (midbrain) — contains cranial nerve nuclei
          - ·· Pons — a respiratory and cranial nerve center
          - ·· Medulla — a respiratory control center
      - The spinal cord
        - Where the 31 spinal nerves originate

A close look at the CNS

This illustration shows a cross section of the brain and spinal cord, which together make up the central nervous system (CNS). The brain joins the spinal cord at the base of the skull and ends near the second lumbar vertebra. Note the H-shaped mass of gray matter in the spinal cord.

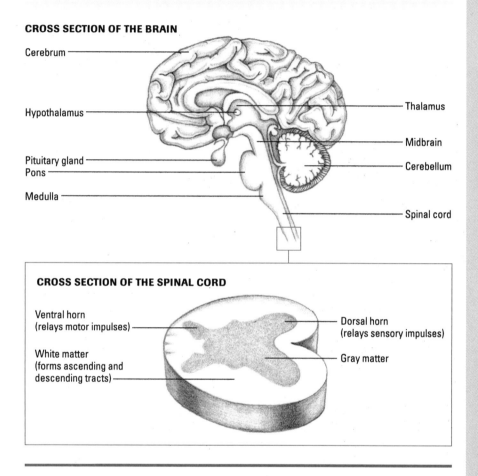

CROSS SECTION OF THE BRAIN

Cerebrum

Hypothalamus

Pituitary gland
Pons

Medulla

Thalamus

Midbrain

Cerebellum

Spinal cord

CROSS SECTION OF THE SPINAL CORD

Ventral horn
(relays motor impulses)

White matter
(forms ascending and
descending tracts)

Dorsal horn
(relays sensory impulses)

Gray matter

- Conducts sensory and motor impulses to and from the brain
- Controls reflexes
- The inner core is the gray matter consisting of nerve cells
- The outer white matter consists of bundles of myelinated nerve fibers
• The peripheral nervous system
  – Composed of the 12 pairs of cranial nerves and 31 pairs of spinal nerves
  – The cranial nerves are the primary motor and sensory pathways among the brain, head, and neck
  – Peripheral sensory nerves transmit stimuli to the dorsal horn of the spinal cord from sensory receptors located in the skin, muscles, sensory organs, and viscera

Key facts about the peripheral nervous system

• Has 12 pairs of cranial nerves and 31 pairs of spinal nerves
• Transmits stimuli from sensory receptors located in the skin, muscles, sensory organs, and viscera to the spinal cord
• Carries impulses that affect movement

Key facts about the autonomic nervous system

- Regulates the activities of the visceral organs
- Affects the smooth muscles and glands
- Controls fight-or-flight responses
- Maintains baseline body functions

Key facts about CT scanning

- Produces three-dimensional image
- May be performed with or without contrast medium
- Requires written, informed consent
- Requires the child to hold still (may require sedation)

Key facts about MRI

- May be performed with or without noniodinated contrast medium
- Provides greater detail than CT scan
- Allows visualization of cerebral arteries and venous sinuses
- Requires the child to hold still (may require sedation)

– The upper motor neurons of the brain and the lower motor neurons of the cell bodies in the ventral horn of the spinal cord carry impulses that affect movement
- The autonomic nervous system
  – Contains motor neurons that regulate the activities of the visceral organs and affect the smooth muscles and glands
  – The sympathetic division controls fight-or-flight responses
  – The parasympathetic division maintains baseline body functions

DIAGNOSTIC TESTS

● Computed tomography (CT) scan
- Purpose
  – Produces a three-dimensional image of the area scanned
  – Performed with or without a contrast medium
- Nursing interventions
  – Explain the purpose of test to the parents and child
  – Obtain written, informed consent
  – Make sure the child holds still during the test; sedation may be necessary
  – If a contrast medium is ordered:
    · Verify that the patient isn't allergic to shellfish or iodine; if he has one of these allergies, consult the physician for premedication or alternative diagnostic test orders
    · Verify that the child doesn't have any renal problems; if he does, consult the physician because contrast medium can be toxic to the kidneys

● Magnetic resonance imaging (MRI)
- Purpose
  – Performed with or without a noniodinated contrast medium
  – Provides greater detail than a CT scan
  – Advances in MRI allow visualization of cerebral arteries and venous sinuses without administration of contrast medium
- Nursing interventions
  – If the child has surgically implanted metal objects (such as pins and clips), notify the radiology department because these may interfere with the picture
  – Explain the procedure to the parents and child
  – Make sure the child holds still during the test; sedation may be necessary

● Electroencephalography (EEG)
- Purpose
  – Shows abnormal electrical activity in the brain (such as from a seizure, metabolic disorder, or drug overdose)

– Is noninvasive
- Nursing interventions
  – Explain the purpose of the test
  – Make sure the child holds still during the test; sedation may be necessary

Ultrasonography

- Purpose
  – Reveals carotid lesions or changes in carotid blood flow and velocity through the use of high-frequency sound waves
  – Reveals intraventricular hemorrhages
- Nursing interventions
  – Explain the purpose of the test to the parents and child
  – Make sure the child holds still during the test

Lumbar puncture

- Purpose
  – Aspirates cerebrospinal fluid (CSF) from the subarachnoid space of the spinal cord between L3 and L4 or L4 and L5
  – Allows for analysis of the CSF and measurement of CSF pressure
- Nursing interventions
  – Before the procedure, obtain written, informed consent
  – Keep the child in a side-lying, knee-chest position during the procedure
  – Monitor the child's condition throughout the procedure
  – Make sure that the child rests for 1 hour after the procedure

Cerebral arteriography (angiography)

- Purpose
  – Radiopaque dye is injected into a catheter that has been inserted into an artery (usually the femoral artery)
  – Provides X-ray visualization of the cerebral vasculature
- Nursing interventions
  – Explain the procedure to the parents and child
  – Obtain written, informed consent
  – Identify allergies before the test
  – Verify the child's current medication regimen; report the use of anticoagulants
  – Make sure the child holds still during the test; sedation may be necessary
  – Monitor for allergic reactions to the dye
  – After the test, immobilize the site and monitor it for pulses and evidence of bleeding or hematoma

ICP monitoring

- Purpose
  – To directly and invasively measure ICP

– A subarachnoid screw and an intraventricular catheter (or a fiber-optic catheter in the ventricle, subarachnoid space, subdural space, or the brain parenchyma) converts CSF pressure readings into waveforms that are digitally displayed on a monitor

- Nursing interventions
  - Before the procedure
    - Explain the procedure to the child and parents
    - Obtain written, informed consent
  - After the procedure
    - Monitor ICP range and waveforms
    - Identify and document trends and alert the physician to changes
    - Maintain sterile technique during care of monitoring equipment
    - Monitor the site for signs of infection

● **Electromyography**
- Purpose
  - Detects lower motor neuron disorders, neuromuscular disorders, and nerve damage
  - A needle is inserted into selected muscles at rest and during voluntary contractions to pick up nerve impulses and measure nerve conduction time
- Nursing interventions
  - Explain the procedure to the parents and child
  - Check the child's medications for those that may interfere with the test (cholinergics, anticholinergics, skeletal muscle relaxants)
  - Obtain written, informed consent
  - Make sure the child holds still during the procedure; sedation may be necessary
  - Monitor the site for infection or bleeding after the procedure

● **Otoscopic examination**
- Purpose
  - Allows visualization of the canal and inner structures of the ear
  - Allows for detection of foreign bodies, cerumen, or stenosis in the external ear canal
- Nursing interventions
  - Use the largest speculum that fits into the ear canal
  - To straighten the ear canal in infants and children younger than age 3, pull the pinna down and back or out; for children older than age 3, pull the pinna up and back
  - Test hearing acuity through play audiometry or through audiometry using earphones in children age 4 and older

● **Ophthalmoscopic examination**
- Purpose
  - Helps visualize internal eye structures

– Allows detection of ocular manifestations of systemic disease
- Nursing interventions
  – Explain the procedure to the parents and child
  – Ensure cooperation during tests by allowing the child to hold a favorite toy, which may decrease anxiety

NURSING DIAGNOSES

● **Probable nursing diagnoses**
- Imbalanced nutrition: Less than body requirements
- Impaired physical mobility
- Delayed growth and development
- Impaired verbal communication
- Risk for aspiration
- Decreased intracranial adaptive capacity
- Acute pain
- Disturbed sensory perception (auditory, tactile)

● **Possible nursing diagnoses**
- Risk for impaired parenting
- Risk for injury
- Ineffective breathing pattern
- Hyperthermia
- Ineffective airway clearance
- Impaired adjustment

CEREBRAL PALSY

● **Definition**
- A nonprogressive neuromuscular disorder of varying degrees resulting from damage or a defect in the part of the brain that controls motor function
- A group of disorders arising from a malfunction of motor centers and neural pathways in the brain
- Types of cerebral palsy (CP)
  – Ataxic
  – Athetoid
  – Spastic
  – Rigid
  – Mixed

● **Causes**
- Mostly unknown
- Anoxia before, during, or after birth
- Infection
- Trauma

Key facts about ophthalmoscopic examination

- Helps visualize internal eye structures
- Allows detection of ocular manifestations of systemic disease

Probable nursing diagnoses for a patient with a neurosensory disorder

- Imbalanced nutrition: Less than body requirements
- Impaired physical mobility
- Delayed growth and development
- Impaired verbal communication
- Risk for aspiration
- Decreased intracranial adaptive capacity
- Acute pain
- Disturbed sensory perception (auditory, tactile)

Key facts about CP

- Nonprogressive neuromuscular disorder
- Caused by damage or defect in part of brain that controls motor function

Types of CP

- Ataxic
- Athetoid
- Spastic
- Rigid
- Mixed

Causes of CP

- Prenatal conditions, such as maternal rubella, toxemia, and anoxia
- Perinatal and birth difficulties
- Infection or trauma during infancy

TOP 2

Assessment findings in all types of CP

1. Abnormal motor performance and coordination
2. Altered muscle tone

Causes of cerebral palsy

Conditions that result in cerebral anoxia, hemorrhage, or other damage may also result in cerebral palsy (CP).

- *Prenatal conditions that may increase the risk of CP:* Maternal infection (especially rubella), maternal drug ingestion, radiation, anoxia, toxemia, maternal diabetes, abnormal placental attachment, malnutrition, and isoimmunization
- *Perinatal and birth difficulties that increase the risk of CP:* Forceps delivery, breech presentation, placenta previa, abruptio placentae, metabolic or electrolyte disturbances, abnormal maternal vital signs from general or spinal anesthesia, pro-

lapsed cord with a delay in the delivery of the head, premature birth, prolonged or unusually rapid labor, and multiple births (especially the infant born last in a multiple birth)
- *Infection or trauma during infancy:* Poisoning, severe kernicterus resulting from erythroblastosis fetalis, brain infection, head trauma, prolonged anoxia, brain tumor, cerebral circulatory anomalies causing blood vessel rupture, and systemic disease resulting in cerebral thrombosis or embolus

- Bilirubin encephalopathy

(See also *Causes of cerebral palsy.*)

● **Pathophysiology**
- No characteristic pathologic picture
- A previous anoxic episode plays the largest role in the pathologic state of brain damage

● **Complications**
- Impaired physical mobility
- Self-care deficits
- Physical injury
- Impaired communication
- Mental impairment

● **Assessment findings**
- All types
  - Delayed gross motor development
  - Abnormal motor performance and coordination; can manifest early in life as poor sucking and feeding difficulty
  - Posture abnormality occurring at rest or when changing position
  - Altered muscle tone
    · Increased or decreased resistance to passive range of motion (ROM)
    · Opisthotonic postures (exaggerated arching of the back)
    · Spasticity of hip muscles and lower extremities, making diapering difficult
  - Abnormal reflexes
  - Persistent primitive reflexes

– Other disabilities
  - Mental retardation of varying degrees in 18% to 50% of patients (most children with CP have at least a normal IQ but can't demonstrate it on standardized tests)
  - Seizures
  - Attention deficit hyperactivity disorder
  - Sensory deficits
    - Vision (strabismus)
    - Hearing
    - Speech
- Ataxic
  – Poor balance and muscle coordination caused by disturbances in movement and balance
  – Unsteady, wide-based gait
- Athetoid
  – Involuntary, uncoordinated motion with varying degrees of muscle tension
  – Slow state of writhing muscle contractions whenever voluntary movement is attempted
  – Facial grimacing
  – Poor swallowing
  – Drooling
  – Poor speech articulation
- Rigid
  – Rigid posture
  – Lack of active movement
- Spastic
  – Hyperactive stretch reflex in associated muscle groups
  – Hyperactive deep tendon reflexes
  – Rapid involuntary muscle contraction and relaxation
  – Contractures affecting the extensor muscles
  – Scissoring
- Mixed
  – Signs of more than one type of CP
  – Severe disability

● **Diagnostic test findings**
- Neuroimaging studies determine the site of brain impairment
- Cytogenic studies (genetic evaluation of the child and other family members) rule out other potential causes
- Metabolic studies rule out other causes

● **Medical management**
- Baclofen (Lioresal) pump insertion
  – Delivers baclofen, a skeletal muscle relaxant, directly to the intrathecal space around the spinal cord

Other disabilities indicating CP

- Mental retardation of varying degrees
- Seizures
- Attention deficit hyperactivity disorder
- Sensory deficits

Findings in CP

Ataxic
- Poor balance and muscle coordination
- Unsteady, wide-based gait

Athetoid
- Involuntary, uncoordinated motion
- Slow state of writhing muscle contractions when voluntary movement is attempted
- Facial grimacing
- Drooling and poor swallowing
- Poor speech articulation

Rigid
- Rigid posture
- Lack of active movement

Spastic
- Hyperactive stretch reflex and deep tendon reflexes
- Rapid involuntary muscle contraction and relaxation
- Contractures of extensor muscles
- Scissoring

Mixed
- Signs of more than one type of CP
- Severe disability

Managing CP with a baclofen pump

- Implanted
- Used to treat spasticity
- Delivers baclofen (Lioresal), a skeletal muscle relaxant, directly to the intrathecal space around the spinal cord
- Replaced every 3 to 5 years

Key nursing interventions for CP

- Institute a high-calorie diet.
- Perform ROM exercises.
- Assist with locomotion, communication, and educational opportunities.
- Promote age-appropriate mental activities and incentives for motor development.
- Provide rest periods.
- Refer the child for speech, nutrition, and physical therapy.

Key facts about Down syndrome

- Congenital condition
- Characterized by mental retardation and multiple associated defects
- Caused by genetic nondisjunction resulting in three chromosomes on the 21st pair or translocation of chromosome 21
- Commonly associated with congenital heart defects and other abnormalities

– Used to treat spasticity
– Pump lasts for 3 to 5 years; after that time, a new pump must be implanted
- Muscle relaxants or neurosurgery to decrease spasticity, if appropriate
- Anticonvulsants, such as phenytoin (Dilantin) and phenobarbital (Luminal), to control seizures
- An artificial urinary sphincter may be indicated for the incontinent child who can use the hand controls
- Orthopedic surgery may be indicated to correct contractures
- Braces or splints and special appliances, such as adapted eating utensils and a low toilet seat with arms, to help the child perform activities independently

● **Nursing interventions**
- Institute a high-calorie diet for the child with increased motor function to help him keep up with increased metabolic demands
- Perform ROM exercises to minimize contractures
- Assist with locomotion, communication, and educational opportunities to enable the child to attain an optimal developmental level
- Make food easy to manage to decrease stress during mealtimes
- Promote age-appropriate mental activities and incentives for motor development to promote growth and development
- Provide rest periods to promote rest and reduce metabolic needs
- Provide a safe environment; for example, have the child use protective headgear or bed pads to prevent injury
- Divide tasks into small steps to promote self-care and activity and increase self-esteem
- Refer the child for speech, nutrition, and physical therapy to maintain or improve functioning
- If the child can't speak, use assistive communication devices to promote a positive self-concept
- Assist family members in setting realistic goals and managing stress

DOWN SYNDROME

● **Definition**
- A congenital condition characterized by mental retardation in varying degrees and multiple associated defects
- Also known as trisomy 21

● **Causes**
- Genetic nondisjunction, with three chromosomes on the 21st pair (total of 47 chromosomes)
- Unbalanced translocation of chromosome 21 in which the long arm breaks and attaches to another chromosome

- A risk factor is maternal age; the older the mother, the greater the risk of nondisjunction

● **Pathophysiology**
- A chromosomal aberration characterized by:
  - Mental retardation
  - Dysmorphic facial features
  - Other distinctive physical abnormalities
- Commonly associated with congenital heart defects (in approximately 60% of patients; up to 44% of these patients die before age 1) and other abnormalities

● **Complications**
- Impaired growth and development
- Physical injury
- Aspiration
- Death

● **Assessment findings**
- Brushfield's spots (marbling and speckling of the iris)
- Flat, broad forehead
- Flat nose
- Hypotonia
- Mild to moderate retardation
- Protruding tongue (due to small oral cavity)
- Short stature with pudgy hands
- Simian crease (a single crease along the palm)
- Small head with slow brain growth
- Upward slanting eyes
- Genital and perineal abnormalities

● **Diagnostic test findings**
- Amniocentesis allows prenatal diagnosis
  - Recommended for women older than age 34, regardless of a negative family history
  - Recommended for a woman of any age if she or the father carries a translocated chromosome
- Karyotype shows the specific chromosomal abnormality
- Fetal ultrasound may reveal varying degrees of abnormalities, but many fetuses have few detectable defects

● **Medical management**
- Provide gavage feedings, if necessary, because the infant's sucking reflex may be poor
- Treat coexisting conditions
  - Congenital heart problems, vision defects, hypothyroidism
  - Skeletal, immunologic, metabolic, biochemical, and oncologic problems treated according to specific problem

---

Key signs of Down syndrome

- Brushfield's spots
- Flat, broad forehead
- Flat nose
- Hypotonia
- Mild to moderate retardation
- Protruding tongue
- Short stature with pudgy hands
- Simian crease
- Small head with slow brain growth
- Upward slanting eyes
- Genital and perineal abnormalities

Prenatal diagnosis of Down syndrome using amniocentesis

- Recommended for women older than age 34, regardless of a negative family history
- Recommended for a woman of any age if she or the father carries a translocated chromosome

Conditions coexisting with Down syndrome

- Congenital heart problems
- Vision defects
- Hypothyroidism
- Skeletal, immunologic, metabolic, biochemical, and oncologic problems

Key nursing interventions for Down syndrome

- Provide activities and toys appropriate for the child.
- Set realistic, reachable goals.
- Provide stimulation and communicate at a level appropriate to the child's mental age.
- Mainstream daily routines to promote normalcy.
- Encourage parents to care for, bond with, and hold their child.

● Nursing interventions

- Provide activities and toys appropriate for the child to support optimal development
- Set realistic, reachable goals; break tasks into small steps to make them easier to accomplish
- Use behavior modification, if applicable, to promote safety and prevent injury to the child and others
- Provide stimulation and communicate at a level appropriate to the child's mental age rather than chronological age to promote a healthy emotional environment
- Provide a safe environment to prevent injury
- Mainstream daily routines to promote normalcy
- Encourage parents to care for, bond with, and hold their child
- Teach parents to perform all of the above interventions because care will mostly be provided at home by the parents
- Refer the parents of an affected child for genetic counseling to explore the cause of the disorder and discuss the risk of recurrence in a future pregnancy
- Refer the parents to a social worker or grief counselor for additional support, if needed

HEAD INJURIES

● Definition

- Traumatic damage to the head (the scalp, skull, meninges, or brain)
- Head injuries are a common cause of death in children older than age 1
- The extent of the brain injury is directly related to the force and location of impact

● Causes

- Motor vehicle–related accidents
- Child abuse
- Vigorous shaking
- Bicycle accidents, especially in those without helmets
- Sports accidents, especially in those without helmets
- Falls

Causes of head injuries

- Motor vehicle–related accidents
- Child abuse
- Vigorous shaking
- Bicycle accident
- Sports accidents
- Falls

● Pathophysiology

- The intracranial components are damaged because of a force too great to be absorbed by the skull, muscles, and ligaments that support the head
- The skulls of infants and children are pliable and can absorb much of the physical impact, providing some level of protection to the intracranial components, but they have a larger head size and less support from muscles and ligaments, making them more prone to acceleration-deceleration injuries

- Types of head injuries
  - Scalp laceration—can cause a child to bleed to death because of the vascularity of the surface area
  - Epidural, intracranial hemorrhage—bleeding into the space between the dura mater and the skull
  - Subdural hemorrhage—bleeding between the dura mater and the arachnoid layer of the meninges
  - Concussion
    - A transient state of neurologic dysfunction caused by a jarring of the brain
    - The most common head injury
  - Contusion
    - A sign of petechial hemorrhage on the superficial aspects of the brain at the site of the impact
    - A lesion that occurs away from the site of direct trauma
  - Skull fracture
    - Linear (simple)
    - Depressed (depression of a bone toward the brain)
    - Basilar (at the skull base)

- **Complications**
  - Hemorrhage
  - Infection
  - Edema
  - Herniation

- **Assessment findings**
  - Change in level of consciousness (LOC) or mental status
  - Confusion
  - Listlessness
  - Irritability
  - Pale skin
  - Vomiting
  - Increased head circumference
  - Bulging fontanels
  - Hemiparesis, quadriplegia
  - Headache
  - Decreased memory
  - Diminished pupillary responses

- **Diagnostic test findings**
  - CT and MRI scans show neurologic trauma and injury
  - ICP monitoring shows increased ICP
  - Skull X-rays show fractures or areas of injury

- **Medical management**
  - Medications, such as diphenhydramine (Benadryl) or chloral hydrate (Aquachloral Supprettes), may be used to decrease restlessness

Types of head injuries

- Scalp laceration
- Epidural, intracranial hemorrhage
- Subdural hemorrhage
- Concussion
- Contusion
- Skull fracture

Complications of head injuries

- Hemorrhage
- Infection
- Edema
- Herniation

TOP 3

Assessment findings in head injuries

1. Change in LOC
2. Headache
3. Diminished pupillary responses

GO WITH THE FLOW

Assessing a head injury

INITIAL ASSESSMENT
- Check airway, breathing, circulation.
- Stabilize and examine neck and spine.
- Check vital signs.
- Perform neurologic examination.

↓

Is child stable?

NO ↓ / YES ↓

NO → Continue to reassess; assessments change

NO ↓ / YES ↓

Continue assessments every 2 hours.

SUSPECT NEUROLOGIC DETERIORATION
Anticipate:
- Testing with computed tomography or magnetic resonance imaging
- Frequent neurologic examinations, including vital signs, level of consciousness, pupil response, grasping ability, signs of posturing, response to stimuli, purposeful movements
- Promoting comfort; providing sedation and analgesics
- Decreasing the family's anxiety and involving them in care and the decision process

RECHECK EVERY 2 HOURS FOR AT LEAST 36 HOURS
- Clean injury.
- Check for bleeding or watery discharge from nose or ears.
- Apply ice for 1 hour to decrease pain and swelling.
- Don't give analgesics or sedatives that may mask clinical assessment.
- Raise head of bed 20 to 30 degrees.

Medications for head injuries

- Diphenhydramine (Benadryl) or chloral hydrate (Aquachloral Supprettes) to decrease restlessness
- Acetaminophen to treat headaches
- Anticonvulsants to control seizures
- Antibiotics (prescribed when the child sustains a laceration or leaks CSF)

- Acetaminophen may be used to treat headaches
- Anticonvulsants are used to control seizures
- Antibiotics are prescribed when the child sustains a laceration or leaks CSF
- Lacerations of the scalp and dura are sutured
- Some fractures require surgery to remove scattered bone fragments

● **Nursing interventions**

(See *Assessing a head injury.*)

• Prepare for surgical evaluation of the injury, if necessary
• Promote bed rest and limit unnecessary body movements; slightly elevate the head of the bed
• Initiate seizure precautions
• Provide a quiet environment
• Awaken the child every 2 hours to check his LOC
• Monitor fluid status carefully; restrict fluids as needed to decrease ICP
• Prevent injury through family and community teaching programs to stress child safety (bicycle helmets, car restraining devices, protective skating equipment)
• Check ear or nose drainage for glucose (CSF tests positive for glucose)
• Note behavioral changes (such as aggression, withdrawal, irritability); watch for alterations in sleep patterns, gait, or school performance

HEARING LOSS

● **Definition**

• The inability to perceive the normal range of sounds that's audible to a person with normal hearing
  – The loss may be the same at all frequencies or may be greater at some frequencies than others
  – Hearing is 1.5% impaired for every decibel that the pure tone average exceeds 25 dB
• Sudden hearing loss
  – Hearing loss in a person with no previous hearing impairment
  – Sudden hearing loss is considered an emergency because prompt treatment may restore full hearing

● **Causes**

• Congenital
  – May be transmitted as a dominant, autosomal recessive, or sex-linked recessive trait
  – Congenital abnormalities of the ears, nose, or throat
• Certain conditions during pregnancy or delivery may cause hearing loss in neonates
  – Trauma—prolonged fetal anoxia during delivery, intracranial hemorrhage causing damage to the cochlea or acoustic nerve
  – Toxicity—ototoxic drugs, serum bilirubin levels greater than 20 mg/dl (toxic to the brain)
  – Infection—rubella, syphilis
• Prematurity or low birth weight neonates—most likely to have structural or functional hearing impairment

---

Key nursing interventions for head injuries

• Prepare for surgical evaluation of the injury, if necessary.
• Promote bed rest and limit unnecessary body movements; slightly elevate the head of the bed.
• Initiate seizure precautions.
• Awaken the child every 2 hours to check his LOC.
• Check ear or nose drainage for glucose (CSF tests positive for glucose).
• Note behavioral changes.

What to monitor for in a patient with a head injury

• Behavioral changes, such as aggression, withdrawal, and irritability
• Alterations in sleep patterns, gait, or school performance

Pregnancy- and birth-related causes of hearing loss

• Trauma – prolonged fetal anoxia during delivery, intracranial hemorrhage damaging the cochlea or acoustic nerve
• Toxicity – ototoxic drugs, serum bilirubin levels greater than 20 mg/dl (toxic)
• Infection – rubella, syphilis

Causes of sudden hearing loss

- Metabolic disorders (diabetes mellitus, hypothyroidism, hyperlipoproteinemia)
- Vascular disorders (hypertension and arteriosclerosis)
- Head trauma or brain tumors
- Ototoxic drugs
- Neurologic disorders (multiple sclerosis, neurosyphilis)
- Blood dyscrasias (leukemia, hypercoagulation)

Ototoxic drugs

- Tobramycin (Nebcin)
- Streptomycin
- Quinine
- Gentamicin (Garamycin)
- Furosemide (Lasix)
- Ethacrynic acid (Edecrin)

Types of hearing loss

- Conductive – interrupted passage of sound from external ear to the junction of the stapes and oval window
- Sensorineural – impaired cochlea or acoustic nerve dysfunction
- Mixed – combined dysfunction of conduction and sensorineural transmission

Findings associated with hearing loss

- Deficient response to auditory stimuli
- Lack of response to sound or verbal commands
- Impaired speech development
- Poor academic performance
- Straining to hear

- Causes specific to sudden hearing loss:
  - Metabolic disorders — diabetes mellitus, hypothyroidism, hyperlipoproteinemia
  - Vascular disorders — hypertension, arteriosclerosis
  - Head trauma or brain tumors
  - Ototoxic drugs — tobramycin (Nebcin), streptomycin, quinine, gentamicin (Garamycin), furosemide (Lasix), ethacrynic acid (Edecrin)
  - Neurologic disorders — multiple sclerosis, neurosyphilis
  - Blood dyscrasias — leukemia, hypercoagulation
- Prolonged exposure to loud noise (85 to 90 dB) or brief exposure to extremely loud noise (greater than 90 dB) causes noise-induced hearing loss
- Repeated otitis media
- Mechanical
  - Foreign objects
  - Cerumen accumulation

Pathophysiology

- Conductive — interrupted passage of sound from the external ear to the junction of the stapes and oval window
- Sensorineural — impaired cochlea or acoustic (eighth cranial) nerve dysfunction, causing failure of transmission of sound impulses within the inner ear or brain
- Mixed — combined dysfunction of conduction and sensorineural transmission

Complications

- Physical injury
- Altered perception

Assessment findings

- A deficient response to auditory stimuli — this generally becomes apparent within 2 to 3 days of life
- No reaction or turning to locate a sound or doesn't respond to being repeatedly called by name unless the speaker's lips are visible
- Lack of response to simple verbal commands or questions
- Not soothed by music or by being read to
- As the child grows older, impaired speech development
  - Doesn't develop recognizable speech
  - Fails to vocalize, remains at the babbling stage, or shows decreased babbling
- Poor academic performance
- Tendency to listen to radio and television at high volumes
- Straining to hear
- History of premature birth, meningitis, maternal prenatal history of rubella or use of ototoxic medication such as gentamicin

Diagnostic test findings

- Abnormal behavioral testing—evaluates a child's behavioral response to sound
- Abnormal auditory brain stem response test
  - A click-type noise is presented to a sedated child via earphones
  - Electrodes measure the response of the hearing nerves to sound
  - This test is done within the first 24 hours of life
- Abnormal otoacoustic emissions test
  - Pulse sounds are presented via a probe in the ear canal of a sleeping child
  - The echo response created in the inner ear is recorded
  - This test is done within the first 24 hours of life
- Abnormal Weber's test
  - A vibrating tuning fork is placed on the top of the child's head
  - If there's a sensorineural hearing loss in one ear, the unaffected ear will hear the sound louder
- Abnormal Rinne test
  - One ear is tested at a time—the ear not being tested is masked
  - A vibrating tuning fork is placed on the mastoid bone, behind the ear and level with the canal
  - When the child can no longer hear the tuning fork, place the fork closer to the ear canal and determine if the child can hear the sound again
  - Normally, the sound is heard longer through the air
  - Negative Rinne test—conduction hearing loss; sound is heard through bone as long or longer than it's heard through the air
  - Positive Rinne test—neural loss; sound is heard longer by air conduction in sensorineural loss
  - Sound is heard longer by bone conduction in conductive hearing loss
- Abnormal audiologic test results

Medical management

- Aggressive immunization against rubella in children and positive titers in pregnant women to prevent congenital hearing loss
- Hyperbilirubinemia can be controlled by phototherapy and exchange transfusions
- Judicious use of ototoxic medications in children
- Overnight rest for children with noise-induced hearing loss (greater than 90 dB)
- Alterations in the location or shape of the ears warrant an evaluation of kidney function because these organs develop simultaneously in utero

Nursing interventions

- Refer a child with suspected hearing loss to an audiologist or otolaryngologist for further evaluation

Diagnostic tests to identify hearing loss

- Behavioral tests
- Auditory brain stem test
- Otoacoustic emissions test
- Weber's test
- Rinne test
- Audiologic test

Caring for the pediatric patient with hearing loss

- Stand directly in front of the child when communicating with him.
- Approach the child within his visual range; get his attention by raising your arm or waving.
- Wait for the child's attention before speaking.

Key nursing interventions for a child with hearing loss

- Refer the child to an audiologist or otolaryngologist.
- Develop the patient's ability to communicate through sign language, lip reading, or other effective means.
- Stand directly in front of the patient with hearing loss when communicating with him.
- Approach the child within his visual range.
- Wait for the child's attention before speaking.
- Use demonstration to explain procedures and treatments.

Key facts about hydrocephalus

- Excess CSF in ventricles and subarachnoid spaces
- Can be noncommunicating (CSF flow is blocked) or communicating (CSF absorbs abnormally)

Causes of noncommunicating hydrocephalus

- Congenital anomalies
- Infection — syphilis, granulomatous diseases, meningitis
- Tumor
- Cerebral aneurysm
- Blood clot after intracranial hemorrhage

- Develop the patient's ability to communicate through sign language, lip reading, or other effective means
- Educate pregnant women about the danger of exposure to drugs, chemicals, or infection and carefully monitor during labor and delivery to prevent fetal anoxia
- Educate parents and children about the dangers of noise exposure and encourage the use of protective devices in a noisy environment
- Stand directly in front of the patient with hearing loss when communicating with him
  - Make sure the light is on your face, and speak slowly and distinctly
  - If possible, speak to him at eye level
- Approach the patient within his visual range, and elicit attention by raising your arm or waving; touching him may be unnecessarily startling
- Wait for the child's attention before speaking
- Decrease additional noise in the room
- Use demonstration to explain procedures and treatments before initiating them

HYDROCEPHALUS

Definition
- An increase in the amount of CSF in the ventricles and subarachnoid spaces of the brain
- Can be noncommunicating or communicating

Causes
- Noncommunicating
  - Congenital anomalies
  - Infection — syphilis, granulomatous diseases, meningitis
  - Tumor
  - Cerebral aneurysm
  - Blood clot after intracranial hemorrhage
- Communicating
  - Surgery to repair a myelomeningocele
  - Adhesions between meninges at the base of the brain or meningeal hemorrhage
  - Rarely, a tumor in the choroid plexus that causes an overproduction of CSF

Pathophysiology
- Noncommunicating hydrocephalus
  - CSF flow is blocked by tumors, hemorrhage, or structural abnormalities
  - Fluid accumulates in the ventricles

Signs of hydrocephalus

In infants, characteristic signs of hydrocephalus include a marked enlargement of the head; distended scalp veins; thin, shiny, and fragile-looking scalp skin; and weak muscles that can't support the head.

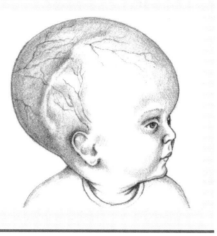

- Communicating hydrocephalus
  - CSF is absorbed abnormally after it reaches the subarachnoid space because of scarring, congenital anomalies, or hemorrhage
  - Fluid isn't blocked
- Arnold-Chiari malformation is the downward displacement of cerebellar components through the foramen magnum into the cervical spinal canal and is common in hydrocephalus with spina bifida

Complications
- Physical injury
- Delayed growth and development
- Decreased intracranial adaptive capacity

Assessment findings
- Increased head circumference, usually increases rapidly in infants
- Full, tense, bulging fontanels
- Widening suture lines
- Distended scalp veins
- Irritability or lethargy; decreased attention span
- High-pitched cry
- Sunset sign (sclera visible above the iris)
- Inability to support the head when upright
- "Cracked pot" sound when the skull is percussed
- Vomiting not related to food intake

(See also *Signs of hydrocephalus*.)

Diagnostic test findings
- Angiography, CT scan, and MRI differentiate hydrocephalus from intracranial lesions and may demonstrate Arnold-Chiari malformation
- Light reflects off the opposite side of the skull with skull transillumination

Types of shunts

- Ventriculoperitoneal — allows CSF to drain from the lateral ventricle to the peritoneal cavity
- Ventriculoatrial — drains fluid from the lateral ventricle into the right atrium of the heart and ultimately directs fluid into the venous circulation

Caring for a shunt

- Have the child lay flat to avoid rapid decompression.
- Observe for shunt blockage and signs of increased ICP.
- Observe for signs of infection.
- If the shunt's caudal end is externalized, keep the CSF drainage bag at ear level to prevent ICP changes.

Types of blindness

- Legal blindness — optimal visual acuity of 20/200 or less in the better eye after correction or visual field of 20 degrees or less in the better eye
- Severe visual impairment — inability to read newsprint even with correction
- Visually impaired — difficulty reading newsprint with correction
- Low vision — impaired vision that isn't improved by conventional eyeglasses, contact lenses, medications, or surgery but in which some usable vision remains

- Skull X-rays show thinning of the skull with separation of the sutures and widening of fontanels

● **Medical management**
- Ventriculoperitoneal shunt insertion — allows CSF to drain from the lateral ventricle in the brain to the peritoneal cavity
- Ventriculoatrial shunt (less common) — drains fluid from the brain's lateral ventricle into the right atrium of the heart, where the fluid makes its way into the venous circulation
- Anticonvulsants for seizures — carbamazepine (Tegretol), phenobarbital (Luminal), diazepam (Valium), phenytoin (Dilantin)
- Removal of tumor, if present

● **Nursing interventions**
- Measure head circumference to aid in diagnosis of hydrocephalus
- Monitor vital signs and intake and output
- Assess neurologic status
- After the shunt is inserted:
  - To promote CSF drainage and prevent shunt occlusions, don't allow the child to lie on the same side of the body as the shunt
  - Instruct the child to lay flat to avoid rapid decompression
  - Observe for shunt blockage and signs of increased ICP (increased head circumference and full fontanel)
  - Observe for signs of infection
  - If the caudal end of the shunt must be externalized because of infection, keep the CFS drainage bag at ear level to prevent an increase or decrease in ICP
- Support the child's head when the child is upright
- Provide proper skin care to the head; turn it frequently
- Teach parents signs of increasing ICP

IMPAIRED VISION

● **Blindness**
- Definition
  - The absence of sight
  - It may describe a total loss of vision or a limitation in vision
    - Legal blindness — optimal visual acuity of 20/200 or less in the better eye after best correction, or a visual field of 20 degrees or less in the better eye
    - Severe visual impairment — describes visual impairment in someone who can't read ordinary newsprint even with correction
    - Visually impaired — impaired vision in someone who has difficulty reading ordinary newsprint even with correction

- Low vision — impaired vision that can't be improved by conventional eyeglasses, contact lenses, medications, or surgery but in which some usable vision remains
- Causes
  - Preventable
    - Trachoma — communicable bacterial eye infection characterized by chronic conjunctivitis
    - Onchocerciasis — microfilaria infection transmitted by a blackfly and other species of Simulium
    - Xerophthalmia — dryness of conjunctiva and cornea from vitamin A deficiency
  - Acquired
    - Glaucoma
      - A group of disorders characterized by high intraocular pressure and optic nerve damage
      - The incidence of blindness is decreasing owing to early detection and treatment
    - Cataracts due to inheritance, prenatal infection, anoxia, or maternal systemic disease
    - Diabetic retinopathy
    - Herpes simplex keratitis
    - Retinal detachment (such as in severe cases of retinopathy of prematurity)
    - Trauma
- Pathophysiology
  - The loss of vision relates directly to the cause
- Complications
  - Physical injury
  - Altered perception
- Assessment findings
  - Eyes may not be at the same level
  - The juncture of the pinna may not form a straight line from the lateral corner of the eye
  - Possible strabismus
  - Possible nystagmus
  - Delayed acquisition of behavior patterns
  - Delayed posture control and acquisition of developmental tasks
  - Disadvantaged in unfamiliar surroundings
  - More dependent than usual
  - Inhibited exploration because of frightening and intimidating experiences (such as the feeling of falling)
  - Self-stimulating behaviors, such as eye-rubbing or body-rocking
  - Inability to fixate on objects, follow a moving light, or reach out to objects

Preventable causes of blindness

- Trachoma
- Onchocerciasis
- Xerophthalmia

Acquired causes of blindness

- Glaucoma
- Cataracts
- Diabetic retinopathy
- Herpes simplex keratitis
- Retinal detachment
- Trauma

Complications of blindness

- Physical injury
- Altered perception

Diagnosing blindness

- Involves Snellen chart
- "Normal" vision is 20/20; ability to clearly read a 1" (2.5-cm) letter at a distance of 20′ (6 m)
- All measurements obtained from Snellen chart are compared to the standard normal vision of 20/20

Managing blindness

- Laser eye surgery
- Traditional surgery
- Medication
- Photodynamic therapy
- Corrective lenses

Key nursing interventions for blindness

- Assist the child in learning to understand the world through the other senses.
- Encourage the parents to treat the child normally and to stimulate the child's other senses with play and touch.
- Encourage exploration and independence; arrange furniture to promote mobility and safety.
- Act as the child's safety advocate.
- Announce yourself on entering the room, and explain intended actions before doing them.
- Explain strange sounds to the child.

- – Lack of initiation of eye contact with the parents
- – Head tilting or frequent blinking or squinting
- – Holding the head very close to books or work
- – Walking or crawling into furniture or people
- Diagnostic test findings
  - – Abnormal Snellen chart and test results
    - · Made up of a series of letters and numbers (for ages 6 and older) or symbols (for ages 3 to 6) of progressively smaller size, the largest at the top
    - · "Normal" vision is 20/20
    - · A person who can clearly read a 1" (2.5-cm) letter at a distance of 20′ (6 m) is considered to have normal vision
    - · All measurements obtained from using the Snellen chart are a comparison to the standard normal vision of 20/20
- Medical management
  - – Dependent on specific cause
  - – Laser eye surgery
  - – Traditional surgery
  - – Medication
  - – Corrective lenses
- Nursing interventions
  - – Assist the child in learning to understand the world through the other senses
  - – Encourage the parents to treat the child normally and to stimulate the child's other senses with play and touch
  - – Encourage exploration and independence; arrange furniture to promote mobility and safety
  - – Act as the child's safety advocate
  - – Announce yourself on entering the room, and explain intended actions before doing them
  - – Explain strange sounds to the child
  - – Teach the parents tips for the child with partial sight
    - · Seat the child at the front of the classroom
    - · Use large-print materials
    - · Use contrasting wall colors

● **Amblyopia (lazy eye)**
- Definition
  - – Reduced unilateral visual acuity despite optical correction in an eye without pathologic defect
  - – It can cause vision loss through disuse
  - – Vision loss doesn't usually occur until age 9 when the retinal system has reached maturity
- Causes
  - – Strabismus, especially if untreated

– Unequal refractive errors
– Cataracts
– Corneal opacities
– Prolonged occlusion of one or both eyes, which is usually the result of patching to treat strabismus
• Pathophysiology
– One eye doesn't receive sufficient stimulation
– Diplopia (double vision) occurs because each retina receives different images
– The brain accommodates by suppressing the less intense image
– Eventually there's a loss of vision because the visual cortex doesn't respond to visual stimulation of that eye
• Complications
– Physical injury
– Altered perception
• Assessment findings
– Decreased visual acuity in the affected eye despite optical correction
– Possible central vision loss in the suppressed eye
• Diagnostic test findings
– Usually easily diagnosed with a complete examination of the eyes
– Special tests aren't usually required
• Medical management
– Treatment of the primary visual defect before age 6
– Patch over the healthy eye or administration of atropine eye drops to the healthy eye
• Nursing interventions
– Provide the child with a safe environment
– Review the components of a safe environment with the child and his family
– Place important objects on the side where the child has better vision
– Promote independence in activities of daily living (ADLs) and self-care
– Teach the patient to utilize assistive devices, as necessary

● **Conjunctivitis (pink eye)**
• Definition
– Inflammation of the conjunctiva
– Usually benign and self-limiting
• Causes
– Neonates
• Infection during birth from *Chlamydia trachomatis*
• If recurrent, it may be because of nasolacrimal duct obstruction
– Children
• Infectious — viral and bacterial (highly contagious)
• Allergic reaction

Key facts about amblyopia

• Also called *lazy eye*
• Can lead to diplopia and vision loss
• Caused by strabismus, unequal refractive errors, cataracts, and corneal opacities

Assessment findings in amblyopia

• Decreased visual acuity in the affected eye despite optical correction
• Possible central vision loss in suppressed eye

Key nursing interventions for amblyopia

• Provide the child with a safe environment.
• Review the components of a safe environment with the child and his family.
• Place important objects on the side where the child has the better vision.
• Promote independence in ADLs and self-care.
• Teach the child to utilize assistive devices, as necessary.

Types of conjunctivitis

- Infectious (bacterial or viral)
- Allergic
- Irritant
- Chemical

Signs of conjunctivitis

Bacterial
- Purulent drainage
- Crusted drainage over eyelid
- Inflamed conjunctiva
- Edematous eyelid
- Generally a bilateral infection

Viral
- Occurrence with upper respiratory infection
- Watery or serous drainage
- Inflamed conjunctiva
- Edematous eyelid

Allergic
- Itching
- Watery or thick discharge
- Inflamed conjunctiva
- Edematous eyelid

Irritant
- Tearing
- Pain
- Inflamed conjunctiva
- Generally a unilateral reaction

Chemical
- Tearing
- Possibly severe eye irritation and pain
- Redness and swelling

- Reaction to a foreign body
- Pathophysiology
  - Infectious — caused by bacteria or viruses
  - Allergic — caused by an allergic reaction
  - Irritant — caused by foreign material in the eye
  - Chemical — caused by a chemical substance
- Complications — injury to eyes from rubbing or itching
- Assessment findings
  - Bacterial
    - Purulent drainage
    - Crusted drainage over the eyelid, especially on awakening
    - Inflamed conjunctiva
    - Edematous eyelid
    - Generally a bilateral infection
  - Viral
    - Generally occurs with an upper respiratory infection
    - Watery or serous drainage
    - Inflamed conjunctiva
    - Edematous eyelid
  - Allergic
    - Itching
    - Watery or thick discharge
    - Inflamed conjunctiva
    - Edematous eyelid
  - Irritant
    - Tearing
    - Pain
    - Inflamed conjunctiva
    - Generally a unilateral reaction
  - Chemical
    - Dependent on chemical irritant
    - Tearing
    - Possibly severe eye irritation and pain
    - Redness and swelling
- Diagnostic test findings
  - Diagnosis is primarily determined by the patient's history and assessment findings
  - Cultures from eye drainage are positive for bacterial strains (in bacterial conjunctivitis)
- Medical management
  - Bacterial conjunctivitis (highly contagious)
    - Topical antibacterial agents shorten the length of the infection and destroy the infectious organism
    - Drops are used during the day

- Ointment, which remains in the eye for a longer period and may blur vision during the day, is used at night
  - Viral conjunctivitis is self-limiting
  - Antihistamines are used to treat symptoms of allergic conjunctivitis
  - The foreign body causing the conjunctivitis is removed
  - For chemical conjunctivitis, the eye is irrigated with copious amounts of tap water for 15 to 20 minutes
- Nursing interventions
  - Follow infection control measures carefully
    - Wash hands thoroughly
    - Use aseptic technique when handling eye secretions because of the high risk of possible infection transmission
  - Don't let the child share pillows, towels, or bed linens with others
  - Administer ophthalmic antibiotics; apply ointment from the inner canthus to the outer canthus
  - Teach parents how to administer ophthalmic medications

INCREASED INTRACRANIAL PRESSURE

- **Definition**
  - Higher than normal pressure within the cranium
  - A persistent increase destroys healthy brain tissue and alters mental function
- **Causes**
  - Tumors or space-occupying lesions
  - Accumulation of fluid within the ventricular system
  - Bleeding or hemorrhage
  - Edematous brain tissue
  - Trauma
- **Pathophysiology**
  - ICP is the pressure exerted within the intact skull by the intracranial volume
    - Brain tissue in water—80%
    - CSF—10%
    - Blood—10%
  - The rigid skull allows very little space for expansion of these substances; when ICP increases to pathologic levels, brain damage can result
  - The brain compensates for increases in ICP by regulating the volumes of the three substances in three ways:
    - Limiting blood flow to the head
    - Displacing CSF into the spinal canal
    - Increasing absorption or decreasing production of CSF by withdrawing water from brain tissue into the blood and excreting it through the kidneys

---

Managing conjunctivitis

- Topical antibacterials (bacterial and viral conjunctivitis)
- Antihistamines (allergic conjunctivitis)
- Removal of foreign body

Causes of increased ICP

- Tumors or space-occupying lesions
- Accumulation of fluid within the ventricular system
- Bleeding or hemorrhage
- Edematous brain tissue
- Trauma

How the brain compensates for increased ICP

- Limits blood flow to the head
- Displaces CSF into the spinal cord
- Increases CSF absorption or decreases CSF production

Complications of increased ICP

- Brain death
- Cardiac arrest
- Respiratory insufficiency or arrest

TOP 3

Signs of increased ICP in infants

1. Bulging fontanels without normal pulsations
2. Shrieking, high-pitched cry
3. Increased head circumference

TOP 3

Signs of increased ICP in children

1. Vomiting
2. Headache
3. Seizures

● **Complications**
- Brain death
- Cardiac arrest
- Respiratory insufficiency or arrest

● **Assessment findings**
- Infants
  - Bulging fontanels without normal pulsations
  - Irritability
  - Shrieking, high-pitched cry
  - Increased head circumference
  - Decreased LOC
  - Altered feeding patterns
  - Distended veins in the scalp
- Children
  - Vomiting with and without nausea
  - Headache
  - Diplopia
  - Seizures
- General
  - Lack of interest
  - Decreased motor activity
  - Increased sleep
  - Weight loss
  - Lethargy that progresses to drowsiness
  - Increased blood pressure, decreased heart rate, and decreased respirations
- Late signs
  - Diminished response to noxious stimuli
  - Altered pupil size and reactivity — sudden and fixed dilated pupils, unilaterally or bilaterally — is a neurosurgical emergency
  - Posturing — decerebrate or decorticate
  - Cheyne-Stokes respirations
  - Papilledema

● **Diagnostic test findings**
- ICP monitoring, a direct, invasive method of identifying trends in ICP, reveals increased ICP
- Nuclear brain scan may show test material accumulation in areas where there are brain lesions
- CT and MRI scanning reveals hemorrhage, tumors, inflammation, or congenital abnormalities

● **Medical management**
- Subdural tap — a needle inserted into the anterior fontanel helps relieve ICP

- Ventricular tap—a needle inserted into lateral ventricle removes CSF and relieves ICP
- Hyperventilation via mechanical ventilation, if possible, to decrease carbon dioxide levels in the blood
- Medications
  - Infectious processes are treated with antibiotics
  - Corticosteroids are used to treat inflammatory conditions and edema
  - Osmotic diuretics such as mannitol (Osmitrol) and diuretics such as furosemide (Lasix) are used to treat cerebral edema
  - Barbiturates or paralyzing agents, such as pancuronium (Pavulon), may be used to help decrease ICP
  - Anticonvulsants are administered to control seizure activity

● **Nursing interventions**
- Monitor neurologic status frequently, including LOC and pupil size and reactivity
- Monitor ICP, report deviations, and maintain patency and calibration of ICP monitor
- Ensure patent airway
  - Clear accumulated secretions, noting that suctioning may elevate ICP
  - Monitor mechanical ventilation
- Minimize ICP
  - Maintain the head of the bed at 15 to 30 degrees
  - Position the child with his head midline to promote drainage of the venous system and avoid pressure on the jugular veins
  - Avoid performing Valsalva's maneuver and prevent painful stimuli
  - Provide a quiet environment
  - Provide pain management
- Monitor fluid and electrolytes
- Provide a safe physical environment and observe seizure precautions
- Provide emotional support to the child and his family and explain all procedures and treatments

INTRAVENTRICULAR HEMORRHAGE

● **Definition**
- Intraventricular hemorrhage (IVH) is the rupture of a part of the vascular network of the germinal matrix, resulting in bleeding in the brain
- IVH is most commonly found in preterm neonates, especially in neonates weighing less than 1,500 g and neonates of less than 32 weeks' gestation

● **Causes**
- Vascular malformation

Managing increased ICP
- Subdural tap
- Ventricular tap
- Hyperventilation via mechanical ventilation
- Medications, including antibiotics, corticosteroids, osmotic diuretics, barbiturates, and anticonvulsants

How to minimize ICP
- Maintain the head of the bed at 15 to 30 degrees.
- Position the child with his head midline to promote drainage of the venous system and to avoid pressure on the jugular veins.
- Avoid performing Valsalva's maneuver and prevent painful stimuli.
- Provide a quiet environment.
- Manage pain.

Key facts about IVH
- Involves the rupture of a part of the vascular network of the germinal matrix
- Results in bleeding in the brain
- Most commonly found in preterm neonates

Causes of IVH

- Vascular malformation
- Tumor
- Trauma
- Birth asphyxia, early gestational age, or low birth weight
- Respiratory distress, metabolic instabilities, or hypertension
- Drug use

Complications of IVH

- Hydrocephalus
- Obliterative arachnoiditis
- Cerebral hemorrhage
- Brain death
- Motor deficits
- Mental retardation

Key signs of IVH

- Increased ICP
- Apnea
- Bradycardia
- Bulging anterior fontanel
- Increased head circumference
- Separated sutures
- Seizures

Diagnostic test findings in IVH

- Ultrasonography, CT scan, and MRI show blood collection in the ventricular system.
- ICP monitoring reveals increased ICP.

- Tumor
- Trauma (may occur before, during, or after birth)
- Birth asphyxia, early gestational age, or low birth weight
- Respiratory distress, metabolic instabilities, or hypertension
- Use of drugs (such as surfactant therapy)

● **Pathophysiology**
- Early in prenatal development, there's a delicate but extensive network of vasculature that develops in the area of the ventricles that receives a disproportionately large quantity of cerebral blood flow
- As term approaches, more blood flows to the periventricular region's germinal matrix
- Events that cause increased cerebral blood flow (hypoxic episodes) cause the vascularized region to rupture

● **Complications**
- Hydrocephalus
- Obliterative arachnoiditis
- Cerebral hemorrhage
- Brain death
- Motor deficits
- Mental retardation

● **Assessment findings**
- Increased ICP
- Sudden deterioration in condition
- Apnea
- Bradycardia
- Cyanosis
- Hypotonia
- Decreased hematocrit
- Bulging anterior fontanel
- Increased head circumference
- Separated sutures
- Twitching
- Stupor
- Seizures

● **Diagnostic test findings**
- Ultrasonography, CT scan, and MRI show blood collection in the ventricular system
- ICP monitoring reveals increased ICP

● **Medical management**
- Ventilatory support as indicated
- Spinal and ventricular taps
- Diuretics
- Seizure suppression

Nursing interventions

- Measure head circumference daily; note increases of 0.5 cm or greater
- Assess fontanels every 8 hours for fullness or bulging; check for widening of suture lines
- Assess for increased incidence of apnea, bradycardia, changes in muscle tone or activity, and unexplained drops in hemoglobin and hematocrit
- Anticipate CT or MRI scans to confirm extent of hemorrhage
- Prevent fluctuations in cerebral blood pressure
- Decrease noxious environmental stimuli; decrease noise, lights, and handling
- Maintain head in midline position to prevent venous congestion that results in hydrostatic pressure changes and increases ICP
- Monitor and treat pain (pain can impede venous return and increase ICP)
- Support the family by teaching developmentally supportive interventions that prevent IVH or prevent it from worsening

MENINGITIS

Definition

- An inflammation of the meninges of the brain and spinal cord
- Characterized by sudden onset
- Causes serious illness within 24 hours

Cause

- Vascular dissemination from focus of infection elsewhere in the body; infections may include or result from:
  - Bacteremia
    - Pneumonia
    - Empyema
    - Osteomyelitis
    - Endocarditis
    - *Borreliosis burgdorferi* (Lyme disease)
  - Sinusitis
  - Otitis media
  - Encephalitis
  - Myelitis
  - Brain abscesses
    - *Neisseria meningitides*
    - *Haemophilus influenzae* (in children and young adults)
    - *Streptococcus pneumoniae*
  - Skull fracture
  - Penetrating head wound
  - Lumbar puncture

Aseptic meningitis

Aseptic meningitis is a benign syndrome characterized by headache, fever, vomiting, and meningeal symptoms. It results from some form of viral infection, including enteroviruses (most common), arboviruses, herpes simplex virus, mumps virus, or lymphocytic choriomeningitis virus.

SIGNS AND SYMPTOMS
Aseptic meningitis begins suddenly with a fever up to 104° F (40° C), alterations in consciousness (drowsiness, confusion, stupor), and neck or spine stiffness, which is slight at first. (The patient experiences such stiffness when bending forward.) Other signs and symptoms include headaches, nausea, vomiting, abdominal pain, poorly defined chest pain, and sore throat.

DIAGNOSTIC TESTS
Patient history of recent illness and knowledge of seasonal epidemics are essential in differentiating among the many forms of aseptic meningitis. Negative bacteriologic cultures and cerebrospinal (CSF) analysis showing pleocytosis and increased protein levels suggest the diagnosis. Isolation of the virus from CSF confirms it.

TREATMENT
Treatment is supportive, including bed rest, maintenance of fluid and electrolyte balance, analgesics for pain, and exercises to combat residual weakness. Isolation isn't necessary once bacterial meningitis is ruled out. Careful handling of excretions and good hand-washing technique prevent spreading the disease.

  – Ventricular shunting procedures
- Aseptic meningitis — viral (see *Aseptic meningitis*)

● **Pathophysiology**
- Inflammation may involve all three meningeal membranes — the dura mater, the arachnoid, and the pia mater
- Viral or bacterial agents are transmitted by the spread of droplets; organisms enter the blood from the nasopharynx or middle ear
- Prognosis is good and complications are rare if the disease is recognized early and the infecting organism responds to antibiotic therapy
- 10% to 15% of bacterial meningitis cases are fatal; sequelae are common when it occurs in the first 2 months of life
- The condition is common in infants and toddlers; its incidence is now greatly decreased with the administration of routine *H. influenzae* type B vaccine

● **Complications**
- Respiratory compromise or respiratory arrest
- Physical injury
- Death

● **Assessment findings**
- Coma
- Delirium

- Fever
- Headache
- High-pitched cry
- Irritability
- Nuchal rigidity that may progress to opisthotonos (arching of the back)
- Gradual or abrupt onset following an upper respiratory infection
- Petechial or purpuric lesions possibly present in bacterial meningitis
- Positive Brudzinski's sign (the child flexes the knees and hips in response to passive neck flexion)
- Positive Kernig's sign (the child is unable to extend the leg when the hip and knee are flexed)
- Projectile vomiting causing dehydration; dehydration may prevent a bulging fontanel and thus mask an important sign of increased ICP
- Seizures
- Bulging fontanels, separated sutures
- Chills
- Malaise
- Sinus arrhythmias
- Diplopia

● **Diagnostic test findings**
- Lumbar puncture shows increased CSF pressure, cloudy color, increased white blood cell (WBC) count and protein level, and decreased glucose level if meningitis is caused by bacteria
- Xpert EV test can quickly detect viral meningitis and distinguish it from bacterial meningitis (in 2½ hours)

● **Medical management**
- Analgesics to treat pain of meningeal irritation
- Corticosteroids — dexamethasone (Decadron)
- Parenteral antibiotics — ceftazidime (Fortaz), ceftriaxone (Rocephin); possibly intraventricular administration of antibiotics
- Burr holes to evacuate subdural effusion, if present
- Oxygen therapy (possible intubation and mechanical ventilation to induce hyperventilation to decrease ICP)

● **Nursing interventions**
- Maintain droplet precautions until at least 24 hours of effective antibiotic therapy have elapsed; continued precautions are recommended for meningitis caused by *H. influenzae* or *N. meningitides*
- Provide a hypothermia blanket, as indicated
- Maintain seizure precautions
- Monitor vital signs and intake and output to assess for excess fluid volume

TOP 3

Signs of meningitis

1. Nuchal rigidity
2. Positive Brudzinski's sign
3. Positive Kernig's sign

Diagnostic findings in bacterial meningitis

- Increased CSF pressure
- Cloudy CSF
- Increased WBC count and protein level
- Decreased glucose level

Managing meningitis

- Analgesics
- Corticosteroids
- Parenteral antibiotics

- Assess the child's neurologic status frequently to monitor for increased ICP
- Provide a dark and quiet environment
- Keep the child flat in bed
- Move the child gently
- Administer parenteral antibiotics

NEURAL TUBE DEFECTS

Definition
- Congenital malformations that produce skull and spinal column defects
- Neural tube defects (NTDs) result from the failure of the neural tube to close during embryonic development at approximately 28 days after conception

Causes
- Exposure to a teratogen
- Isolated birth defects
- Multiple malformation syndrome—chromosomal abnormalities such as trisomy 18 or 13 syndrome
- Lack of folic acid in the maternal diet around the time of conception

Pathophysiology
- Spina bifida occulta
  - Incomplete closure of one or more vertebrae without protrusion of the spinal cord or meninges
  - In severe forms, a protrusion of the spinal contents in an external sac or cystic lesion occurs because of the incomplete closure
- Spina bifida cystica
  - Myelomeningocele
    - External sac contains meninges, CSF, and a portion of the spinal cord or nerve roots distal to the conus medullaries
    - When the spinal nerve roots end at the sac, motor and sensory functions below the sac are terminated
  - Meningocele—external sac contains meninges and CSF
- Encephalocele
  - Saclike portion of the meninges and brain protrudes through a defective opening in the skull
  - Usually in the occipital area but may occur in the parietal, nasopharyngeal, or frontal area
- Anencephaly
  - The closure defect occurs at the cranial end of the neuroaxis and, as a result, part of or the entire top of the skull is missing, severely damaging the brain
  - Portions of the brain stem and spinal cord may also be missing
  - Invariably fatal

Causes of NTDs

- Exposure to teratogens
- Isolated birth defects
- Multiple malformation syndrome
- Lack of folic acid in the maternal diet at the time of conception

Types of NTDs

- Spina bifida occulta – Incomplete closure of one or more vertebrae without protrusion of spinal cord or meninges
- Spina bifida cystica – External sac can contain meninges, CSF and, possibly, a portion of the spinal cord or nerve roots
- Encephalocele – Saclike portion of meninges and brain protrudes through a defective opening in the skull
- Anencephaly – Closure defect at the cranial end of the neuroaxis; part of or the entire top of the skull is missing; fatal

Complications
- Death
- Multiple handicaps
- Decreased motor activity below the sac or paralysis
- Neurogenic bladder and bowel
- CNS infection
- Hydrocephalus

Assessment findings
- Spina bifida occulta
  - Skin abnormalities over the spinal defect; may appear alone or in combination with each other
    - Depression or dimple
    - Tuft of hair
    - Soft fatty deposits
    - Port wine nevi
  - Occasionally, foot weakness
  - Occasionally, bowel and bladder disturbances
- Spina bifida cystica
  - A saclike structure protruding over the spine
  - Trophic skin disturbances
    - Ulcerations
    - Cyanosis
  - Clubfoot
  - Knee contractures
  - Hydrocephalus
  - Possible mental retardation
  - Possible Arnold-Chiari formation
  - Curvature of the spine
  - Permanent neurologic dysfunction (myelomeningocele)
    - Flaccid or spastic paralysis
    - Bowel or bladder incontinence
- Encephalocele
  - Vary with the degree of tissue involvement and location of the defect
  - Paralysis
  - Hydrocephalus
  - Mental retardation
- Anencephaly
  - Exposed neural tissue
  - Skull has a froglike appearance when viewed from the front

Diagnostic test findings
- Amniocentesis can detect elevated alpha-fetoprotein (AFP) levels in amniotic fluid, which may indicate the presence of an open NTD

Complications of NTDs
- Death
- Multiple handicaps
- Decreased motor activity below the sac or paralysis
- Neurogenic bladder and bowel
- CNS infection
- Hydrocephalus

Assessment findings in spina bifida occulta
- Skin abnormalities over the spinal defect
- Foot weakness (occasionally)
- Bowel and bladder disturbances (occasionally)

Assessment findings in spina bifida cystica
- Trophic skin disturbances
- Clubfoot
- Knee contractures
- Hydrocephalus
- Possible mental retardation
- Possible Arnold-Chiari formation
- Permanent neurologic dysfunction

Assessment findings in encephalocele
- Paralysis
- Hydrocephalus
- Mental retardation

Assessment findings in anencephaly
- Exposed neural tissue
- Froglike skull

- Elevated acetylcholinesterase levels can confirm the diagnosis
- Increased maternal serum AFP and serum markers, such as human chorionic gonadotropin or unconjugated estriol
  - Offered to women who aren't scheduled for amniocentesis, such as those with a lower risk of NTDs and those who will be younger than age 34½ at the time of delivery
  - Doesn't diagnose an open NTD or a chromosomal abnormality; only estimates the fetus's risk of such a defect
- Ultrasound may be used to detect open NTDs or ventral wall defects
- In spina bifida occulta, spinal X-ray may show the bone defect
- Myelography can differentiate NTDs from other spinal abnormalities such as spinal cord tumors
- Transillumination of a protruding spinal sac can sometimes distinguish between myelomeningocele and meningocele
  - Meningocele — the sac transluminates
  - Myelomeningocele — the sac doesn't transluminate
- A pinprick examination of the legs and trunk in myelomeningocele shows the level of sensory and motor involvement
- Skull X-rays, cephalic measurements, and CT scan demonstrate associated hydrocephalus
- X-rays in encephalocele show a basilar bony skull defect; CT scan and ultrasonography further define the defect

Medical management

- Surgical correction and closure of a protruding sac usually occurs within 48 hours of birth; surgery doesn't reverse neurologic deficits
- A shunt may be needed to relieve related hydrocephalus
- Surgery to correct associated craniofacial abnormalities in encephalocele

Nursing interventions

- Prenatal
  - Refer the prospective parents to a genetic counselor, who can provide information and support the couple's decision on how to manage the pregnancy
  - Urge all women of childbearing age to take a folic acid supplement until menopause or the end of childbearing potential (see *Folic acid supplement recommendations*)
  - Provide psychological support to the parents to help them accept the diagnosis and preoperative and postoperative care
- Preoperative
  - Check for leakage from the sac
  - Check for infection around the sac
  - Assess for signs and symptoms of CNS infection
  - Assess for motor activity below the sac
  - Measure the head circumference to establish baseline data

Folic acid supplement recommendations

These recommendations for folic acid supplement dosages have been endorsed by the Centers for Disease Control and Prevention, the U.S. Public Health Service, the March of Dimes Birth Defects Foundation, and the Spina Bifida Association of America, among other groups.

ALL WOMEN OF CHILDBEARING AGE

All women who are capable of becoming pregnant should:
- consume 0.4 mg of folic acid daily to reduce the risk of having a child with spina bifida or another neural tube defect (NTD)
- continue to consume 0.4 mg of folic acid daily when pregnant until their health care provider prescribes other prenatal vitamins.

WOMEN AT HIGH RISK

Women with a previous pregnancy affected by an NTD should:
- receive genetic counseling before their next pregnancy
- consume 0.4 mg of folic acid daily
- when actively trying to become pregnant (at least 1 month before conception), increase their dosage of folic acid to 4 mg daily (by taking a separate folic acid supplement, not by increasing their intake of multivitamins)
- continue to take 4 mg of folic acid daily through the first 3 months of pregnancy.

- Assess bowel and bladder function and patterns and monitor intake and output
- Provide emotional support to the parents; be aware that surgery usually occurs 24 to 48 hours after birth
- Teach parents and family measures to prevent contractures, pressure ulcers, urinary tract infections, and other complications
- Prevent trauma by keeping pressure off the sac; keep the child on one side with the knees flexed, or on the abdomen
- Institute measures to keep the sac free from infection; avoid contamination from urine and stool
- Prevent the sac from drying; cover it with saline-soaked sterile dressings
- Institute latex precautions (there's an increased incidence of latex allergies in this population)
- Postoperative
  - Provide routine postoperative care
  - Provide thorough skin care if paralysis occurs; place the child on sheepskin
  - Provide orthopedic appliances, if necessary
  - Prevent constipation
  - Promote ROM
  - Teach clean intermittent catheterization

– Assess motor ability and sensation below the level of the lesion; paralysis is possible

Types of otitis media

- Suppurative otitis media — caused by nasopharyngeal flora that reflux through the eustachian tube and colonize the middle ear (can be acute or chronic)
- Secretory otitis media — caused by obstruction of the eustachian tube (can be acute or chronic)

Predisposing factors for suppurative otitis media in children

- Wider, shorter, more horizontal eustachian tubes
- Increased lymphoid tissue
- Anatomic anomalies

OTITIS MEDIA (MIDDLE EAR INFECTION)

Definition
- Inflammation of the middle ear
- Can be suppurative or secretory (acute or chronic)

Causes
- Disruption of eustachian tube patency
- Bacteria
  – *S. pneumoniae*
  – *H. influenzae*
  – *Moraxella catarrhalis*
  – Staphylococci
  – Gram-negative bacteria

Pathophysiology
- Suppurative otitis media occurs when nasopharyngeal flora reflux through the eustachian tube and colonize the middle ear
  – Risk factors
    · Respiratory tract infection
    · Allergic reaction
    · Nasotracheal intubation
  – Predisposing factors
    · Wider, shorter, more horizontal eustachian tubes and increased lymphoid tissue in children
    · Anatomic anomalies
- Chronic suppurative otitis media
  – Inadequate treatment of acute otitis episodes
  – Infections by resistant strains of bacteria
  – Rarely, tuberculosis
- Secretory otitis media results from obstruction of the eustachian tube
  – A buildup of negative pressure in the middle ear promotes sterile serous fluid from blood vessels to pass through the membrane of the middle ear
  – Effusion may be secondary to eustachian tube dysfunction from viral infection or allergy
  – Effusion may follow barotraumas (pressure injury caused by inability to equalize pressures between the environment and the middle ear)
    · Occurs during rapid aircraft descent in a person with an upper respiratory tract infection
    · Occurs during rapid underwater ascent in scuba diving (barotitis media)

- Chronic secretory otitis media follows persistent eustachian tube dysfunction
    - Mechanical obstruction (adenoidal tissue overgrowth, tumors)
    - Edema (allergic rhinitis, chronic sinus infection)
    - Inadequate treatment of acute suppurative otitis media

● Complications

- Tympanic membrane retraction (the tympanic membrane is drawn inward and retraction pockets develop)
- Tympanosclerosis (eardrum scarring)
- Ruptured tympanic membrane (perforated eardrum)—when it occurs in a child, there's generally an immediate relief or cessation of pain, a decrease in temperature, and visible purulent drainage in the external auditory canal
- Abscesses (brain, subperiosteal, and epidural)
- Septicemia
- Meningitis
- Suppurative labyrinthitis
- Facial paralysis
- Otitis externa
- Mastoiditis

● Assessment findings

- Suppurative otitis media
    - Severe, deep, throbbing pain (from pressure behind the tympanic membrane)
    - Signs of upper respiratory tract infection (sneezing and coughing)
    - Mild to very high fever
    - Hearing loss (usually mild and conductive)
    - Tinnitus
    - Dizziness
    - Nausea
    - Vomiting
    - Bulging of the tympanic membrane with erythema
    - Purulent drainage in the ear canal if tympanic membrane ruptures
    - Some patients are asymptomatic
    - Ruptured tympanic membrane accompanied with sudden stopping of pain
- Acute secretory otitis media
    - Acute secretory otitis media may not cause any symptoms in the first few months of life; irritability may be the only indication of earache
    - Severe conductive hearing loss; varies from 15 to 35 dB, depending on the thickness and amount of fluid in the middle ear cavity

Key signs and symptoms of chronic otitis media

- Thickening and scarring of the tympanic membrane
- Decreased or absent tympanic membrane mobility
- Cholesteatoma
- Painless purulent discharge
- Hearing loss

Common diagnostic tests for otitis media

- Otoscopy
- Pneumatoscopy
- Culture of ear drainage

Managing acute suppurative otitis media

- Antibiotics
- Myringotomy
- Single dose of ceftriaxone (for very sick infants)

Managing acute secretory otitis media

- Valsalva's maneuver to inflate eustachian tube
- Nasopharyngeal decongestant therapy
- Possible myringotomy and aspiration of middle ear fluid

– A sensation of fullness in the ear and popping, crackling, or clicking sounds on swallowing or with jaw movement
– Echo when speaking and vague feeling of top-heaviness due to the accumulation of fluid
– Ruptured tympanic membrane accompanied with sudden stopping of pain

- Chronic otitis media
  – Thickening and scarring of the tympanic membrane
  – Decreased or absent tympanic membrane mobility
  – Cholesteatoma (a cystlike mass in the middle ear)
  – Painless purulent discharge
  – Hearing loss
  – Ruptured tympanic membrane accompanied with sudden stopping of pain

● Diagnostic test findings

- Acute suppurative otitis media
  – Otoscopy—obscured or distorted bony landmarks of the tympanic membrane
  – Pneumatoscopy—decreased tympanic membrane mobility
  – Culture of ear drainage—identifies the causative organism
- Acute secretory otitis media
  – Using otoscopy, bony landmarks appear more prominent because of tympanic membrane retraction
  – Clear or amber fluid appears behind the tympanic membrane
  – Membrane is blue-black if there was a hemorrhage
- Chronic otitis media
  – Otoscopy—thickening, sometimes scarring, and decreased mobility of the tympanic membrane
  – Pneumatoscopy—decreased or absent tympanic membrane movement

● Medical management

- Acute suppurative otitis media
  – Antibiotic therapy—ampicillin (Omnipen) or amoxicillin (Amoxil)
  – Myringotomy to treat severe, painful bulging of the tympanic membrane
  – A single dose of ceftriaxone (Rocephin) is effective against major pathogens, but it's expensive and is reserved for very sick infants
  – In recurring infection, antibiotics must be used with discretion to prevent the development of resistant strains of bacteria
- Acute secretory otitis media
  – Inflation of the eustachian tube using Valsalva's maneuver several times a day
  – Nasopharyngeal decongestant therapy

– Possible myringotomy and aspiration of middle ear fluid followed by insertion of a polyethylene tube into the tympanic membrane for immediate and prolonged equalization of pressure

• Chronic otitis media

– Broad-spectrum antibiotics, such as amoxicillin/clavulanate potassium (Augmentin) or cefuroxime (Ceftin)
– Elimination of eustachian tube obstruction
– Treatment of otitis externa
– Myringoplasty and tympanoplasty to reconstruct middle ear structures when thickening and scarring are present
– Possibly, mastoidectomy
– Excision of cholesteatoma

● **Nursing interventions**

• Explain all diagnostic tests and procedures to the child and his parents
• After myringotomy
  – Maintain drainage flow
    · Don't place cotton or plugs deeply into the ear canal
    · Place sterile cotton loosely in the external ear to absorb drainage
  – Prevent infection
    · Change the cotton whenever it becomes damp
    · Wash hands before and after giving ear care
  – Watch for and report headache, fever, severe pain, or disorientation
• After tympanoplasty
  – Reinforce dressings
  – Observe for excessive bleeding from the ear canal
  – Administer analgesics as needed
  – Warn the child against blowing his nose or getting the ear wet when bathing
• Encourage the child and parents to complete the prescribed course of antibiotic treatment; if nasopharyngeal decongestants are ordered, teach correct instillation
• Suggest applying heat to the ear to relieve pain
• Advise the child and parents to watch for and immediately report pain and fever (signs of secondary infection) in children with acute secretory otitis media
• To prevent otitis media
  – Teach the child and parents how to recognize upper respiratory tract infections, and encourage early treatment
  – To prevent nasopharyngeal flora reflux, instruct parents not to feed their infant in a supine position or put him to bed with a bottle
  – To promote eustachian tube patency, instruct the child to perform Valsalva's maneuver several times daily
  – Identify and treat allergies
  – Avoid secondhand smoke exposure

Managing chronic otitis media

● Broad-spectrum antibiotics
● Elimination of eustachian tube obstruction
● Treatment of otitis externa
● Myringoplasty and tympanoplasty (when thickening and scarring are present)
● Mastoidectomy
● Excision of cholesteatoma

Ways to prevent otitis media

● Teach the child and parents how to recognize upper respiratory tract infections, and encourage early treatment.
● To prevent nasopharyngeal flora reflux, instruct parents not to feed their infant in a supine position or put him to bed with a bottle.
● To promote eustachian tube patency, instruct the child to perform Valsalva's maneuver several times daily.
● Identify and treat allergies.
● Avoid secondhand smoke exposure.

Definitions related to seizure disorders

- **Seizure** – sudden, episodic, involuntary alteration in consciousness, motor activity, behavior, sensation, or autonomic function
- **Epilepsy** – common, intermittent CNS disorder resulting in many types of recurrent seizures

Causes of epilepsy

- Excessive neuronal discharges
- Birth trauma
- Perinatal infection
- Anoxia
- Infectious diseases (meningitis, encephalopathy, or brain abscess)
- Ingestion of toxins (mercury, lead, or carbon monoxide)
- Brain tumors
- Inherited disorders or degenerative disease, such as phenylketonuria or tuberous sclerosis
- Head injury or trauma
- Metabolic disorders, such as hypoglycemia or hypoparathyroidism
- Idiopathic causes

Complications of seizure disorders

- Respiratory insufficiency or arrest
- Physical injury

SEIZURE DISORDERS

Definitions
- Seizure—a sudden, episodic, involuntary alteration in consciousness, motor activity, behavior, sensation, or autonomic function (see *Classifying seizures*)
- Epilepsy—a common, intermittent CNS disorder resulting in many types of recurrent seizures

Causes
- Half of all seizure disorder cases are idiopathic
- Hyperexcitable nerve cells that surpass the seizure threshold
- Neurons overfiring without regard to stimuli or need
- Alcohol withdrawal
- Causes specific to epilepsy
  - Excessive neuronal discharges
  - Birth trauma—inadequate oxygen supply to the brain, blood incompatibility, hemorrhage
  - Perinatal infection
  - Anoxia
  - Infectious diseases—meningitis, encephalopathy, or brain abscess
  - Ingestion of toxins—mercury, lead, or carbon monoxide
  - Brain tumors
  - Inherited disorders or degenerative disease, such as phenylketonuria or tuberous sclerosis
  - Head injury or trauma
  - Metabolic disorders, such as hypoglycemia or hypoparathyroidism
  - Idiopathic causes

Pathophysiology
- Electric discharges
  - Come from central areas in the brain that immediately affect consciousness
  - May be localized in one area of the brain and cause responses specific to the anatomic focus controlled by that area
  - May be initiated in a localized area of the brain and spread to other areas, resulting in a generalized response
  - Are spontaneously released by hyperexcitable cells termed the epileptogenic focus
    - In response to physiologic stimuli (dehydration, increased or decreased blood glucose, altered electrolyte levels, stress), the focus activates normal cells in the surrounding area

Complications
- Respiratory insufficiency or arrest
- Physical injury

Classifying seizures

Seizures can take various forms, depending on their origin and whether they're localized to one area of the brain, as occurs in partial seizures, or occur in both hemispheres, as happens in generalized seizures. This chart describes each type of seizure and lists common signs and symptoms.

TYPE	DESCRIPTION	SIGNS AND SYMPTOMS
Partial		
Simple partial	Symptoms confined to one hemisphere	May have motor (change in posture), sensory (hallucinations), or autonomic (flushing, tachycardia) symptoms; no loss of consciousness
Complex partial	Begins in one focal area but spreads to both hemispheres (more common in adults)	Loss of consciousness; aura of visual disturbances; postictal symptoms
Generalized		
Absence (petit mal)	Sudden onset; lasts 5 to 10 seconds; can have 100 daily; precipitated by stress, hyperventilation, hypoglycemia, fatigue; differentiated from daydreaming	Loss of responsiveness but continued ability to maintain posture control and not fall; twitching eyelids; lip smacking; no postictal symptoms
Myoclonic	Movement disorder (not a seizure); seen as child awakens or falls asleep; may be precipitated by touch or visual stimuli; focal or generalized; symmetrical or asymmetrical	No loss of consciousness; sudden, brief, shocklike involuntary contraction of one muscle group
Clonic	Opposing muscles contract and relax alternately in rhythmic pattern; may occur in one limb more than others	Mucus production
Tonic	Muscles are maintained in continuous contracted state (rigid posture)	Variable loss of consciousness; pupils dilate; eyes roll up; glottis closes; possible incontinence; may foam at mouth
Tonic-clonic (grand mal, major motor)	Violent total body seizure	Aura; tonic first (20 to 40 seconds); clonic next; postictal symptoms
Atonic	Drop and fall attack; needs to wear protective helmet	Loss of posture tone
Akinetic	Sudden brief loss of muscle tone or posture	Temporary loss of consciousness

(continued)

● **Assessment findings**
- Aura just before the seizure's onset (child reports unusual tastes, feelings, or odors)
- Eye deviation to a particular side or blinking

Signs of seizure disorders

- Aura just before seizure onset (report of unusual taste, feeling, or odor)
- Eye deviation or blinking
- Unresponsiveness during muscular contractions
- Incontinence
- Disorientation to time and place, drowsiness, and lack of coordination immediately after seizure

Classifying seizures *(continued)*

TYPE	DESCRIPTION	SIGNS AND SYMPTOMS
Miscellaneous		
Febrile	Seizure threshold lowered by elevated temperature; only one seizure per fever; common in 4% of population under age 5; occurs when temperature is rapidly rising	Lasts less than 5 minutes; generalized, transient, and nonprogressive; doesn't generally result in brain damage; EEG is normal after 2 weeks
Status epilepticus	Prolonged or frequent repetition of seizures without interruption; results in anoxia and cardiac and respiratory arrest	Consciousness not regained between seizures; lasts more than 30 minutes

Managing seizure disorders

- Anticonvulsants
- Surgical removal of focal lesion

Anticonvulsants

- Diazepam (Valium)
- Lorazepam (Ativan)
- Phenobarbital (Luminal)
- Fosphenytoin (Cerebyx)
- Phenytoin (Dilantin)

How to intervene during a seizure

- Stay with the child.
- Move the child to a flat surface that's out of danger.
- Provide a patent airway; place the child on his side to let saliva drain.
- Don't try to interrupt the seizure.
- Gently support the child's head.
- Keep the child's hands from inflicting self-harm but don't restrain them.
- Don't use tongue blades.
- Loosen tight clothing.
- Record seizure activity and assess neurologic status and vital signs.

- Usually, unresponsiveness during tonic-clonic muscular contractions; possible incontinence
- Possible disorientation to time and place, drowsiness, and lack of coordination immediately after seizure

● **Diagnostic test findings**
- EEG results help differentiate epileptic from nonepileptic seizures; each seizure has a characteristic EEG tracing
- Abnormal findings on CT or MRI scan

● **Medical management**
- Anticonvulsants—I.V. diazepam (Valium) or lorazepam (Ativan), phenobarbital (Luminal) or fosphenytoin (Cerebyx), phenytoin (Dilantin) to keep neuron excitability below the seizure threshold
- Surgical removal of a focal lesion to attempt to stop seizures

● **Nursing interventions**
- Stay with the child during a seizure
- Move the child to a flat surface that's out of danger
- Provide a patent airway; place the child on his side to let saliva drain out
- Don't try to interrupt the seizure
- Gently support the child's head
- Keep the child's hands from inflicting self-harm but don't restrain them
- Don't use tongue blades (they add stimuli) and reduce external stimuli
- Loosen tight clothing
- Record seizure activity and assess neurologic status and vital signs
- Pad the crib or bed
- Administer seizure medications
  - Phenytoin keeps neuron excitability below the seizure threshold; side effects include gum hyperplasia, hirsutism, ataxia, gastric distress, nystagmus, anemia, and sedation
  - Other seizure medications include phenobarbital, carbamazepine (Tegretol), and valproic acid (Depakene)

TIME-OUT FOR TEACHING

Seizure disorders

Be sure to include these points in your teaching plan for the parents of a child with a seizure disorder:

- type of seizure and possible cause, if known
- medication regimen, including dose, frequency, times of administration, and possible adverse effects
- safety measures during seizure
- compliance with follow-up laboratory tests and physician visits
- promotion of as normal a life as possible for the child
- reinforcement of positive self-image.

- Monitor serum levels of anticonvulsant medications, such as phenytoin, to ensure therapeutic levels and prevent toxicity
- Instruct the patient and his parents in all aspects of seizure control measures (see *Seizure disorders*)

NCLEX CHECKS

It's never too soon to begin your NCLEX preparation. Now that you've reviewed this chapter, carefully read each of the following questions and choose the best answer. Then compare your responses to the correct answers.

1. A 3-month-old is admitted to the facility with a diagnosis of bacterial meningitis. Which sign of meningeal irritation occurs with this condition?

☐ **1.** Marked irritability
☐ **2.** Overriding sutures
☐ **3.** Prominent scalp veins
☐ **4.** Depressed anterior fontanel

2. Which assessment finding would lead you to suspect Down syndrome in an infant?

☐ **1.** Single palmar crease and hypotonia
☐ **2.** Cleft lip and palate and high-pitched cry
☐ **3.** Flat maxillary area and short palpebral fissures
☐ **4.** Hyperactivity, microcephaly, and persistent postnatal growth lag

3. A nurse is teaching a class of pregnant women about diet. Which nutrient decreases the incidence of NTDs?

☐ **1.** Vitamin A
☐ **2.** Vitamin C
☐ **3.** Vitamin D
☐ **4.** Folic acid

TOP 9

Items to study for your next test on the neurosensory system

1. Structures and functions of the CNS
2. Nursing interventions for lumbar puncture
3. Assessment findings and complications of Down syndrome
4. The difference between conductive and sensorineural hearing loss
5. Medical management of hydrocephalus
6. Assessment findings for increased ICP
7. Ways to minimize ICP
8. Types of neural tube defects
9. Types of seizures

4. Which assessment finding suggests that a neonate has spina bifida occulta?

☐ **1.** Bilateral hip dislocation
☐ **2.** Bulging anterior fontanel
☐ **3.** Noticeable dimpling above the separation of the buttocks
☐ **4.** No movement in the lower extremities

5. Which type of conjunctivitis is highly contagious?

☐ **1.** Allergic
☐ **2.** Irritant
☐ **3.** Chemical
☐ **4.** Bacterial

6. A preterm neonate is diagnosed with IVH. Which nursing intervention should be questioned?

☐ **1.** Rocking the baby
☐ **2.** Assessing the fontanels
☐ **3.** Observing for apnea
☐ **4.** Measuring head circumference daily

7. Why are younger children more prone to otitis media?

☐ **1.** Exposure to other children at day care centers
☐ **2.** Allergies
☐ **3.** Wider, shorter horizontal eustachian tubes
☐ **4.** Increased use of cotton-tipped swabs for ear cleaning

8. Which condition would be highly suspected in an infant who has persistent primitive reflexes?

☐ **1.** Down syndrome
☐ **2.** Cerebral palsy
☐ **3.** Hearing loss
☐ **4.** Aseptic meningitis

9. A nurse is assessing a child following a head injury. Which nursing action is appropriate?

☐ **1.** Placing the child in Trendelenburg's position
☐ **2.** Encouraging fluids every hour
☐ **3.** Checking the nose and ears for watery drainage
☐ **4.** Administering opiate sedation

10. Identify the area of the spinal cord that relays sensory impulses.

ANSWERS AND RATIONALES

1. CORRECT ANSWER: 1

Marked irritability, vomiting, bulging fontanels, and seizures are commonly seen in bacterial meningitis. Separated sutures, not overriding sutures, may occur because of increased intracranial pressure. Scalp veins normally bulge when an infant is crying. A depressed fontanel is a sign of dehydration.

2. CORRECT ANSWER: 1

A single transverse palmar crease, called a simian line, is a characteristic of Down syndrome. Children with Down syndrome also show hypotonia (diminished muscle tone) and muscle weakness. Cleft lip and palate aren't related to Down syndrome. A high-pitched cry is a sign of neurologic illness. Such physical findings as a flat maxilla, microcephaly (an abnormally small head), hyperactivity, and persistent postnatal growth delays result from fetal alcohol syndrome.

3. CORRECT ANSWER: 4

Women can decrease the risk of NTDs by increasing their dietary intake of foods that contain folic acid, such as spinach and other green leafy vegetables. Vitamins A, C, and D are important during pregnancy but aren't directly related to NTDs.

4. CORRECT ANSWER: 3

Spina bifida occulta is a type of neural tube defect of the vertebral canal. Assessment findings commonly include a noticeable dimple and tufts of hair over the affected area on the lower back. Bilateral hip dislocation and a bulging anterior fontanel aren't associated with spina bifida occulta. No movement of the lower extremities is associated with spina bifida cystica and encephalocele.

5. CORRECT ANSWER: 4

Bacterial and viral conjunctivitis are caused by organisms and are highly contagious. Allergic conjunctivitis is related to the particular client's allergies, whether they are aware of them or not. Conjunctivitis caused by irritants or chemicals needs attention to remove them from the conjunctiva.

6. CORRECT ANSWER: 1

Rocking the baby or other stimulation may cause an increase in blood flow and blood pressure to the germinal matrix. The blood vessels in this area are fragile and if blood flow is increased by any source, they may rupture. Neonatal intensive care units are making a concentrated effort to minimize stimulation to premature neonates to prevent IVHs. Assessing the fontanels and measuring head circumference daily are necessary interventions to detect signs of IVH as early as possible. Apnea can be a sign of IVH and is part of the needed assessment.

7. CORRECT ANSWER: 3

Children, especially younger children, have wider, shorter horizontal eustachian tubes. This normal characteristic allows easier access for bacteria that may cause otitis media. Although exposure to organisms at daycare centers can be a potential problem, it is a less likely cause. Although some children do have allergies, an organism causes otitis media. Having allergies does not specifically cause an infection. Use of cotton-tipped swabs, which can easily rupture the ear drum, is not recommended in any age group, but should receive particular attention in children.

8. CORRECT ANSWER: 2

Persistent primitive reflexes (such as the Moro reflex) are an indication of needed further assessment. CP is one condition in which these reflexes persist beyond the normal time variation. Persistent primitive reflexes aren't characteristic of Down syndrome, hearing loss, or aseptic meningitis. Children with Down syndrome may be hypotonic. Hearing loss may be diagnosed if the infant is not babbling or interacting. Signs of aseptic meningitis resemble bacterial meningitis (irritability, vomiting, and other signs). This disease is caused by a virus and is self-limiting.

9. CORRECT ANSWER: 3

Watery drainage from the nose or ears following a head injury may indicate the presence of spinal fluid. The fluid should be reported and checked for glucose. Placing the child in Trendelenburg's position can increase intracranial pressure and blood flow in the presence of a head injury. Fluids shouldn't be encouraged; they will most likely be restricted to decrease the risk of increased ICP. Administering an opioid can mask signs of deteriorating neurologic function.

10. CORRECT ANSWER:

The dorsal horn, indicated by the "x," relays sensory impulses.

8

Altered respiratory functioning

---

1. Abdominal breathing is usually present in a child until what age?

☐ 1. 2

☐ 2. 4

☐ 3. 6

☐ 4. 8

CORRECT ANSWER: 3

2. A neonate who has been exposed to ventilatory support with high positive airway pressure and oxygen during the first 2 weeks of life is at risk for developing which disorder?

☐ 1. Bronchiolitis

☐ 2. Bronchopulmonary dysplasia

☐ 3. Asthma

☐ 4. Cystic fibrosis

CORRECT ANSWER: 2

3. Cystic fibrosis is genetically transferred as which type of trait?

☐ 1. Autosomal dominant

☐ 2. Sex-linked

☐ 3. Multifactorial

☐ 4. Autosomal recessive

CORRECT ANSWER: 4

4. Surfactant is a lipoprotein that lowers surface tension in what part of the lung?

☐ 1. Alveoli

☐ 2. Bronchioles

☐ 3. Bronchi

☐ 4. Trachea

Correct answer: 1

5. What's the peak age for sudden infant death syndrome?

☐ 1. 1 month

☐ 2. 3 months

☐ 3. 12 months

☐ 4. 18 months

CORRECT ANSWER: 2

LEARNING OBJECTIVES

After studying this chapter, you should be able to:

● Describe the conditions or complications related to immature lung development in the child.

● Explain the common treatments for respiratory conditions.

● Differentiate among various childhood respiratory conditions and plan appropriate nursing interventions.

CHAPTER OVERVIEW

The child's respiratory tract differs anatomically from an adult's in ways that predispose the child to numerous respiratory problems. A thorough assessment and prompt interventions—whether at home or in a health care facility—are essential to prevent complications and maximize oxygenation. Preventing infection and educating the parents are also important components of patient care.

KEY CONCEPTS

⬤ **Structures and functions**
(See *Structures of the respiratory system.*)
  • Nose and nasal passages

Functions of the nasal passages
  • Serve as a conduit for air to and from lungs
  • Filter, warm, and moisten air

Structures of the respiratory system

This illustration shows the structures of the respiratory system.

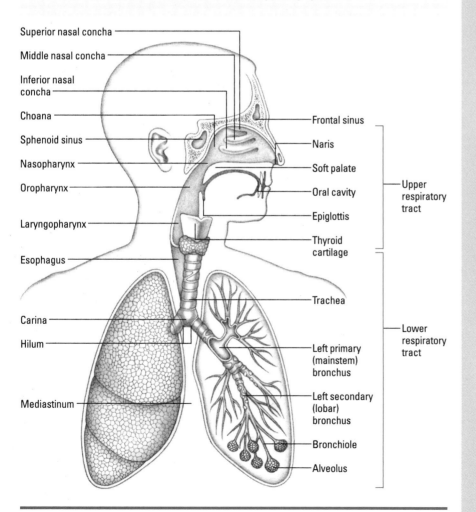

Superior nasal concha
Middle nasal concha
Inferior nasal concha
Choana
Sphenoid sinus
Nasopharynx
Oropharynx
Laryngopharynx
Esophagus
Carina
Hilum
Mediastinum

Frontal sinus
Naris
Soft palate
Oral cavity
Epiglottis
Thyroid cartilage

Upper respiratory tract

Trachea

Lower respiratory tract

Left primary (mainstem) bronchus
Left secondary (lobar) bronchus
Bronchiole
Alveolus

Complications of narrow nasal passages

- Increased airway resistance
- Airway obstruction
- Respiratory distress

Key facts about the pharynx

- Also called the *throat*
- Cylindrical structure that runs from the base of the skull to the esophagus
- Composed of smooth muscle and mucous membranes
- Conduit for the respiratory and digestive tracts

Key facts about the larynx

- Upper end of trachea
- Consists of rigid framework of cartilage
- Contains epiglottis and glottis
- Reflexes are sensitive in infants

Key facts about the trachea

- Made up of C-shaped rings of cartilage
- Supported by smooth muscle
- Passageway for air into lungs

Key facts about the bronchi

- Two bronchi branch off of the trachea
- Composed of the same cartilaginous rings and smooth muscle as the trachea
- Passageway for air into the alveoli

    – Lined with ciliated mucous membranes that filter, warm, and moisten the air

    – Serve as a conduit for air to and from the lungs

    – Infants have narrow nasal passages that make them prone to complications

        · Increased airway resistance because they are nose breathers

        · Airway obstruction and respiratory distress from inflammation

- Pharynx
  - Also called the *throat*
  - Cylindrical structure that runs from the base of the skull to the esophagus, anterior to the cervical vertebrae
  - Composed of smooth muscle and mucous membranes
  - Serves as a conduit for the respiratory and digestive tracts
- Larynx
  - The upper end of the trachea
  - Consists of a rigid framework of cartilage
  - Contains the epiglottis and glottis
    - Prevent solids and fluids from entering the air passages during swallowing
    - In infants, the epiglottis is longer and located higher and further back than in older children
  - The reflexes of the larynx are very sensitive in infants
- Trachea
  - Made up of C-shaped rings of cartilage
  - Supported by smooth muscle
  - Acts as a passageway for air into the lungs
- Bronchi
  - The right (shorter, wider, and more vertical) and left bronchi branch off of the trachea
  - Composed of the same cartilaginous rings and smooth muscle as in the trachea
    - The cartilage in infants is soft and very reactive to stimuli, allowing the airway to become easily obstructed because of edema and bronchospasms
    - The amount of smooth muscle in an infant age 4 to 5 months is enough to cause constriction in response to external stimuli; by age 1 year, the smooth muscle is like that of an adult
  - Act as a passageway for air into the alveoli
    - Alveoli are the smallest branches of the bronchi
    - The primary function of the respiratory system is to distribute air to the alveoli
    - Gas exchange — oxygen and carbon dioxide diffusion — takes place in the alveoli

- The cartilaginous rings disappear as the bronchioles get smaller, leaving the smallest divisions with a lining of a single layer of cells
  - The number of alveoli increase with age; there are nine times as many in a 12-year-old child as in an infant
- Lungs
  - The main component in the body's system that inspires air, extracts oxygen, and exhales the waste product carbon dioxide
  - The right lung has three lobes
  - The left lung has two lobes
  - The mediastinum is the space between the two lungs
  - The lungs aren't fully developed at birth
- The thoracic cavity
  - Surrounded by a framework of the ribs, vertebrae, and sternum
  - The shape and angles of the framework allow the thoracic cavity to change its size during each inspiration and expiration
    - In an infant, the angles of the framework aren't fully developed, forcing infants to depend on abdominal breathing; abdominal breathing is usually present until age 6
    - It's normal for infants to have slightly irregular breathing patterns
  - Pleura
    - The membrane that totally encloses the lung
    - Consists of two layers
      - The visceral layer hugs the entire lung surface
      - The parietal layer lines the inner surface of the chest wall and the upper surface of the diaphragm
  - Pleural cavity
    - The tiny area between the visceral and parietal pleural layers
    - Contains a thin film of serous pleural fluid
      - Lubricates the pleural surfaces so that they slide smoothly against each other as the lungs expand and contract
      - Creates a bond between the layers that causes the lungs to move with the chest wall during breathing
- Respiratory muscles
  - Forced inspiration
    - Pectoral muscles
      - Located in the upper chest
      - They raise the chest to increase the anteroposterior diameter
    - Sternocleidomastoid muscles
      - Located in the side of the neck
      - They raise the sternum
    - Scalene muscles
      - Located in the neck
      - They elevate, fix, and expand the upper chest

Key facts about the alveoli

- Smallest branches of the bronchi
- Site of gas exchange
- Number of alveoli increases with age

Lung functions

- Inspires air
- Extracts oxygen
- Exhales carbon dioxide

Pleural layers of the thoracic cavity

- Visceral layer – hugs the entire lung surface
- Parietal layer – lines the inner surface of the chest wall and the upper surface of the diaphragm

Respiratory muscles and their locations

- Pectoral – upper chest
- Sternocleidomastoid – side of neck
- Scalene – neck
- Posterior trapezius – upper back
- Intercostal – within ribs
- Abdominal rectus – abdomen

Pulmonary circulation

- Oxygen-depleted blood enters the lungs from the pulmonary artery of the right ventricle.
- Blood flows through the main pulmonary arteries into the vessels of the pleural cavities and the main bronchi; it then flows to the capillary networks in the alveoli.
- Oxygenated blood enters the main pulmonary vein and flows into the left atrium for distribution throughout the body.

Respiratory function definitions

- **Tachypnea** – a fast respiratory rate (greater than 60 breaths/minute)
- **Hyperpnea** – deep respirations
- **Apnea** – unintentional cessation in spontaneous breathing for more than 20 seconds

Common diagnostic tests for respiratory disorders

- ABG analysis
- Pulse oximetry
- Pulmonary function tests
- Chest X-rays
- Computed tomography scan
- Magnetic resonance imaging
- Sputum specimen analysis
- Bronchoscopy

- Posterior trapezius muscles
  - Located in the upper back
  - They raise the thoracic cage
- – Active expiration
  - Intercostal muscles
    - Within the ribs
    - Contract to shorten the chest's transverse diameter
  - Abdominal rectus muscles
    - Located in the abdomen
    - Pull down the lower chest, thus depressing the lower ribs

Pulmonary circulation

- Oxygen-depleted blood enters the lungs from the pulmonary artery of the heart's right ventricle
- Blood flows through the main pulmonary arteries into the smaller vessels of the pleural cavities and the main bronchi, through the arterioles and, eventually, to the capillary networks in the alveoli
- The oxygenated blood then flows through progressively larger vessels, enters the main pulmonary vein, and flows into the left atrium for distribution throughout the body

Respiratory quantity and quality

- Tachypnea — a fast respiratory rate (greater than 60 breaths/minute)
- Hyperpnea — deep respirations
- Apnea — unintentional cessation in spontaneous breathing for more than 20 seconds with or without bradycardia and color change

DIAGNOSTIC TESTS

Arterial blood gas (ABG) analysis

- Purpose
  - – Assesses pH, bicarbonate level, level of oxygen, and the carbon dioxide level in the blood to determine how well the lungs are working
    - *Partial pressure of oxygen* (PaO_2) indicates how well oxygen can move from the lungs to the blood
    - *Partial pressure of carbon dioxide* ($PaCO_2$) indicates how well carbon dioxide can move out of the blood to the lungs and its ability to be exhaled
    - *Bicarbonate* is a chemical buffer that maintains the blood's pH within normal levels
    - *pH* indicates the acid or base level of the blood; blood pH is usually about 7.4
  - – Decreased PaO_2 may indicate hypoventilation, ventilation-perfusion mismatch, or shunting of blood away from gas exchange sites
  - – Increased $PaCO_2$ reflects hypoventilation or marked ventilation-perfusion mismatch

– Decreased $Paco_2$ reflects increased alveolar ventilation

– Changes in pH may reflect metabolic or respiratory dysfunction

• Nursing interventions

– Explain the procedure to the parents and child

– Check arterial circulation before the arterial puncture is made

– After the sample is obtained, apply firm pressure to the arterial site

– Note on the sample if the child is on oxygen

– Keep the sample on ice and transport it immediately to the laboratory

– Assess the puncture site for bleeding or hematoma formation

Pulse oximetry

• Purpose

– A painless method to measure oxygen saturation

• Nursing interventions

– Place the oximeter on a site with adequate circulation, such as the finger, foot, or toe

– Periodically rotate sites to prevent skin breakdown

– Ensure that pulse readings in the site used for oximetry correlate with the child's heart rate before performing oximetry

Pulmonary function tests (PFTs)

• Purpose

– Measures lung volume, flow rates, and compliance of the lungs

• Nursing interventions

– Note that results may not be accurate because the young child has trouble following directions

– Explain the procedure to the child and his parents

– Instruct the child and his parents that he should have only a light meal before the test

– If appropriate, tell the child that he shouldn't smoke for 4 to 6 hours before the tests

– Tell the parents to withhold bronchodilators and intermittent positive-pressure breathing therapy

– Just before the test, tell the child to void and loosen tight clothing, and obtain the child's height and weight

Chest X-rays

• Purpose

– To show conditions, such as atelectasis, pleural effusions, infiltrates, pneumothorax, lesions, mediastinal shifts, and pulmonary edema

• Nursing interventions

– Ensure adequate protection by covering the child's gonads and thyroid gland with a lead apron

– Explain the purpose of the test to the parents and child

– Make sure the child holds still during the test; assist the child, if necessary

---

Interpreting ABG analysis results

• **Decreased Pao_2:** may indicate hypoventilation, ventilation-perfusion mismatch, or shunting of blood away from gas exchange sites

• **Increased $Paco_2$:** indicates hypoventilation or marked ventilation-perfusion mismatch

• **Decreased $Paco_2$:** indicates increased alveolar ventilation

• **Changes in pH:** may reflect metabolic or respiratory dysfunction

What PFTs measure

• Lung volume
• Flow rates
• Lung compliance

Key facts about CT scanning

- Provides three-dimensional picture
- 100 times more sensitive than chest X-ray
- Requires written, informed consent

Key facts about sputum specimen analysis

- Studies sputum quantity, color, viscosity, and odor
- Can identify infectious organisms
- Can detect respiratory tract neoplasms

Key facts about bronchoscopy

- Allows direct visualization of the trachea and part of the bronchi
- Allows collection of respiratory tract secretions
- Allows an opportunity for brush biopsy or lesion biopsy

● Computed tomography (CT) scan
- Purpose
  - Provides a three-dimensional picture that's 100 times more sensitive than a chest X-ray
- Nursing interventions
  - Explain the purpose of the test to the parents and child
  - Obtain written, informed consent
  - Make sure that the child holds still during the test; sedation may be necessary

● Magnetic resonance imaging
- Purpose
  - Identifies obstructed arteries and tissue perfusion
- Nursing interventions
  - If the child has surgically implanted objects, notify the radiology department because these may interfere with the picture
  - Explain the procedure to the parents and child
  - Make sure the child holds still during the test; sedation may be necessary

● Sputum specimen analysis
- Purpose
  - Permits the study of sputum quantity, color, viscosity, and odor
  - Microbiological stains and culture of sputum can identify infectious organisms
  - Cytologic preparations can detect respiratory tract neoplasms
- Nursing interventions
  - Explain the collection procedure to the child and parents
    - Have the child expectorate into a sterile collection cup
    - If the child can't expectorate, he may need nasotracheal or endotracheal (ET) tube suctioning
  - Ensure that the specimen is sent to the laboratory for evaluation in a timely fashion

● Bronchoscopy
- Purpose
  - Allows direct visualization of the trachea and part of the bronchi
    - Localizes the site of lung hemorrhage
    - Visualizes masses in the airways
  - Allows collection of respiratory tract secretions
  - Allows an opportunity for brush biopsy or lesion biopsy
  - May be used to remove foreign objects
- Nursing interventions
  - Explain the procedure to the child and parents
  - Administer premedications as ordered (to relax or sedate the child as necessary)

NURSING DIAGNOSES

● **Probable nursing diagnoses**
  • Impaired gas exchange
  • Ineffective airway clearance
  • Ineffective breathing pattern
  • Risk for infection
  • Ineffective tissue perfusion: Cardiopulmonary
  • Impaired spontaneous ventilation

● **Possible nursing diagnoses**
  • Anxiety
  • Delayed growth and development
  • Imbalanced nutrition: Less than body requirements
  • Risk for deficient fluid volume

ASTHMA

● **Definition**
  • A reversible, diffuse, obstructive pulmonary disease

● **Causes**
  • Hyperresponsiveness of the lower airway
  • May be idiopathic or intrinsic; may be caused by a hyperresponsive reaction to an allergen, exercise, or environmental change

● **Pathophysiology**
  • The obstructive symptoms of asthma are caused by three mechanisms
    – Inflammation of the mucous membranes
    – Smooth muscle bronchospasm
    – Increased mucus secretion, leading to airway obstruction and air trapping (see *The asthmatic bronchus,* page 200)

● **Complications**
  • Respiratory insufficiency
  • Death

● **Assessment findings**
  • Alteration in chest contour from chronic air trapping; barrel chest
  • Altered cerebral function
  • Diaphoresis
  • Dyspnea
  • Exercise intolerance
  • Fatigue and apprehension
  • Prolonged expiration with an expiratory wheeze; in severe distress, possible inspiratory wheeze
  • Unequal or decreased breath sounds

Probable nursing diagnoses for a patient with a respiratory disorder

- Impaired gas exchange
- Ineffective airway clearance
- Ineffective breathing pattern
- Risk for infection
- Ineffective tissue perfusion: Cardiopulmonary
- Impaired spontaneous ventilation

Key facts about asthma

- Reversible, diffuse, obstructive pulmonary disease
- Caused by hyperresponsiveness of lower airway in reaction to allergen, exercise, or environment
- May be idiopathic or intrinsic

How asthma affects the airways

- Inflammation of the mucous membranes
- Smooth muscle bronchospasm
- Increased mucus secretion, leading to airway obstruction and air trapping

The asthmatic bronchus

This illustration shows the effects of asthma on the airways.

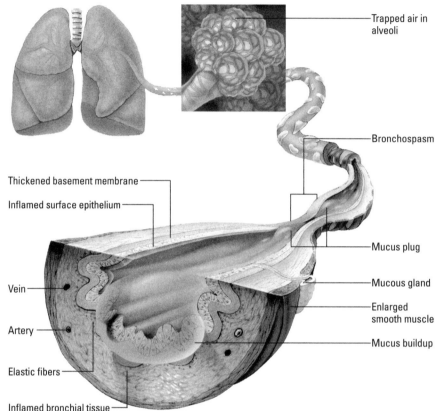

Trapped air in alveoli

Bronchospasm

Thickened basement membrane

Inflamed surface epithelium

Mucus plug

Mucous gland

Vein

Enlarged smooth muscle

Artery

Mucus buildup

Elastic fibers

Inflamed bronchial tissue

TOP 7

Assessment findings in asthma

1. Diaphoresis
2. Dyspnea
3. Prolonged expiration with expiratory wheeze
4. Possible inspiratory wheeze
5. Unequal or decreased breath sounds
6. Use of accessory muscles, intercostal retractions, and nasal flaring
7. Cough

Diagnostic test findings in asthma

- Decreased oxygen saturation
- Increased $Paco_2$ from respiratory acidosis
- Hyperexpansion of airways
- Air trapping
- Decreased expiratory flow

- Use of accessory muscles (intercostal retractions and nasal flaring)
- Cough
- Increased capillary refill time

● **Diagnostic test findings**
- Pulse oximetry may show decreased oxygen saturation
- ABG measurements may show increased $Paco_2$ from respiratory acidosis
- Skin test identifies the source of the allergy
- Sputum analysis rules out respiratory infection
- Chest X-ray shows hyperexpansion of airways
- PFTs indicate air trapping and decreased expiratory flow

● **Medical management**
- Chest physiotherapy (after edema has abated)
- Hyposensitization through the use of allergy shots, if appropriate
- Parenteral fluids to thin mucus secretions
- Oxygen therapy, as tolerated

- Medications
  - Beta-adrenergic blockers, bronchodilators (short-acting)
  - Bronchodilator — albuterol (Proventil), salmeterol (Serevent)
  - Mast cell stabilizer — cromolyn (Intal) to prevent the release of mast cell products after an antigen-antibody union has taken place
  - Inhaled corticosteroids to decrease edema of the mucous membranes (for chronic asthma, daily doses to control chronic inflammation); also oral and I.V. steroids are used in severe cases
  - Anticholinergic — ipratropium (Atrovent) to inhibit bronchoconstriction
  - Leukotriene modifiers or leukotriene receptor antagonists — zileuton (Zyflo), montelukast (Singulair), zafirlukast (Accolate) to inhibit bronchoconstriction and inflammation

- **Nursing interventions**
- Assess respiratory and cardiovascular status; tachycardia, tachypnea, and quiet breath sounds signal worsening respiratory status
- Monitor vital signs to detect changes and prevent complications
- Assess the nature of the child's cough (hacking, unproductive progressing to productive), especially at night in the absence of infection; early detection and treatment lessens respiratory distress
- Modify the environment to avoid an allergic reaction
  - Remove the offending allergen
  - Allergens can trigger an asthma attack
- Rinse the child's mouth after he inhales medication to promote comfort and prevent irritation to the oral mucosa
- For exercise-induced asthma, give prophylactic treatments of beta-adrenergic blockers or cromolyn 10 to 15 minutes before the child exercises; premedication before exercise may prevent an asthma attack
- Forbid smoking in the child's environment; secondhand smoke can trigger an asthma attack
- During an acute attack
  - Allow the child to sit upright to promote chest expansion and ease breathing; provide moist oxygen, if necessary, to promote mobilization of secretions
  - Monitor for alterations in vital signs (especially cardiac stimulation and hypotension) to detect signs of impending respiratory arrest and cardiac decompensation
  - Administer medications through a metered dose inhaler (MDI) or a nebulizer
    - A child as young as age 4 can use an MDI if a spacer (chamber) is attached
    - The child can puff the medication into the spacer and then inhale, avoiding the problem of trying to coordinate the activities of pressing the MDI and inhaling slowly

Asthma medications

- Bronchodilators
- Mast cell stabilizers
- Inhaled corticosteroids
- Anticholinergics
- Leukotriene modifiers and leukotriene receptor antagonists

How to respond to an acute asthma attack

- Allow the child to sit upright.
- Provide moist oxygen, if necessary.
- Monitor for alterations in vital signs.
- Monitor for hyperglycemia.
- Administer medications.
- Maintain a calm environment.
- Monitor peak flow rates.
- Monitor effectiveness of drug therapy.

- Monitor peak flow rates, which indicate the degree of lung impairment (baseline values need to be established when the child is healthy to set comparison rates)
- Maintain a calm environment; provide emotional support and reassurance to decrease anxiety and oxygen demands
- Monitor effectiveness of drug therapy; failure to respond to drugs during an acute attack can result in status asthmaticus, a potentially fatal complication that arises when impaired gas exchange and heightened airway resistance increase the work of breathing

BRONCHIOLITIS

- **Definition**
  - A lower respiratory infection in infants
- **Causes**
  - Respiratory syncytial virus (RSV)
  - Other causative viruses include parainfluenza, adenovirus, and influenza viruses
- **Pathophysiology**
  - Swollen bronchiole mucosa, lumina filled with exudates, bronchi and bronchiole walls infiltrated with inflammatory cells, necrosis of epithelial cells lining the small airways, and the presence of peribronchiolar interstitial pneumonitis characterize this infection
  - The infection is spread by respiratory secretions, rather than droplets
  - It typically affects infants and children under age 2 in the winter and spring
- **Complications**
  - Respiratory insufficiency
  - Obstructed airway
- **Assessment findings**
  - Possible air trapping and atelectasis
  - Sternal retractions
  - Nasal flaring
  - Tachypnea
  - Thick mucus
  - Wheezes and crackles
  - Cough
- **Diagnostic test results**
  - Bronchial mucus culture shows RSV
  - Chest X-ray
- **Medical management**
  - Humidified oxygen
  - I.V. fluids

Viruses that cause bronchiolitis

- Respiratory syncytial virus
- Parainfluenza
- Adenovirus
- Influenza

Signs of bronchiolitis

- Possible air trapping and atelectasis
- Sternal retractions
- Tachypnea
- Thick mucus
- Wheezes and crackles

Managing bronchiolitis

- Humidified oxygen
- I.V. fluids
- Isolation

- Isolation to prevent health care–associated infection
- Medication (for children at risk for chronic disease or severely affected infants)
  - Epinephrine may improve airway resistance in some cases; should only be continued if improvements appear
  - Palivizumab (Synagis) may prevent RSV in high-risk infants
- Prevent exposure to secondhand smoke

● **Nursing interventions**
- Monitor vital signs and pulse oximetry to determine oxygenation needs and to detect deterioration or improvement in the child's condition
- Assess respiratory and cardiovascular status; tachycardia may result from hypoxia or effects of bronchodilator use
- Use gloves, gowns, and aseptic hand washing as secretion precautions to prevent spread of infection
- Administer chest physiotherapy after edema has abated; it helps loosen mucus that may be blocking small airways
- Administer humidified oxygen therapy to liquefy secretions and reduce bronchial edema
- Administer and maintain I.V. therapy to promote hydration and replace electrolytes
- Administer fluids by mouth after acute crisis

BRONCHOPULMONARY DYSPLASIA

● **Definition**
- Bronchopulmonary dysplasia (BPD) is a chronic lung disease that begins in infancy

● **Causes**
- Ventilatory support with high positive airway pressure and oxygen in the first 2 weeks of life
- Possibly genetic factors
- Prematurity

● **Pathophysiology**
- An acute insult to the neonate's lungs requires positive-pressure ventilation and a high concentration of oxygen over time
  - Respiratory distress syndrome (RDS)
  - Pneumonia
  - Meconium aspiration
- These therapies result in tissue and cellular injury and damage to the bronchiolar epithelium in the immature lung
- Ciliary activity is inhibited, so the child has trouble clearing mucus from the lungs

TOP 3

Interventions for bronchiolitis

1. Monitor vital signs and pulse oximetry.
2. Assess respiratory and cardiovascular status.
3. Administer humidified oxygen therapy.

Causes of BPD

- Ventilatory support with high positive airway pressure and oxygen in the first 2 weeks of life
- Possibly genetic factors
- Prematurity

Complications of BPD

- Respiratory insufficiency
- Lower respiratory tract infections
- Hypertension
- Death

TOP 4

Assessment findings in BPD

1. Atelectasis
2. Crackles, rhonchi, or wheezing
3. Dyspnea
4. Sternal retractions

Pulmonary changes on X-ray in BPD

- Bronchiolar metaplasia
- Interstitial fibrosis

Managing BPD

- Chest physiotherapy
- Continued ventilatory support and oxygen
- Enteral nutrition or TPN
- Supportive measures to enhance respiratory function
- Medications (bronchodilators or diuretics)

- Recovery usually occurs in 6 to 12 months; however, the child may remain ventilator-dependent for years

● **Complications**
- Respiratory insufficiency
- Lower respiratory tract infections
- Hypertension
- Death

● **Assessment findings**
- Atelectasis
- Crackles, rhonchi, or wheezing
- Delayed development
- Dyspnea
- Hypoxia without ventilator assistance
- Fatigue
- Delayed muscle growth
- Pallor
- Circumoral cyanosis
- Prolonged capillary filling time
- Respiratory distress
- Right-sided heart failure
- Sternal retractions
- Weight loss or difficulty feeding

● **Diagnostic test findings**
- ABG analysis reveals hypoxemia
- Chest X-ray reveals pulmonary changes
  - Bronchiolar metaplasia
  - Interstitial fibrosis

● **Medical management**
- Chest physiotherapy
- Continued ventilatory support and oxygen
- Enteral or total parenteral nutrition (TPN)
- Supportive measures to enhance respiratory function
- Medications
  - Bronchodilators—albuterol to counter increased airway resistance
  - Diuretics—furosemide (Lasix)

● **Nursing interventions**
- Assess respiratory and cardiovascular status; children with BPD are susceptible to lower respiratory tract infections, hypertension, and respiratory failure
- Monitor vital signs, pulse oximetry, and intake and output to assess and maintain adequate hydration, which is necessary to liquefy secretions and to detect early signs of respiratory compromise

- Anticipate continued ventilatory support and oxygen
- Continue supportive measures to enhance respiratory function
- Administer bronchodilators to counter increased airway resistance
- Be aware that because of a tendency to accumulate interstitial fluid in the lung, diuretics are given
- Perform chest physiotherapy
- Provide adequate time for rest; increased oxygen consumption results in a higher need for calories without increasing the amount of fluid
- Provide nutritional support, including increased caloric density
- Begin an intensive program to promote normal development
- Encourage the parents to visit and become involved in care; the child may require lengthy hospitalization

CROUP

Definition
- A severe inflammation and obstruction of the upper airway (see *How croup affects the upper airway*)

Causes
- Viral-induced edema around the larynx
  - Parainfluenza viruses (two-thirds of the infections)
  - Adenoviruses
  - RSV
  - Influenza viruses
  - Measles virus

Key facts about croup

- Severe inflammation and obstruction of the upper airway
- Caused by virus or bacterium
- Affects boys more than girls
- Usually occurs between ages 3 months and 5 years during winter
- Results in respiratory insufficiency

How croup affects the upper airway

In croup, inflammatory swelling and spasms constrict the larynx, thereby reducing airflow. This cross-sectional drawing (from chin to chest) shows the upper airway changes caused by croup. Inflammatory changes almost completely obstruct the larynx (which includes the epiglottis) and significantly narrow the trachea.

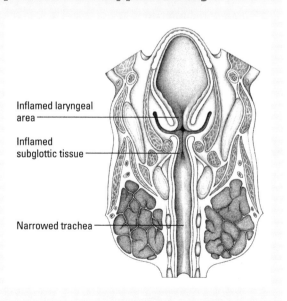

Inflamed laryngeal area

Inflamed subglottic tissue

Narrowed trachea

- Bacterial
  - Pertussis
  - Diphtheria
  - Mycoplasma

Pathophysiology

- Spasmodic laryngitis — typically involves paroxysmal attacks of laryngeal obstruction generally occurring at night
- Acute obstructive laryngitis — a sudden narrowing of the upper airway that results from vocal cord edema
- Acute laryngotracheobronchitis — inflammation of the mucosal lining of the larynx and trachea results in a constricted airway
- A childhood disease that affects boys more than girls, usually between ages 3 months and 5 years, in the winter

Complications

- Respiratory insufficiency

Assessment findings

- Barking cough or hoarseness, sometimes described as a "seal bark" cough
- Usually begins with coldlike symptoms for 1 to 2 days
- Worse at night and can last 5 to 6 days
- Crackles and decreased breath sounds (indicate condition has progressed to bronchi)
- Increased dyspnea and lower accessory muscle use
- Inspiratory stridor with varying degrees of respiratory distress
- Sudden or gradual onset
- Muffled vocal sounds

Diagnostic test findings

- If bacterial infection is the cause, throat cultures may identify the organism and its sensitivity to antibiotics as well as rule out diphtheria
- Laryngoscopy may reveal inflammation and obstruction in epiglottal and laryngeal areas
- Neck X-ray shows areas of upper airway narrowing and edema in subglottic fold and rules out the possibility of foreign body obstruction as well as masses and cysts

Medical management

- Cool humidification during sleep with a cool mist tent or room humidifier
- Exposure of child to cool air
- Oxygen administration, if necessary
- Medications
  - Antipyretics such as acetaminophen (Tylenol)

Signs of croup

- Barking cough or hoarseness
- Crackles and decreased breath sounds
- Increased dyspnea
- Increased lower accessory muscle use
- Inspiratory stridor with varying degrees of respiratory distress
- Muffled vocal sounds

Managing croup

- Cool humidification during sleep
- Exposure to cool air
- Oxygen administration
- Medications, including antipyretics, racemic epinephrine, and corticosteroids
- I.V. fluids
- Tracheostomy or ET intubation for impending airway failure

- – Inhaled racemic epinephrine (AsthmaNefrin) and corticosteroids, such as methylprednisolone (Solu-Medrol), to alleviate respiratory distress
  - – Antibiotics if the infection is bacterial
- I.V. fluids to prevent dehydration
- Tracheostomy or ET intubation for impending airway failure in very severe cases

Nursing interventions
- Keep the child calm to ease respiratory effort and conserve energy
- Take the child into the bathroom, close the door, turn on the shower's hot-water spigot full-force, and sit with the child as the room fills with steam; this should decrease laryngeal spasm
- Take the child outside into cool air
- Use a cool-mist vaporizer near the child's bed after an acute episode (after a crisis, mucus production increases, and the child may vomit large amounts; this vomiting doesn't require medical treatment)
- Encourage clear liquid intake to keep mucus thin
- Anticipate that the child may need hospitalization for tracheostomy, oxygen, or mist if the crisis doesn't resolve
- Assess respiratory and cardiovascular status to detect any indications that obstruction is worsening
- Monitor vital signs and pulse oximetry to detect early signs of respiratory compromise
- Administer medications, as ordered, and note effectiveness to maintain or improve the child's condition
- Provide emotional support for the parents to decrease anxiety
- Monitor for rebound obstruction when administering racemic epinephrine; the drug's effects are short term and may result in rebound obstruction

TOP 4

Interventions for croup

1. Keep the child calm.
2. Use a cool-mist vaporizer near the child's bed.
3. Monitor vital signs and pulse oximetry.
4. Take the child outside into cool air.

CYSTIC FIBROSIS

Definition
- A generalized dysfunction of the exocrine glands
- Affects multiple organ systems

Causes
- Genetic inheritance
- Transmitted as an autosomal recessive trait
  - – One of the most common inherited diseases in children
  - – One of the most common causes of childhood death
- Research suggests that there may be as many as 300 genes that code for cystic fibrosis (CF)

Key facts about CF
- Disease that causes generalized dysfunction of exocrine glands
- Characterized by airway obstruction caused by increased mucus production and decreased pancreatic enzyme production
- Transmitted as an autosomal recessive trait
- One of the most common causes of childhood death

Three pancreatic enzymes absent in CF

1. Lipase
2. Amylase
3. Trypsin

Key assessment findings in CF

- History of chronic, productive cough and recurrent respiratory infection
- Report of salty taste on the child's skin
- Bulky, greasy, foul-smelling stools
- Failure to thrive
- Meconium ileus (in neonate)

Managing CF

- Oral pancreatic enzymes with meals to offset pancreatic enzyme deficiencies
- Fat-soluble vitamin A, D, E, and K supplements
- Chest physiotherapy
- Postural drainage
- Breathing exercises
- Aerosol therapy
- Dornase alfa
- High-protein formula, if needed

● **Pathophysiology**
- The disease is characterized by airway obstruction caused by the increased and constant production of mucus and little or no release of pancreatic enzymes (lipase, amylase, and trypsin) due to mucus blocking ducts in the pancreas; without these enzymes, the body can't absorb fats and proteins

● **Complications**
- Respiratory insufficiency
- Death

● **Assessment findings**
- Bulky, greasy, foul-smelling stools that contain undigested food
- Thin arms and legs from steatorrhea
- Distended abdomen
- Failure to thrive from malabsorption
- History of chronic, productive cough and recurrent respiratory infections commonly due to *Pseudomonas* infections
- Meconium ileus in the neonate from a lack of pancreatic enzymes
- Parents' report of a salty taste on the child's skin
- Sweat that contains two to five times the normal levels of sodium and chloride
- Voracious appetite from undigested food lost in stools

● **Diagnostic test findings**
- Chest X-ray indicates early signs of obstructive lung disease
- Sweat test using pilocarpine iontophoresis is greater than 60 mEq/L
- Stool specimen analysis indicates the absence of trypsin
- Deoxyribonucleic acid testing
  - Locates the presence of the delta F 508 deletion (found in about 70% of patients with CF, although the disease can cause more than 100 other mutations)
  - Allows prenatal diagnosis in families with a previously affected child
- PFTs
  - Reveal decreased vital capacity, elevated residual volume due to air entrapments, and decreased forced expiratory volume in 1 second
  - This test is used if pulmonary exacerbation already exists
- Liver enzyme tests may reveal hepatic insufficiency
- Sputum culture reveals organisms that the patient with CF typically and chronically colonizes such as *Staphylococcus*
- Serum albumin measurement helps assess nutritional status
- Electrolyte analysis assesses hydration status
- Immunoreactive trypsin isn't a diagnostic test for CF, but part of the neonatal screening program; an elevated level must be followed up with additional testing

Medical management

- Oral pancreatic enzymes with meals and snacks to offset pancreatic enzyme deficiencies
- Fat-soluble vitamin A, D, E, and K supplements
- Chest physiotherapy
- Postural drainage
- Breathing exercises
- Aerosol therapy (bronchodilators, mucolytics)
- Dornase alfa (Pulmozyme) (a genetically engineered pulmonary enzyme)
  - Given by aerosol nebulizer
  - Helps thin airway mucus
  - Improves lung function and reduces the risk of pulmonary infection
- A high-protein formula, such as Probana, if needed
- For pulmonary infection
  - Broad-spectrum antimicrobials
  - Oxygen therapy, as needed
  - Antihistamines are contraindicated because they have a drying effect on mucous membranes, making expectoration of mucus difficult or impossible
- Single or double lung transplants and heart and lung transplantation

Nursing interventions

- Teach the child and parents not to restrict salt to maintain appropriate electrolyte balance; in hot weather, a sodium supplement may be necessary
- Administer pancreatic enzymes with meals and snacks
- Provide high-calorie, high-protein foods; the infant may need predigested formula such as Pregestimil
- Give multivitamins twice a day, especially fat-soluble vitamins
- Perform pulmonary hygiene (chest percussion and postural drainage) 2 to 4 times per day after mucolytic, bronchodilator, or antibiotic nebulizer inhalation treatment; inhaled deoxyribonuclease is used to thin mucus before chest physiotherapy
- Encourage physical activity or creative breathing exercises
- Teach the parents to avoid administering cough suppressants and antihistamines; the child must be able to cough and expectorate
- Administer I.V. antibiotics for a *Pseudomonas* infection only when the infection interferes with daily functioning
- Initiate genetic counseling for the family
- Promote as normal a life as possible (see *Teaching parents about cystic fibrosis*, page 210)

Managing pulmonary infection

- Broad-spectrum antimicrobials
- Oxygen therapy, as needed
- Bronchodilators
- Chest physiotherapy

Key facts about epiglottiditis

- Inflammation of the epiglottis that may rapidly progress to complete airway obstruction
- Caused by *H. influenzae* or pneumococci or group A beta-hemolytic streptococci
- Most commonly occurs in children ages 2 to 7
- Abrupt onset
- Rapidly progressive
- Requires immediate medical attention

Key assessment findings in epiglottiditis

- Difficult and painful swallowing
- Increased drooling
- Restlessness
- Stridor

EPIGLOTTIDITIS

- **Definition**
  - Inflammation and edema of the epiglottis
- **Causes**
  - Bacterial *H. influenzae*
  - Pneumococci and group A beta-hemolytic streptococci
- **Pathophysiology**
  - A serious obstructive inflammatory process of the lidlike cartilaginous structure overhanging the entrance to the larynx and serving to prevent food from entering the larynx and trachea while swallowing
  - Most commonly occurs in children ages 2 to 7; incidence has greatly decreased since the introduction of the *H. influenzae* type B conjugate vaccine
  - This infection has an abrupt onset, is rapidly progressive to respiratory distress, and requires immediate medical attention
  - Laryngeal obstruction results from inflammation and edema of the epiglottis
  - Epiglottiditis may rapidly progress to complete upper airway obstruction within 2 to 5 hours and requires prompt recognition and intervention
- **Complications**
  - Respiratory insufficiency
  - Death
- **Assessment findings**
  - Cough

- Difficult and painful swallowing
- Extending the neck in a sniffing position
- Fever
- Increased drooling
- Irritability
- Lower rib retractions
- Pallor
- Tachycardia
- Tachypnea
- Refusal to drink or eat
- Restlessness
- Sore throat
- Stridor
- Tripod sitting positions
- Use of accessory muscles

● **Diagnostic test findings**
- Lateral neck X-ray shows an enlarged epiglottis
- Throat examination reveals a large, edematous, bright red epiglottis

● **Medical management**
- Emergency ET intubation or tracheotomy, as necessary, to secure a patent airway
- Oxygen therapy or cool mist tent
- I.V. fluids to prevent dehydration
- A 10-day course of parenteral antibiotics — usually a second- or third-generation cephalosporin (if the child is allergic to penicillin, a quinolone or sulfa drug may be substituted)

● **Nursing interventions**
- Don't inspect the throat of a child with epiglottiditis without emergency personnel and supplies (such as an anesthesiologist, a laryngoscope, and an ET tube) on hand because inspection could stimulate a spasm of the epiglottis and cause respiratory occlusion
- Decrease the number of examining personnel to decrease the child's anxiety
- Allow the child to sit on a parent's lap; the sitting position makes breathing easier
- Administer antibiotics as ordered
- Monitor vital signs and pulse oximetry for changes in oxygenation
- Maintain oxygen therapy, if necessary
- Provide emotional support to the child and family

FOREIGN BODY ASPIRATION

● **Definition**
- The passage of a foreign body into the lung

Managing epiglottiditis

- Emergency ET intubation or tracheotomy, as necessary
- Oxygen therapy or cool mist tent
- I.V. fluids
- Ten-day course of parenteral antibiotics

Key nursing interventions for epiglottiditis

- Inspect the throat of a child with epiglottiditis only with emergency personnel and supplies on hand.
- Allow the child to sit on a parent's lap (sitting eases breathing).
- Administer antibiotics, as ordered.
- Monitor vital signs and pulse oximetry.
- Maintain oxygen therapy, if necessary.
- Provide emotional support to the child and family.

Risk factors for foreign body aspiration

- Altered level of consciousness
- Tracheoesophageal fistula
- CNS abnormalities

Complications of foreign body aspiration

- Respiratory insufficiency
- Pneumonitis
- Death

Signs of foreign body aspiration

- Coughing
- Stridor
- Wheezing
- Foreign object in the mouth or throat

● **Causes**
- Inhalation of a foreign body
- Risk factors
  - Altered level of consciousness
    · Sedation
    · Anesthesia
    · Seizure disorders
    · Stroke
  - Tracheoesophageal fistula
  - Central nervous system (CNS) abnormalities

● **Pathophysiology**
- Occurs in children with an impaired swallowing mechanism and cough reflex
- Common in infants and toddlers because they have narrow airways and high levels of curiosity
- Dried bean aspiration poses the greatest danger because beans absorb respiratory moisture and form an obstruction; peanuts cause an immediate emphysema reaction
- Most small objects end up in the right bronchus because it's straighter and wider than the left

● **Complications**
- Respiratory insufficiency
- Pneumonitis
- Death

● **Assessment findings**
- Coughing
- Stridor
- Wheezing
- Foreign object in the mouth or throat

● **Diagnostic test findings**
- Bronchoscopy allows visualization of the foreign object
- Neck or chest X-ray reveals the location of the object

● **Medical management**
- Tracheotomy or intubation, if necessary
- Bronchoscopy to identify and remove the foreign object
- Abdominal thrust to dislodge the object if it's obstructing the airway

● **Nursing interventions**
- Examine the mouth and throat to locate the foreign body
- Be aware that the object may be expelled spontaneously
- Perform the abdominal thrust if the child's airway is occluded; for infants, back blows and chest thrusts are used to relieve obstruction and to prevent injury to abdominal organs

RESPIRATORY DISTRESS SYNDROME (RDS)

● **Definition**
- A respiratory dysfunction in neonates
- Related to a developmental delay in lung maturation
- The disease was previously called *hyaline membrane disease*

● **Causes**
- Prematurity, especially in neonates with low birth weight

● **Pathophysiology**
- By 27 weeks' gestation, airways and alveoli of the fetus's respiratory system are present, but the intercostal muscles are weak and the alveoli and capillary blood supply are immature
- A preterm neonate with RDS develops widespread alveolar collapse from lack of surfactant
  - Surfactant
    - A lipoprotein present in alveoli and respiratory bronchioles
    - Lowers surface tension
    - Helps maintain alveolar patency
    - Prevents alveolar collapse, particularly at end expiration
  - Lack of surfactant results in widespread atelectasis
    - Leads to inadequate alveolar ventilation with shunting of blood through collapsed areas of the lung
    - Causes hypoxemia and acidosis
- RDS occurs almost exclusively in neonates born before 37 weeks' gestation
  - Neonates commonly afflicted
    - Those born to diabetic mothers
    - Those delivered by cesarean birth
    - Second-born twins
    - Those with perinatal asphyxia
    - Those delivered suddenly after antepartum hemorrhage
  - RDS is the most common cause of neonatal mortality
- If untreated, RDS is fatal within 72 hours of birth

● **Complications**
- Respiratory insufficiency
- Death

● **Assessment findings**
- Breathing may be normal at first
- Rapid, shallow respirations within minutes or hours of birth
- Intercostal, subcostal, or sternal retractions
- Nasal flaring
- Audible expiratory grunting—a natural compensatory mechanism designed to produce positive end-expiratory pressure and prevent further alveolar collapse

Key facts about RDS

- Respiratory dysfunction in neonates
- Related to delay in lung maturation
- Caused by prematurity

Key facts about surfactant

- Lipoprotein present in alveoli and respiratory bronchioles
- Lowers surface tension
- Helps maintain alveolar patency
- Prevents alveolar collapse
- Lack of surfactant results in widespread atelectasis, which leads to inadequate alveolar ventilation and shunting of blood through collapsed lung areas

Neonates commonly afflicted with RDS

- Those born before 37 weeks' gestation
- Those born to diabetic mothers
- Those delivered by cesarean birth
- Second-born twins
- Those with perinatal asphyxia
- Those delivered suddenly after antepartum hemorrhage

TOP 3

Assessment findings in RDS

1. Intercostal, subcostal, or sternal retractions
2. Nasal flaring
3. Audible expiratory grunting

Chest X-ray findings in RDS

- May be normal for the first 6 to 12 hours
- Ground glass appearance and air-filled bronchi after 24 hours

Special ventilation techniques used to manage RDS

- High-frequency jet ventilation
- High-frequency oscillatory ventilation
- Extracorporeal membrane oxygenation
- Nasal CPAP

Managing RDS

- Vigorous respiratory support
- Radiant infant warmer or isolette for thermoregulation
- I.V. fluids and sodium bicarbonate to control acidosis and maintain fluid and electrolyte balance
- Tube feedings or TPN if the neonate is too weak to eat
- Surfactant administration by ET tube within the first 24 hours

- Hypotension
- Peripheral edema
- Oliguria
- Apnea
- Bradycardia
- Cyanosis secondary to hypoxemia, left-to-right shunting through the foramen ovale, or right-to-left intrapulmonary shunting through atelectatic regions of the lung
- Pallor
- Frothy sputum
- Low body temperature as a result of an immature nervous system and the absence of subcutaneous fat

● Diagnostic test findings

- Chest X-ray may be normal for the first 6 to 12 hours (in 50% of neonates with RDS), but 24 hours after birth it will show a characteristic ground glass appearance and air-filled bronchi
- ABG analysis shows decreased PaO_2; normal, decreased, or increased $PaCO_2$; and decreased pH (from respiratory or metabolic acidosis or both)
- Chest auscultation reveals normal or diminished air entry and crackles (rare in early stages)

● Medical management

- Vigorous respiratory support
  - Warm, humidified, oxygen-enriched gases are administered by oxygen hood or, if such treatment fails, by continuous positive airway pressure (administered by nasal prongs or mask) or mechanical ventilation via ET intubation
  - Special ventilation techniques are used on patients who don't respond to conventional mechanical ventilation
    - High-frequency jet ventilation
    - Nasal continuous positive airway pressure (CPAP) used in less severe cases to prevent BPD and tracheal malasia
    - High-frequency oscillatory ventilation
  - Extracorporeal membrane oxygenation
    - The last choice for ventilation
    - Only available in certain specialized institutions
- A radiant infant warmer or isolette for thermoregulation
- I.V. fluids and sodium bicarbonate to control acidosis and maintain fluid and electrolyte balance
- Tube feedings or TPN if the neonate is too weak to eat
- Administration of surfactant by an ET tube within the first 24 hours

● Nursing interventions

- Expect the neonate to be on a ventilator or nasal CPAP to keep the alveoli open

– Administer oxygen as needed
– In neonates, mechanical ventilation is usually done in a pressure-limited mode rather than the volume-limited mode used in adults
– Watch for signs of barotrauma
  · Increase in respiratory distress
  · Subcutaneous emphysema
* Organize care to ensure minimal handling
* Control the neonate's temperature to reduce stress and decrease additional energy use
* Use aseptic technique to reduce the risk of infection
* Administer I.V. fluids to ensure adequate hydration, but withhold oral food and fluids if the neonate has a high respiratory rate; anticipate possible nasogastric tube feedings
* Turn the neonate every 2 hours; raise the head of the bed; perform chest percussion before suctioning
* Closely monitor blood gases as well as fluid intake and output
  – If the neonate has an umbilical catheter (arterial or venous), check for arterial hypotension or abnormal central venous pressure
  – Watch for complications, such as infection, thrombosis, or decreased circulation to the legs
  – If the neonate has a transcutaneous oxygen monitor, change the site of the lead placement every 2 to 4 hours to avoid burning the skin
* Weigh the neonate once or twice daily
* To evaluate the neonate's progress, assess skin color, rate and depth of respirations, severity of retractions, nasal flaring, frequency of expiratory grunting, frothing at the lips, and restlessness
* Teach the parents about their neonate's condition and let them participate in his care (using aseptic technique) to encourage normal parent-neonate bonding
* Advise parents that full recovery may take up to 12 months; when the prognosis is poor, prepare the parents for the neonate's impending death, and offer emotional support

SUDDEN INFANT DEATH SYNDROME (SIDS)

Definition
* The sudden death of an infant in which a postmortem examination fails to confirm the cause of death
* Also called *crib death* or *cot death*

Causes
* Unknown (see *Risk factors for SIDS,* page 216)

Pathophysiology
* Almost always occurs during sleep
* The major cause of postneonatal death

What to assess when evaluating progress in RDS

* Skin color
* Rate and depth of respirations
* Severity of retractions
* Nasal flaring
* Frequency of expiratory grunting
* Frothing at the lips
* Restlessness

Key facts about SIDS

* Also called *crib death* or *cot death*
* Exact cause is unknown
* A major cause of postneonatal death
* Almost always occurs during sleep without noise or struggle
* Peak age of occurrence is 3 months; 90% of cases occur before age 6 months
* Higher incidence during winter
* Can't be prevented

SIDS risk factors

- Young mother (< age 20)
- Low-birth-weight neonate
- Premature birth
- Multiple pregnancy
- Family history of SIDS
- Maternal smoking
- Prone sleeping

Autopsy findings in SIDS deaths

- Pulmonary edema
- Intrathoracic petechiae
- Chronic hypoxia (suggested by other changes)

Risk factors for SIDS

These risk factors may contribute to sudden infant death syndrome (SIDS):
- mother who's younger than age 20, poor, or unmarried
- low birth weight
- prematurity
- multiple pregnancies
- siblings who died of SIDS
- maternal smoking
- prone sleeping.

- May result from an abnormality in the control of ventilation, causing prolonged apneic periods with profound hypoxia and cardiac arrhythmias
- May result from undetected abnormalities, such as an immature respiratory system and respiratory dysfunction
- The peak age is 3 months; 90% of cases occur before age 6 months, especially during the winter and early spring months
- The syndrome can't be prevented or explained; the infant usually dies during sleep without noise or struggle

Complications
- Death

Assessment findings
- History of low birth weight
- History of siblings with SIDS

Diagnostic test findings
- Autopsy findings
  - Pulmonary edema
  - Intrathoracic petechiae
  - Other minor changes suggesting chronic hypoxia

Medical management
- Resuscitation as ordered by the physician
  - If attempted, drugs are administered according to pediatric advanced life support protocols
    - Epinephrine
    - Atropine
    - Sodium bicarbonate, as indicated by ABG analysis
  - If successfully resuscitated, the infant is temporarily placed on mechanical ventilation
  - After infant is extubated
    - Infant is tested for infantile apnea
    - Parents are given a home apnea monitor
    - Parents are taught infant cardiopulmonary resuscitation

Nursing interventions
- Be aware that assessment, planning, and implementation related to the parents needs to begin as soon as the parents arrive in the emergency department

- Provide the family with a room and a staff member who can stay with them; support them and reinforce the fact that the death wasn't their fault
- Stay calm and let the parents express their feelings; they may express anger at emergency department personnel, each other, or anyone involved with the child's care
- Prepare the family for how the infant will look and feel
- Let the parents touch, hold, and rock the infant, if desired; allow them to say good-bye
- Prepare the parents for the need for an autopsy, which is the only way to diagnose SIDS
- Contact spiritual advisors, significant others, support systems, and the local SIDS organization
- Provide literature on SIDS and support groups
- Suggest psychological support for the surviving children
- Encourage the mother to participate in a prenatal or postnatal smoking-cessation program, as appropriate, and provide emotional support
- Provide a hand print, foot print, and lock of hair
- Promote the "back to sleep" campaign — research indicates a decreased incidence of SIDS in infants maintained in a supine position while sleeping

TONSILLITIS

- **Definition**
  - Acute or chronic inflammation of the tonsils
- **Causes**
  - Group A beta-hemolytic streptococcal infection
  - Other bacterial infections
  - Virus
  - Oral anaerobes
- **Pathophysiology**
  - Waldeyer's tonsillar ring — a mass of lymphoid tissue around the nasal and oral pharynx that consists of three pairs of tonsils
    - Palatine tonsils
      - Also known as the *faucial tonsils*
      - Located on both sides of the oropharynx, behind and below the opening of the mouth
      - Surface is visible on oral examination
      - Removed during tonsillectomy
    - Pharyngeal tonsils
      - Also known as the *adenoids*
      - Located on the back wall of the nasopharynx above the palatine tonsils

---

Support for parents coping with SIDS-related death

- Reinforce the fact that the death wasn't their fault.
- Allow them to touch, hold, and rock the infant, if desired.
- Allow them to say good-bye to the infant.
- Contact spiritual advisors, significant others, support systems, and the local SIDS organization.

Structures of Waldeyer's tonsillar ring

- Palatine tonsils
- Pharyngeal tonsils
- Lingual tonsils

Complications of tonsillitis

- Obstruction from tonsillar hypertrophy
- Peritonsillar abscess

Signs and symptoms of acute tonsillitis

- Mild to severe sore throat
- Decreased food intake
- Dysphagia
- Abdominal pain
- Vomiting
- Fever
- Swelling
- Tenderness in the lymph glands in the submandibular area
- Muscle and joint pain
- Chills
- Malaise
- Headache
- Pain that commonly refers to the ears
- Excess secretions that cause a constant urge to swallow
- A feeling of constriction in the back of the throat

Managing tonsillitis

- Antibiotics for bacterial infections
- Possible tonsillectomy for chronic tonsillitis
- Lozenges, analgesics, or antipyretics for comfort

- Close to the nares and eustachian tubes, which causes problems when they become inflamed
  - Lingual tonsils
    - Located at the base of the tongue
    - Rarely removed

Complications
- Obstruction from tonsillar hypertrophy
- Peritonsillar abscess

Assessment findings
- Acute tonsillitis
  - Mild to severe sore throat
  - Decreased food intake
  - Dysphagia
  - Abdominal pain
  - Vomiting
  - Fever
  - Swelling
  - Tenderness in the lymph glands in the submandibular area
  - Muscle and joint pain
  - Chills
  - Malaise
  - Headache
  - Pain that commonly refers to the ears
  - Excess secretions that cause a constant urge to swallow
  - A feeling of constriction in the back of the throat
- Chronic tonsillitis
  - Recurrent sore throat
  - Purulent drainage in the tonsillar crypts

Diagnostic test findings
- Throat culture determines the infecting organism
- Serum analysis reveals leukocytosis

Medical management
- Antibiotics for bacterial infections
  - Penicillin or another broad-spectrum antibiotic are the drugs of choice for a group A beta-hemolytic streptococcus infection
  - Most oral anaerobes also respond to penicillin
  - To prevent complications, antibiotic therapy should continue for 10 to 14 days
- Chronic tonsillitis or the development of complications may require tonsillectomy, but only after the patient has been free from tonsillar or respiratory tract infection for 3 to 4 weeks
- Lozenges, analgesics, and antipyretics may be used to maintain comfort

Nursing interventions

- Preoperative
  - Explain why the child is coming to the hospital
  - Encourage the parents to stay with the child until surgery
  - Prepare the child for the sights and sounds of surgery; explain that the child will be asleep during surgery
  - Allow the child to play with the equipment
  - Provide reassurance that the child will never be alone and won't feel the procedure
  - Put a transitional object in the recovery room for the child
  - Prepare the child for a sore throat
  - Maintain a soft to liquid diet
  - The child may breathe through his mouth; a vaporizer (cool mist) may help to keep mucous membranes from drying out
- Postoperative
  - Place the child in a prone or side-lying position to facilitate drainage
  - Don't suction except to remove an obstruction; this will prevent trauma to the site
  - Check for signs of hemorrhage, which require immediate attention
    - Frequent swallowing
    - Restlessness
    - Fast, thready pulse
    - Vomiting bright red blood; however, be aware that vomiting dried blood is common
  - Provide an ice collar for comfort and for reducing edema
  - Provide clear, cool, non-citrus fluids (don't offer red fluids, which can be mistaken for blood if vomited)
  - Engage the child in therapeutic doll play to help deal with feelings and confusion about the procedure after recovery
  - Administer pain medications as needed

UPPER RESPIRATORY INFECTION (NASOPHARYNGITIS)

Definition

- The "common cold"

Causes

- Rhinoviruses
- RSV
- Adenovirus
- Influenza virus
- Parainfluenza virus

Pathophysiology

- An infectious process involving the upper respiratory tract

Signs of hemorrhage after tonsillectomy

- Frequent swallowing
- Restlessness
- Fast, thready pulse
- Vomiting bright red blood

Key facts about upper respiratory infection

- Also known as *the common cold*
- Severity of symptoms is worse in children and infants
- Generally self-limited and resolves without complications in 4 to 10 days
- Occurs six to nine times per year in children

- Symptoms are more severe in infants and children than in adults
- Generally self-limited and resolves without complications in 4 to 10 days
- The child generally has six to nine colds per year

● **Complications**
- Otitis media
- Pneumonia

● **Assessment findings**
- Fever, especially in young children; older children experience low-grade fevers
- Irritability
- Restlessness
- Decreased appetite
- Decreased activity
- Mouth breathing
- Vomiting
- Diarrhea
- Dry, irritated nasal passages
- Sneezing
- Chills
- Aching muscles
- Nasal discharge
- Cough

● **Diagnostic test findings**
- Clinical assessment and examination reveals signs and symptoms of nasopharyngitis
- Allergy testing is negative (see *Differentiating respiratory allergies from the common cold*)

● **Medical management**
- Medications
  - Antipyretics to treat fever and discomfort
  - Decongestants to decrease swelling in the nasal passages
  - Cough suppressants

● **Nursing interventions**
- Place the child in a prone position, unless contraindicated, and provide a cool-mist vaporizer to relieve nasal obstruction
- Use saline nose drops and a bulb syringe on the infant
- Ensure adequate fluid intake to prevent dehydration and to keep secretions as thin as possible
- Encourage rest and increased fluid intake
- Explain to the child and family that nasopharyngitis is spread by secretions and that contact with others should be avoided

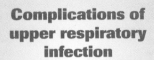

Complications of upper respiratory infection

- Otitis media
- Pneumonia

Signs of upper respiratory infection

- Fever
- Irritability
- Restlessness
- Decreased appetite
- Decreased activity
- Mouth breathing
- Vomiting
- Diarrhea
- Dry, irritated nasal passages
- Sneezing
- Chills
- Aching muscles
- Nasal discharge
- Cough

Medications for upper respiratory infection

- Antipyretics
- Decongestants
- Cough suppressants

Differentiating respiratory allergies from the common cold

The chart below highlights some of the distinguishing features of respiratory allergies and the common cold.

RESPIRATORY ALLERGIES	COMMON COLD
Usually not accompanied by fever	Fever may or may not be present
Usually occur in a seasonal pattern	No pattern
Child may constantly sneeze	Sneezing may be sporadic
Presence of allergic shiners and nasal crease	No corresponding signs
Mucus usually clear and watery	Mucus may be purulent, yellow, or green
Pruritus of the nasal passage, back of the throat, and inner ear	May be accompanied by sore throat; usually not accompanied by pruritus of eyes and nose
Family history of allergies	History of contagion among friends and family
Eosinophils present in nasal smear	Eosinophils absent in nasal smear

Features of respiratory allergies

- Seasonal pattern
- Constant sneezing
- Allergic shiners and nasal crease
- Clear, watery mucus
- Pruritus of nasal passage, back of throat, and inner ear
- Increased risk with family history of allergies
- Eosinophils in nasal smear

NCLEX CHECKS

It's never too soon to begin your NCLEX preparation. Now that you've reviewed this chapter, carefully read each of the following questions and choose the best answer. Then compare your responses to the correct answers.

1. A child with difficulty breathing and a "barking cough" is displaying signs associated with which condition?
- ☐ **1.** Cystic fibrosis
- ☐ **2.** Asthma
- ☐ **3.** Epiglottiditis
- ☐ **4.** Croup

2. Which instruction about preventing SIDS should a nurse include when teaching the parents of an infant?
- ☐ **1.** Position the infant on his stomach to sleep.
- ☐ **2.** Position the infant in an infant seat to sleep.
- ☐ **3.** Position the infant on his back to sleep.
- ☐ **4.** Position the infant in a side-lying position to sleep.

TOP 6

Items to study for your next test on the respiratory system

1. Structures and functions of the respiratory system
2. Asthma medications
3. Signs of croup
4. Cystic fibrosis
5. Assessment findings in RDS
6. Risk factors for SIDS

3. Which test result is a key finding in a child with CF?
- [ ] **1.** Chest X-ray revealing interstitial fibrosis
- [ ] **2.** Neck X-ray showing areas of upper airway narrowing
- [ ] **3.** Lateral neck X-ray revealing an enlarged epiglottis
- [ ] **4.** Positive pilocarpine iontophoresis sweat test

4. A nurse is assessing the lung sounds of a child with asthma. Which sound is the nurse most likely to hear?
- [ ] **1.** Vesicular sound
- [ ] **2.** Wheezing
- [ ] **3.** Crackles
- [ ] **4.** Pleural friction rub

5. Which nursing interventions is appropriate when providing care for a client after a tonsillectomy?
- [ ] **1.** Place the client in a side-lying position.
- [ ] **2.** Suction the client every hour.
- [ ] **3.** Offer the child fruit punch.
- [ ] **4.** Provide heat for comfort.

6. Which of these assessment findings, if identified in a young infant with bronchopulmonary dysplasia, should a nurse immediately report to the physician?
- [ ] **1.** Pulse oximetry of 94% while receiving oxygen by nasal cannula
- [ ] **2.** Decreased intake with last feeding
- [ ] **3.** Respiratory rate greater 60 breaths/minute with moderate sub-sternal retractions
- [ ] **4.** Sleeping more than 3 hours at a time

7. A child receiving albuterol (Proventil), two puffs every 3 hours, for asthma exacerbation is at risk for developing which adverse effects?
- [ ] **1.** Tachycardia, insomnia, and restlessness
- [ ] **2.** Constipation, rash, and blurred vision
- [ ] **3.** Bradypnea, lethargy, and tinnitus
- [ ] **4.** Increased appetite, increased risk for superinfection, and gum hyperplasia

8. Which outcome is important to include in the care plan for a child who has CF?
- [ ] **1.** The child's "barrel chest" will be less prominent.
- [ ] **2.** The child's fingertips won't become "clubbed."
- [ ] **3.** The child gains weight appropriately for his age.
- [ ] **4.** The child will have tutoring available in the home.

9. When an infant has an upper respiratory infection, which action should a nurse take before feeding the child?

☐ **1.** Perform chest physiotherapy and postural drainage.
☐ **2.** Place the child in an infant seat to elevate the head.
☐ **3.** Give an antitussive to reduce the risk of GI upset.
☐ **4.** Instill normal saline solution and suction the nares with a bulb syringe.

10. A child with CF should receive which vitamin supplements in his daily diet? Select all that apply.

☐ **1.** A
☐ **2.** C
☐ **3.** D
☐ **4.** E
☐ **5.** K
☐ **6.** B_{12}

ANSWERS AND RATIONALES

1. CORRECT ANSWER: 4
A "seal bark" cough and difficulty breathing indicate croup. CF produces a chronic productive cough and recurrent respiratory infections. Asthma may cause prolonged expiration with an expiratory wheeze on auscultation, dyspnea, and accessory muscle use. Epiglottiditis results in increased drooling, difficulty swallowing, tachypnea, and stridor.

2. CORRECT ANSWER: 3
The parents should be instructed to position the infant on his back to sleep to decrease the risk of SIDS. An infant may be positioned in an infant seat during periods of respiratory distress to encourage lung expansion, but it shouldn't be encouraged as a routine position for sleep. Research demonstrates an increased incidence of SIDS in an infant positioned on his stomach to sleep. The side-lying position should be avoided because the infant can reposition himself into a prone (stomach-lying) position.

3. CORRECT ANSWER: 4
A child with CF has a positive pilocarpine iontophoresis sweat test. The child sweats normally, but this sweat contains two to five times the normal levels of sodium and chloride. Chest X-ray findings that reveal bronchiolar metaplasia and interstitial fibrosis are associated with bronchopulmonary dysplasia. A neck X-ray that reveals upper airway narrowing and edema in the subglottic folds indicates croup. A lateral neck X-ray that reveals an enlarged epiglottis indicates epiglottiditis.

4. CORRECT ANSWER: 2
When listening to the lung sounds of a client with asthma, the most commonly heard adventitious sound is wheezing. Wheezing sounds like a musical note. Vesicular sounds are soft, low-pitched, normal breath sounds heard

over the periphery of the lungs. Crackles are discontinuous high-pitched popping noises and are usually heard in a client with pulmonary edema. Pleural friction rub is coarse and low-pitched; it may be heard in a client with pneumonia or tuberculosis.

5. CORRECT ANSWER: 1

Placing the client in a side-lying position, checking for signs of hemorrhage, and providing an ice collar (not heat) for comfort are all appropriate interventions after a tonsillectomy. To prevent trauma to the site, the client should only be suctioned to remove obstructions. Cool, clear, noncitrus fluids should be offered to the client. Red fluids, such as fruit punch, may be mistaken for blood if vomited.

6. CORRECT ANSWER: 3

Infants with bronchopulmonary dysplasia are commonly maintained on a low dose of oxygen, even at home. One decreased feeding wouldn't warrant a call to the physician, but the nurse should closely monitor intake and output. A respiratory rate greater than 60 breaths/minute indicates respiratory distress, especially when coupled with moderate retractions. Infants, especially preterm neonates, normally sleep 2 to 3 hours at a time.

7. CORRECT ANSWER: 1

The most common adverse effects seen with albuterol (Proventil) include nausea, vomiting, increased heart rate, restlessness, insomnia, and tachycardia.

8. CORRECT ANSWER: 3

Children with CF commonly experience failure to thrive and have difficulty gaining weight due to steatorrhea, even in the presence of a voracious appetite. Once clubbed fingers and barrel chest develop, they're always present. Parents should strive to keep the child in school and a normal environment.

9. CORRECT ANSWER: 4

Infants are obligatory nose breathers. In order for infants to be able to suck, breathe, and swallow effectively, the nares must be clear. Chest physiotherapy and postural drainage aren't necessary because infants need to be held during feedings. Antitussives aren't given because of sedative property, and children need to cough effectively.

10. CORRECT ANSWER: 1, 3, 4, 5

Children with CF should receive daily supplements of the fat-soluble vitamins (A, D, E, and K). Although vitamins C and B_{12} are important, they aren't fat-soluble vitamins and, unlike the fat-soluble vitamins, are easily absorbed by the child with CF.

9

Altered cardiac functioning

PRETEST

1. What's the function of the Purkinje fibers?

☐ 1. Delays impulses to keep ventricles from contracting too quickly

☐ 2. Controls the heart rate rhythm

☐ 3. Conducts impulses into the muscle

☐ 4. Resumes rapid conduction of impulses through the ventricle

CORRECT ANSWER: 3

2. What's the purpose of the foramen ovale?

☐ 1. Carries oxygenated blood from placenta to fetus

☐ 2. Allows blood to pass between the atria and bypass the lungs

☐ 3. Carries deoxygenated blood from fetus to placenta

☐ 4. Connects pulmonary artery to the aorta

CORRECT ANSWER: 2

3. Which disorder is an example of a mixed congenital heart defect?

☐ 1. Ventricular septal defect

☐ 2. Tetralogy of Fallot

☐ 3. Patent ductus arteriosus

☐ 4. Transposition of the great vessels

CORRECT ANSWER: 4

4. What type of congenital defect occurs when the endocardial cushions fail to fuse completely?

- ☐ 1. Atrioventricular canal defect
- ☐ 2. Atrial septal defect
- ☐ 3. Coarctation of the aorta
- ☐ 4. Aortic stenosis

CORRECT ANSWER: 1

5. Which diagnostic finding indicates tetralogy of Fallot?

- ☐ 1. Boot-shaped cardiac silhouette on X-ray
- ☐ 2. Oblong appearance of heart on X-ray
- ☐ 3. Increased pulmonary vascular markings
- ☐ 4. Left ventricular hypertrophy

CORRECT ANSWER: 1

LEARNING OBJECTIVES

After studying this chapter, you should be able to:

- Distinguish between the four categories of congenital heart defects.
- Plan care for a child with a congenital heart defect.
- Describe the criteria for determining rheumatic fever.

CHAPTER OVERVIEW

Four major classifications of cardiac anomalies are associated with altered cardiac function in the pediatric patient: defects that increase pulmonary blood flow, obstructive defects, mixed defects, and defects that decrease pulmonary blood flow. Interventions are geared toward palliative treatment or correction of the defect. Rheumatic fever, an autoimmune disorder that can affect the heart's tissues, commonly follows a group A beta-hemolytic streptococcal infection of the pharynx. Nursing care focuses on immediate patient needs and those associated with long-term convalescence.

KEY CONCEPTS

● **Structures and functions**
- Circulatory system
  - Pulmonary circulation
    - Blood picks up new oxygen
    - Blood liberates the waste product carbon dioxide
  - Systemic circulation
    - Blood carries oxygen and nutrients to all active cells
    - Blood transports waste products to the kidneys, liver, and skin for excretion
    - Blood carries hormones from one part of the body to another
- Heart
  - Located behind the sternum
  - Propels blood through the system by continuous rhythmic contractions (see *Inside the heart,* page 228)
  - Made up of three layers
    - Endocardium — the smooth inner layer
    - Myocardium — the thick, muscular middle layer that contracts in rhythmic beats
    - Epicardium — the thin, serous membrane or outer surface of the heart
  - Four chambers
    - Two atria
      - Thin-walled chambers
      - Serve as reservoirs during ventricular contraction (systole) and as pumps during ventricular relaxation (diastole)
      - Separated by an atrial septum
    - Two ventricles
      - Thick-walled chambers
      - The left ventricle propels blood through the aorta
      - The right ventricle, which is much thinner than the left ventricle because it meets only one-sixth of the resistance, forces blood through the pulmonary artery

How circulation works

- Pulmonary
- Blood picks up oxygen
- Blood releases carbon dioxide
- Systemic
- Blood carries oxygen and nutrients to active cells
- Blood transports waste products to kidneys, liver, and skin for excretion
- Blood carries hormones from one part of the body to another

Three heart layers

- Endocardium — smooth, inner layer
- Myocardium — thick, muscular layer
- Epicardium — thin, serous, outer membrane

What's in the heart

- Four chambers: two atria (thin-walled) and two ventricles (thick-walled)
- Four valves: two atrioventricular and two semilunar
- Blood vessels (carry blood to and from heart)

Inside the heart

Within the heart lie four chambers (two atria and two ventricles) and four valves (two atrioventricular and two semilunar valves). A system of blood vessels carries blood to and from the heart.

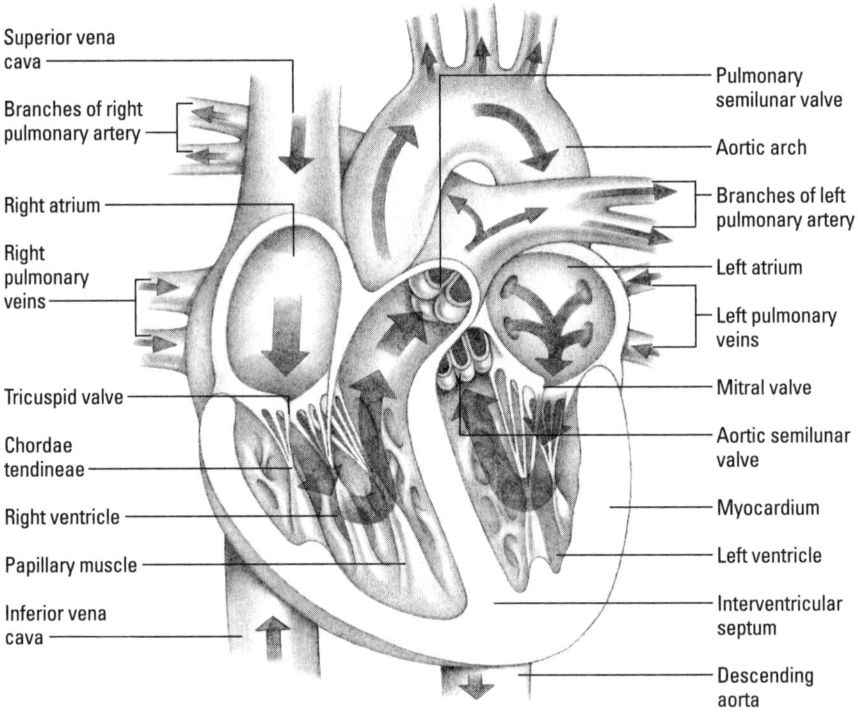
Superior vena cava
Branches of right pulmonary artery
Right atrium
Right pulmonary veins
Tricuspid valve
Chordae tendineae
Right ventricle
Papillary muscle
Inferior vena cava
Pulmonary semilunar valve
Aortic arch
Branches of left pulmonary artery
Left atrium
Left pulmonary veins
Mitral valve
Aortic semilunar valve
Myocardium
Left ventricle
Interventricular septum
Descending aorta

- Separated by a ventricular septum
- Valves
  - Atrioventricular
    - Tricuspid
      - The valve between the right atrium and ventricle
      - Has three leaflets, or cusps, and three papillary muscles
    - Mitral
      - The valve between the left atrium and ventricle
      - Consists of two cusps shaped like a bishop's miter and two papillary muscles
    - Atrioventricular valves prevent blood backflow from the ventricles to the atria during ventricular contraction
    - The leaflets of both valves are attached to the papillary muscles of the ventricle by thin, fibrous bands called chordae tendineae; the leaflets separate and descend funnel-like into the ventricles during diastole and are pushed upward and togeth-

Types of valves and their functions

- Atrioventricular
  - Tricuspid and mitral
  - Prevent blood backflow from ventricles to atria during ventricular contraction
- Semilunar
  - Aortic and pulmonic
  - Prevent blood backflow from aorta and pulmonary artery during ventricular relaxation

er during systole to occlude the mitral and tricuspid orifices
- Papillary muscles contract during systole and prevent the leaflets from prolapsing into the atria during ventricular contraction
  - Semilunar
    - Aortic — the valve between the left ventricle and the aorta
    - Pulmonic — the valve between the right ventricle and pulmonary artery
    - Prevent blood backflow from the aorta and pulmonary artery into the ventricles during ventricular relaxation
- Pericardium
  - Sac that covers the entire heart
  - Made of two layers
    - Visceral layer — in contact with the heart
    - Parietal layer — the outer layer
  - Fluid lubricates the parietal pericardium to prevent irritation when the heart moves against this layer
- Conduction system
  - The sinoatrial (SA) node
    - Within the right atrial wall near the opening of the superior vena cava
    - Also called the pacemaker of the heart
    - Normally controls the heart rate rhythm at 60 to 100 beats/minute
  - The atrioventricular (AV) node
    - Located within the right atrium near the lower end of the septum
    - Delays impulses to keep the ventricles from contracting too quickly
    - Has a rate of 40 to 60 beats/minute
  - The AV bundle (bundle of His)
    - Extends from the AV node to each side of the interventricular septum and divides into right and left bundle branches
    - Resumes rapid conduction of the impulses through the ventricles
    - Has a rate of 30 to 40 beats/minute
  - The Purkinje fibers
    - Extend from the AV bundle into the walls of the ventricles
    - Conduct impulses rapidly through the muscle
    - Have a rate of 20 to 30 beats/minute
- Arteries
  - Large, thick-walled blood vessels that carry blood away from the heart
  - Artery walls have three layers
    - The tunica adventitia — the outer layer

Components of the conduction system

- SA node – pacemaker; controls heart rhythm
- AV node – delays impulses
- AV bundle (bundle of His) – resumes rapid conduction of the impulses
- Purkinje fibers – conduct impulses rapidly through the muscle

Major arteries

- Pulmonary artery – carries deoxygenated blood to the lungs to be oxygenated
- Aorta – the first artery involved in the process of delivering oxygenated blood to the body

Major veins

- Superior and inferior vena cava – collect blood from systemic circulation and return it to the right atrium
- Pulmonary veins – bring oxygenated blood from the lungs to the left atrium

Key facts about capillaries

- Small network of thin-walled vessels
- Pass blood from arteries to veins, returning it to the heart

Key facts about the lymphatic system

- Complex network of capillaries, vessels, valves, ducts, nodes, and organs
- Protect and maintain the internal fluid environment of the body
- Produce, filter, and transport lymph
- Produce blood cells

- The tunica media — the middle layer
- The tunica intima — the inner layer
  - Distribute highly oxygenated blood to the capillaries
  - Pulmonary artery
    - Stems from the right ventricle and carries deoxygenated blood to the lungs to be oxygenated
    - The only artery in the body that doesn't specifically carry oxygenated blood
  - Aorta
    - Stems from the left ventricle
    - The first artery in the process of delivering oxygenated blood to the body
- Veins
  - Smaller, thinner-walled blood vessels that carry deoxygenated blood from the capillaries to the heart
  - Function as collectors and reservoirs
  - The superior and inferior vena cava collect blood from systemic circulation and return it to the right atrium
  - The pulmonary veins bring oxygenated blood from the lungs to the left atrium; they're the only veins in the body that carry oxygenated blood
  - Semilunar valves at various intervals within the vein control blood flow back to the heart
  - Vein walls contain the same three layers as the arterial walls
  - Deep veins course through the more internal parts of the body
  - Superficial veins lie near the surface of the body
- Capillaries
  - The smallest network of thin-walled vessels
  - Pass blood from arteries to veins, which return it to the heart
- Lymphatic system
  - A complex network of capillaries, vessels, valves, ducts, nodes, and organs
  - Protect and maintain the internal fluid environment of the body
  - Produce, filter, and transport lymph
  - Produce blood cells
  - Transport fats, protein, and substances to the blood
- Fetal circulation structures
  - Umbilical vein — carries oxygenated blood from the placenta to the fetus
  - Umbilical arteries — carry deoxygenated blood from the fetus to the placenta
  - Foramen ovale — serves as the septal opening between the atria of the fetal heart, helping blood bypass the fetal lungs

– Ductus arteriosus—connects the pulmonary artery to the aorta, allowing blood to shunt around the fetal lungs

– Ductus venosus—carries oxygenated blood from the umbilical vein to the inferior vena cava, bypassing the liver

● **Cardiac pressures**

- Pressure on the left side of the heart is higher than on the right side after birth, with the highest internal pressure in the left ventricle
- In most cardiac anomalies involving communication between chambers, blood will flow from areas of high pressure to areas of low pressure; this is called a left-to-right shunt
- In communicating structures that don't involve chambers, such as patent ductus arteriosus (PDA), blood will also flow from high-pressure to low-pressure areas
- Increased flow to the right side of the heart causes tissue hypertrophy from increased pressure and increased blood flow
- The pressure eventually equalizes between chambers, and the right side may fail in its attempt to compensate

DIAGNOSTIC TESTS

● **Cardiac catheterization**

- Purpose
  - Evaluates ventricular function
  - Measures heart pressures
  - Measures the blood's oxygen saturation level
  - Method of obtaining cardiac muscle biopsy
  - Used to obtain electrophysiologic studies
- Nursing interventions
  - Before the procedure
    - Describe the procedure to the child and his parents
    - Weigh the child and take vital signs
    - Check the color and temperature of the child's extremities, and assess pedal pulses
    - Check the child's developmental and activity level
    - Prepare the child by using doll play and hospital play
      - Show the child where the catheter is inserted
      - Make a security object (for example, a teddy bear or toy) available
  - After the procedure
    - Keep the affected extremity immobile after catheterization to prevent hemorrhage
    - Keep the catheter site clean and dry and monitor for bleeding, hematoma formation, and diminished pulse

What ECG can detect

- Ischemia
- Injury
- Necrosis
- Bundle-branch blocks
- Fascicular blocks
- Conduction delay
- Chamber enlargement
- Arrhythmias

Types of echocardiography

- Doppler
- Transesophageal

Diagnostic tests requiring nothing-by-mouth status

- Transesophageal echocardiography
- Electrophysiologic studies

- Compare postcatheterization assessment data to precatheterization baseline data
- Ensure adequate intake (I.V. and oral) to compensate for blood loss during the procedure, nothing-by-mouth status, and diuretic action of some dyes used

● **Electrocardiography (ECG)**
  - Purpose
    – Detects the presence of ischemia, injury, necrosis, bundle-branch blocks, fascicular blocks, conduction delay, chamber enlargement, and arrhythmias
  - Nursing interventions
    – Explain to the child and parents that the child may have to lie on his left side, inhale and exhale slowly, or hold his breath at intervals during the test

● **Chest X-ray**
  - Purpose
    – Evaluates cardiac silhouette and size
    – Assesses pulmonary circulation
  - Nursing interventions
    – Explain to the child that he will be standing or sitting upright and will need to take a deep breath and hold it and stay still while the picture is being taken

● **Echocardiography**
  - Purpose
    – Evaluates cardiac structures and functions using echoes from pulsed high-frequency sound waves
  - Nursing interventions
    – Doppler
      - Explain to the child that he will have to lie still during the procedure
      - Explain that the procedure is painless
    – Transesophageal
      - Explain to the child and family that the child will be given a medication to relax him before the procedure
      - Explain the procedure to the child and family — ultrasound combined with endoscopy
      - Maintain nothing-by-mouth status before the procedure

● **Electrophysiologic studies**
  - Purpose
    – Diagnoses conduction system disease
    – Diagnoses serious arrhythmias
  - Nursing interventions
    – Before the procedure

- Weigh the child and obtain vital signs
- Prepare the child for cardiac catheterization
- Maintain nothing-by-mouth status before the procedure
- Withhold antiarrhythmics and anticoagulants as ordered
- Explain the procedure to the child and family
  - After the procedure
    - Perform neurovascular checks distal to the catheter insertion site
    - Assess the puncture site for bleeding and hematoma
    - Restart antiarrhythmics and anticoagulants as ordered

● **Magnetic resonance imaging (MRI)**
- Purpose
  - Performed with or without a noniodinated contrast medium to define heart structure
  - Provides greater detail than a computed tomography scan
- Nursing interventions
  - Note if the child has surgically implanted metal objects (such as pins or clips), which would be a contraindication for the procedure
  - Explain the procedure to the parents and child
  - Make sure the child holds still during the test; sedation may be necessary

NURSING DIAGNOSES

● **Probable nursing diagnoses**
- Decreased cardiac output
- Impaired gas exchange

● **Possible nursing diagnoses**
- Anxiety
- Imbalanced nutrition: Less than body requirements

CONGENITAL HEART DEFECTS — DEFECTS THAT INCREASE PULMONARY BLOOD FLOW

● **Overview**
- Includes PDA, atrial septal defect, ventricular septal defect, and AV canal defect (see *Cardiac defects that increase pulmonary blood flow*, page 234)

● **Patent ductus arteriosus**
- Definition
  - The lumen of the duct between the aorta and pulmonary artery remains open after birth
- Causes
  - Unknown

Probable nursing diagnoses for a patient with a cardiovascular disorder

- Decreased cardiac output
- Impaired gas exchange

Defects that increase pulmonary blood flow

- PDA
- Atrial septal defect
- Ventricular septal defect
- AV canal defect

Cardiac defects that increase pulmonary blood flow

These illustrations depict three congenital heart defects that increase pulmonary blood flow: patent ductus arteriosus, atrial septal defect, and ventricular septal defect.

PATENT DUCTUS ARTERIOSUS

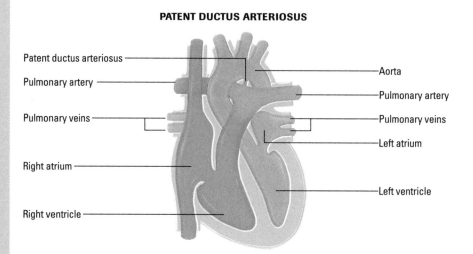

Patent ductus arteriosus

Pulmonary artery

Pulmonary veins

Right atrium

Right ventricle

Aorta

Pulmonary artery

Pulmonary veins

Left atrium

Left ventricle

ATRIAL SEPTAL DEFECT

VENTRICULAR SEPTAL DEFECT

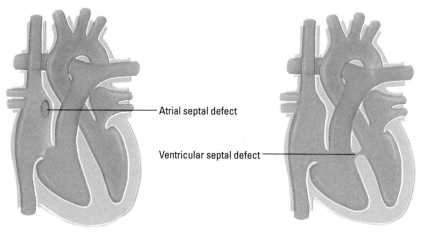

Atrial septal defect

Ventricular septal defect

Conditions associated with PDA

- Premature birth
- Maternal exposure to rubella during the first trimester
- Coarctation of the aorta
- Ventricular septal defect
- Pulmonary and aortic stenosis
- Living at high altitude, long-term exposure to low-blood oxygen tension
- Down syndrome

– May be a defect on one or more genes
– May be associated with:
  · Premature birth
  · Maternal exposure to rubella during the first trimester
  · Coarctation of the aorta
  · Ventricular septal defect

- Pulmonary and aortic stenosis
- Living at high altitude, long-term exposure to low-blood oxygen tension
- Infants with genetic abnormalities such as Down syndrome (trisomy 21)
- Pathophysiology
  - Persistent patency of the ductus arteriosus exists after birth
  - Aortic pressure shunts oxygenated blood from the aorta through the ductus arteriosus to the pulmonary artery
  - The blood returns to the left side of the heart and is again pumped into the aorta
  - Systemic hypoxia results
  - Most prevalent in premature neonates, probably as a result of abnormalities in oxygenation or the relaxant action of prostaglandin E, which prevents the ductal spasm and contracture necessary for closure
- Complications
  - Heart failure
  - Recurrent pneumonia
  - Bacterial endocarditis
  - Pulmonary hypertension
  - Pulmonary vascular disease
- Assessment findings
  - Respiratory distress with signs of heart failure (tachypnea, sweating, poor feeding, poor weight gain)
  - Bounding pulses and a wide pulse pressure
  - Hyperdynamic precordium
  - A continuous "machinery" murmur best heard at the left infraclavicular area or the upper left sternal border
- Diagnostic test findings
  - Chest X-ray
    - Prominent pulmonary vasculature
    - Varying degrees of cardiomegaly, with enlargement of the left atrium, left ventricle, and ascending aorta
  - ECG
    - Normal or left ventricular hypertrophy
    - Right ventricular hypertrophy if pulmonary vascular disease develops
  - Echocardiography
    - Detects and helps estimate the size of the PDA and provides visualization of the shunt
    - Shows an enlarged left atrium and ventricle or right ventricular hypertrophy if pulmonary vascular disease develops
- Medical management
  - Medications

Key assessment findings in PDA

- Respiratory distress with signs of heart failure
- Bounding pulses
- Wide pulse pressure
- Hyperdynamic precordium
- A continuous "machinery" murmur best heard at the left infraclavicular area or the upper left sternal border

How to monitor fluid status

- Enforce fluid restrictions as appropriate to prevent fluid overload.
- Weigh the child daily.
- Weigh soiled diapers.

Key nursing interventions for PDA

- Monitor vital signs, pulse oximetry, and intake and output.
- Assess cardiovascular and respiratory statuses.
- Monitor fluid status, enforcing fluid restriction as appropriate.
- Organize physical care and anticipate the need to reduce the child's oxygen demands.

Key facts about ASD

- Blood flows from left atrium to right atrium, rather than left atrium to left ventricle
- Caused by failure of the atrial septum to completely close by the 7th week of gestation
- Can result in atrial flutter or fibrillation
- Can result in heart failure or pulmonary hypertension in the 3rd or 4th decade of life
- Isolated defects smaller than 8 mm likely to close spontaneously by age 18 months

- • Anticongestive therapy: diuretics and fluid restriction
  - • Indomethacin (Indocin): prostaglandin synthetase inhibitor to achieve pharmacological closure of the PDA (only useful in premature neonates)
  - • Prophylactic antibiotics to prevent bacterial endocarditis
  - – Nonpharmacologic closure
    - • Surgical ligation, performed without bypass through a left posterolateral thoracotomy
    - • Catheter closure of the PDA with coils, done in the cardiac catheterization laboratory
- • Nursing interventions
  - – Explain the heart defect to the child and parents and answer any questions to prepare the child for cardiac catheterization or surgery
  - – Monitor vital signs, pulse oximetry, and intake and output to assess renal function and detect changes
  - – Assess cardiovascular and respiratory statuses to detect early signs of decompensation
  - – Monitor fluid status, enforcing fluid restriction as appropriate to prevent fluid overload
  - – Weigh the child daily to determine fluid overload or deficit
  - – Weigh soiled diapers to monitor fluid output
  - – Organize physical care and anticipate the need to reduce the child's oxygen demands
  - – Give the child high-calorie foods that are easy to ingest and digest
  - – Raise the head of the bed to ease respiratory status

● Atrial septal defect (ASD)

- • Definition
  - – An opening between the left and right atria permits blood flow from left atrium to right atrium, rather than left atrium to left ventricle
- • Causes
  - – Unknown
  - – May be associated with Down syndrome
- • Pathophysiology
  - – Failure of the atrial septum to completely close by the 7th week of gestation
  - – Blood shunts from the left atrium to the right atrium because left atrial pressure is normally slightly higher than right atrial pressure
- • Complications
  - – Heart failure, pulmonary hypertension (in the 3rd to 4th decade of life)
  - – Atrial flutter or fibrillation
  - – Stroke (rare)
- • Assessment findings
  - – Fatigue

– Early to midsystolic murmur and low-pitched diastolic murmur
– Fixed, widely split S_2
– Systolic click or late systolic murmur at the apex
– Clubbing of nails and cyanosis, if right-to-left shunt develops
• Diagnostic test findings
  – Chest X-ray
    · Enlargement of the right atrium and ventricle
    · Prominent pulmonary vasculature
  – ECG
    · Right axis deviation
    · Varying degrees of right bundle-branch block
    · Right ventricular hypertrophy
  – Echocardiography
    · Determines the anatomical location and size of the ASD
    · Provides visualization of the shunt
    · Right ventricular enlargement
    · Volume overload on the right side of the heart
• Medical management
  – Patients with isolated defects 3 to 8 mm in size have spontaneous closure rates of 80% by age 18 months
  – Patients with isolated defects less than 3 mm in size diagnosed by age 3 months have spontaneous closure rates of 100% by age 18 months
  – ASDs greater than 8 mm in size rarely close spontaneously
  – Medications: digoxin (Lanoxin) and diuretics if signs and symptoms of heart failure are present
  – Surgical closure
    · Direct closure of the defect with a patch or stitch closure
    · Procedure is performed under cardiopulmonary bypass through an atrial approach
  – Placement of an atrial occluder (done in the cardiac catheterization laboratory) is emerging as a prominent medical intervention for ASD closure
• Nursing interventions
  – Explain the heart defect to the child and parents and answer any questions to prepare the child for cardiac catheterization or surgery (see *Teaching about cardiac surgery,* page 238)
  – Monitor vital signs, pulse oximetry, and intake and output to assess renal function and detect changes
  – Assess cardiovascular and respiratory statuses to detect early signs of decompensation
  – Take the child's apical pulse for 1 minute before giving digoxin, and withhold the drug to prevent toxicity if the child's heart rate is below 100 beats/minute

Key assessment findings in ASD

• Fatigue
• Early to midsystolic murmur and low-pitched diastolic murmur
• Fixed, widely split S_2
• Systolic click or late systolic murmur at the apex
• Clubbing of nails and cyanosis, if right-to-left shunt develops

Managing ASD

• Possible spontaneous closure (80% chance by age 18 months in patients with isolated defects 3 to 8 mm; 100% chance by age 18 months in patients with isolated defects less than 3 mm in size diagnosed by age 3 months)
• Medication administration
• Surgical closure (patch or stitch)
• Placement of atrial occluder

Key nursing interventions for ASD

• Monitor vital signs, pulse oximetry, and intake and output.
• Assess cardiovascular and respiratory statuses.
• Take the child's apical pulse for 1 minute before giving digoxin; withhold the drug to prevent toxicity if the child's heart rate is below 100 beats/minute.
• Monitor fluid status, enforcing fluid restriction as appropriate to prevent fluid overload.
• Organize physical care and anticipate the need to reduce the child's oxygen demands.

TIME-OUT FOR TEACHING

Teaching about cardiac surgery

Be sure to include these points in your teaching plan for the parents of a child who has undergone cardiac surgery:
- dietary restrictions, if any
- fluid requirements and restrictions
- activity and exercise restrictions
- operative site care and inspection
- medication regimen
- follow-up tests and physician visits
- home care needs
- signs and symptoms of infection.

Key facts about VSD

- Involves an opening in the septum that allows blood to shunt between the left and right ventricle
- Occurs when closure of the ventricular septum is delayed
- Causes right ventricular hypertrophy and, eventually, biventricular heart failure if uncorrected

- Monitor fluid status, enforcing fluid restrictions as appropriate to prevent fluid overload
- Weigh the child daily to determine fluid overload or deficit
- Weigh soiled diapers to monitor fluid output
- Organize physical care and anticipate the need to reduce the child's oxygen demands
- Give the child high-calorie foods that are easy to ingest and digest
- Raise the head of the bed to ease respiratory status

● **Ventricular septal defect (VSD)**
- Definition
  - An opening in the septum between the ventricles that allows blood to shunt between the left and right ventricle
- Causes
  - Unknown
  - May be associated with:
    · Down syndrome or other autosomal trisomies
    · Renal anomalies, prematurity, fetal alcohol syndrome
    · PDA, coarctation of the aorta
- Pathophysiology
  - Delay in closure of the ventricular septum after the 7th week of gestation
  - As the pulmonary vasculature gradually relaxes (between 4 and 8 weeks after birth), right ventricular pressure decreases, allowing blood to shunt from the left to the right ventricle
  - Initially, large VSD shunts cause left atrial and left ventricular hypertrophy
  - Later, an uncorrected VSD causes right ventricular hypertrophy due to increasing pulmonary resistance; eventually biventricular heart failure occurs

- Complications
  - Bacterial endocarditis
  - Heart failure or pulmonary hypertension
  - Acquired left ventricular outflow tract obstruction
  - Aneurysm of the ventricular septum
  - Failure to thrive
  - Arrhythmia
- Assessment findings
  - Weight loss or absence of weight gain
  - Drop in height and head circumference percentile
  - Loud, harsh systolic murmur (along the left sternal border at the third or fourth intercostal space), palpable thrill
  - Loud, widely split pulmonic component of S_2
  - Displacement to left of point of maximal impulse
  - Prominent anterior chest
  - Liver, heart, and spleen enlargement
  - Diaphoresis
  - Tachycardia
  - Rapid, grunting respirations
- Diagnostic test findings
  - Chest X-ray
    - May be normal for small defects or show cardiomegaly with a large left atrium and ventricle
    - In a large defect, it may show prominent pulmonary vasculature
  - ECG
    - In a large defect, shows left and right ventricular hypertrophy, suggesting pulmonary hypertension
  - Echocardiography
    - Demonstrates the anatomic location, size, and number of VSDs and provides visualization of the shunt
  - Cardiac catheterization
    - Helps determine the size and exact location of the VSD
    - Helps determine the degree of shunting
- Medical management
  - Spontaneous closure of the VSD may occur in some infants by age 6 months
  - Medications
    - Digoxin and diuretics if signs and symptoms of heart failure develop
    - Prophylactic antibiotics to prevent bacterial endocarditis
    - Oral iron therapy if anemia develops
  - Surgical closure
    - Direct closure of the defect with a patch or stitch closure

Key nursing interventions for VSD

- Monitor vital signs, pulse oximetry, and intake and output.
- Assess cardiovascular and respiratory statuses.
- Take the child's apical pulse for 1 minute before giving digoxin; withhold the drug to prevent toxicity if the child's heart rate is below 100 beats/minute.
- Organize physical care and anticipate the need to reduce the child's oxygen demands.
- Raise the head of the bed to ease breathing.

Facts about AV canal defects

- Occurs when endocardial cushions fail to fuse completely
- Blood is shunted from left to right
- Frequently associated with Down syndrome

Assessment findings in AV canal defects

- Drop in weight, height, or head circumference percentile
- Signs of heart failure (usually present 6 to 8 weeks after birth)
- Tachycardia
- Tachypnea
- Systolic regurgitant murmur heard at the left lower sternal border

• Performed under cardiopulmonary bypass or deep hypothermia, preferably through an atrial approach

- Nursing interventions
  - Explain the heart defect to the child and parents and answer any questions to prepare the child for cardiac catheterization or surgery
  - Monitor vital signs, pulse oximetry, and intake and output to assess renal function and detect changes
  - Assess cardiovascular and respiratory statuses to detect early signs of decompensation
  - Take the child's apical pulse for 1 minute before giving digoxin, and withhold the drug to prevent toxicity if the child's heart rate is below 100 beats/minute
  - Monitor fluid status, enforcing fluid restrictions as appropriate to prevent fluid overload
  - Weigh the child daily to determine fluid overload or deficit
  - Weigh soiled diapers to monitor fluid output
  - Organize physical care and anticipate the need to reduce the child's oxygen demands
  - Give the child high-calorie foods that are easy to ingest and digest
  - Raise the head of the bed to ease respiratory status

Atrioventricular canal defect

- Definition
  - A defect occurring when the endocardial cushions fail to fuse completely
  - The defect includes a low ASD continuous with a high VSD, with clefts in the mitral and tricuspid valves (creating a common AV valve)
- Causes
  - Unknown
  - Frequently associated with Down syndrome
- Pathophysiology
  - Results from incomplete fusion of the endocardial cushions
  - Generally, blood is shunted from left to right once pulmonary vascular resistance drops; however, depending on the extent of the defect, blood may flow between all four heart chambers
- Complications
  - Bacterial endocarditis
  - Recurrent pneumonia
  - Pulmonary vascular disease
  - Failure to thrive
- Assessment findings
  - Weight loss or absence of weight gain
  - Drop in height or head circumference percentile

- Signs of heart failure (usually present 6 to 8 weeks after birth due to the fall in pulmonary vascular resistance that normally occurs)
- Tachycardia
- Tachypnea
- Systolic regurgitant murmur heard at the left lower sternal border due to mitral insufficiency
- Diagnostic test findings
  - Chest X-ray
    - Cardiomegaly
    - Increased pulmonary vascular markings and prominent pulmonary artery segment
  - ECG shows right ventricular hypertrophy or right bundle branch block
  - Echocardiography can determine the anatomy and functional significance of the atrioventricular canal defect and provides visualization of shunting and any regurgitation
- Medical management
  - Frequent feedings of high-calorie formula, orally or through a nasogastric tube, to help reverse growth failure
  - Medications
    - Digoxin and diuretics if signs of heart failure develop
    - Prophylactic antibiotics to prevent bacterial endocarditis
  - Surgical repair is indicated for all children with an AV canal defect
    - Patch closure of the ASD and VSD, with reconstruction of the AV valves
    - Procedure is performed under cardiopulmonary bypass or deep hypothermia
- Nursing interventions
  - Explain the heart defect to the child and parents and answer any questions to prepare the child for surgery
  - Monitor vital signs, pulse oximetry, and intake and output to assess renal function and detect changes
  - Assess cardiovascular and respiratory statuses to detect early signs of decompensation
  - Take the child's apical pulse for 1 minute before giving digoxin, and withhold the drug to prevent toxicity if the heart rate is below 100 beats/minute
  - Monitor fluid status, enforcing fluid restrictions as appropriate to prevent fluid overload
  - Weigh the child daily to determine fluid overload or deficit
  - Weigh soiled diapers to monitor fluid output
  - Organize physical care and anticipate the need to reduce the child's oxygen demands
  - Give the child high-calorie foods that are easy to ingest and digest
  - Raise the head of the bed to ease respiratory status

Managing AV canal defects

- Frequent feedings of high-calorie formula
- Medication administration
- Surgical repair (patch closure of ASD and VSD, with reconstruction of the AV valves)

Key nursing interventions for AV canal defects

- Monitor vital signs, pulse oximetry, and intake and output.
- Assess cardiovascular and respiratory statuses.
- Take the child's apical pulse for 1 minute before giving digoxin; withhold the drug to prevent toxicity if the child's heart rate is below 100 beats/minute.
- Monitor fluid status, enforcing fluid restrictions as appropriate to prevent fluid overload.
- Organize physical care and anticipate the need to reduce the child's oxygen demands.

Obstructive congenital heart defects

- Coarctation of the aorta
- Aortic stenosis
- Pulmonic stenosis

Key signs and symptoms of coarctation of the aorta

- Signs of heart failure
- Greater blood pressure in upper extremities than in lower extremities
- Pink upper extremities and cyanotic lower extremities
- Absent or diminished femoral pulses
- Continuous midsystolic murmur

CONGENITAL HEART DEFECTS — OBSTRUCTIVE DEFECTS

● Overview

- Defects that obstruct the flow of blood out of the heart, including coarctation of the aorta, aortic stenosis, and pulmonic stenosis

● Coarctation of the aorta

- Definition
  - A narrowing of the aorta just opposite the site of insertion of the ductus arteriosus (see *Recognizing coarctation of the aorta*)
- Causes
  - Unknown
  - May be associated with Turner's syndrome
  - May be associated with other heart defects, such as bicuspid aortic valve, VSD, PDA, and aortic or mitral valve stenosis
- Pathophysiology
  - Obstruction causes hypertension in the aortic branches before the constriction and diminished pressure in the vessel after the constriction
- Complications
  - Rupture of the aorta
  - Systemic hypertension
  - Stroke
  - Heart failure or shock in infancy
  - Left ventricular failure
  - Cerebral aneurysm
- Assessment findings
  - Signs of heart failure
  - Blood pressure greater in upper extremities than in lower extremities
  - Pink upper extremities and cyanotic lower extremities
  - Absent or diminished femoral pulses
  - Continuous midsystolic murmur
  - Chest and arms may be more developed than legs
- Diagnostic test findings
  - Chest X-ray
    - Left ventricular hypertrophy
    - Pulmonary edema
    - Wide ascending and descending aorta
    - Rib-notching from collateral circulation
  - ECG
    - Right ventricular hypertrophy or right bundle branch block in infants
    - Left ventricular hypertrophy in children with long-standing coarctation of the aorta

Recognizing coarctation of the aorta

Collateral circulation develops to bypass the occluding aortic lumen and can be seen on X-ray as notching of the ribs. By adolescence, palpable, visible pulsations may be evident.

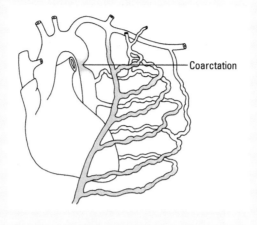

Coarctation

Medications used to manage coarctation of the aorta

- Prostaglandin E
- Inotropic agents
- Diuretics
- Prophylactic antibiotics

– Echocardiography
  • Demonstrates the location, size, and extent of the coarctation
  • Increased left ventricular muscle thickness
  • Coexisting aortic valve abnormalities
– MRI
  • Reveals location of the coarctation of the aorta and determines whether other vessels are affected
• Medical management
  – Medications
    • Prostaglandin E infusion to reopen or maintain a patent ductus arteriosus
    • Inotropic agents: dopamine, dobutamine
    • Diuretics
    • Prophylactic antibiotics to prevent bacterial endocarditis
  – Surgical correction
    • Performed without bypass through a left posterolateral thoracotomy
    • Types of repair
      – End-to-end anastomosis: the area of coarctation is resected and the distal and proximal aorta are anastomosed end to end
      – Patch aortoplasty: the area of coarctation is incised and an elliptical Dacron patch is sutured in place to widen the diameter
      – Subclavian flap aortoplasty: the distal subclavian artery is divided and the flap of the proximal portion of this vessel is used to expand the coarcted area
      – Bypass graft repair is performed by inserting a graft between the ascending and descending portion of the aorta

Types of surgical repair for coarctation of the aorta

- End-to-end anastomosis: the area of coarctation is resected and the distal and proximal aorta are anastomosed end to end
- Patch aortoplasty: the area of coarctation is incised and an elliptical Dacron patch is sutured in place to widen the diameter
- Subclavian flap aortoplasty: the distal subclavian artery is divided and the flap of the proximal portion of this vessel is used to expand the coarcted area
- Bypass graft repair: graft insertion between the ascending and descending portions of the aorta

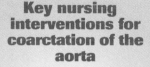

- The ductus arteriosus is always ligated with each of these surgical techniques
- Balloon angioplasty may be performed if recoarctation occurs
- Nursing interventions
  - Explain the heart defect to the child and parents and answer any questions to prepare the child for surgery
  - Monitor vital signs, pulse oximetry, and intake and output to assess renal function and detect changes
  - Assess cardiovascular and respiratory statuses to detect early signs of decompensation
  - Monitor fluid status, enforcing fluid restrictions as appropriate to prevent fluid overload
  - Weigh the child daily to determine fluid overload or deficit
  - Weigh soiled diapers to monitor fluid output
  - Organize physical care and anticipate the need to reduce the child's oxygen demands
  - Give the child high-calorie foods that are easy to ingest and digest
  - Raise the head of the bed to ease respiratory status

Aortic stenosis

- Definition
  - Narrowing or fusion of the aortic valve that interferes with left ventricular outflow to the aorta
- Causes
  - Unknown
  - Rheumatic fever
- Pathophysiology
  - Left ventricular pressure rises to overcome the resistance of the narrowed valvular opening
  - The added workload increases the demand for oxygen, and diminished cardiac output causes poor coronary artery perfusion, ischemia of the left ventricle, and left-sided heart failure
- Complications
  - Bacterial endocarditis
  - Pulmonary edema
  - Heart failure
  - Sudden death due to myocardial ischemia
- Assessment findings
  - Rough, systolic murmur heard loudest at the second intercostal space
  - Diminished carotid pulses
  - Systolic thrill
  - Syncope
  - Hypotension
  - Poor feeding

Key nursing interventions for coarctation of the aorta

- Monitor vital signs, pulse oximetry, and intake and output.
- Assess cardiovascular and respiratory statuses.
- Monitor fluid status, enforcing fluid restrictions as appropriate to prevent fluid overload.
- Organize physical care and anticipate the need to reduce the child's oxygen demands.

Complications of aortic stenosis

- Bacterial endocarditis
- Pulmonary edema
- Heart failure
- Sudden death

Key signs and symptoms of aortic stenosis

- Rough, systolic murmur at second intercostal space
- Diminished carotid pulses
- Systolic thrill
- Syncope
- Hypotension
- Angina-like chest pain on activity

– Angina-like chest pain on activity
- Diagnostic test findings
  – Chest X-ray
    · Left ventricular hypertrophy
    · Prominent pulmonary vasculature
  – ECG shows left ventricular hypertrophy
  – Echocardiography
    · Thickened aortic valve
    · Thickened left ventricular wall
  – Cardiac catheterization demonstrates the degree of the stenosis
- Medical management
  – Medications
    · Digoxin and diuretics for signs of heart failure
    · Anticoagulant therapy to prevent thrombus formation around the stenotic or replaced valve
    · Prophylactic antibiotics to prevent bacterial endocarditis
  – Surgical repair
    · Aortic valvulotomy or prosthetic valve replacement
    · Balloon angioplasty may be used to dilate the stenotic valve
- Nursing interventions
  – Explain the heart defect to the child and parents and answer any questions to prepare the child for cardiac catheterization or surgery
  – Monitor vital signs, pulse oximetry, and intake and output to assess renal function and detect changes
  – Assess cardiovascular and respiratory statuses to detect early signs of decompensation
  – Take the child's apical pulse for 1 minute before giving digoxin and withhold the drug to prevent toxicity if the child's heart rate is below 100 beats/minute
  – Monitor fluid status, enforcing fluid restrictions as appropriate to prevent fluid overload
  – Weigh the child daily to determine fluid overload or deficit
  – Weigh soiled diapers to monitor fluid output
  – Organize physical care and anticipate the need to reduce the child's oxygen demands
  – Give the child high-calorie foods that are easy to ingest and digest
  – Raise the head of the bed to ease respiratory status

Pulmonic stenosis
- Definition
  – A narrowing or fusing of pulmonic valve leaflets at the entrance of the pulmonary artery that interferes with right ventricular outflow to the lungs
- Causes
  – Congenital

– Rheumatic fever
- Pathophysiology
  – Obstructed right ventricular outflow causes right ventricular hypertrophy, resulting in right-sided heart failure
- Complications
  – Bacterial endocarditis
  – Heart failure
- Assessment findings
  – May be asymptomatic
  – Signs of heart failure
  – Systolic murmur heard loudest at the upper left sternal border, split S_2
- Diagnostic test findings
  – Chest X-ray, ECG, and echocardiography may show evidence of right ventricular hypertrophy
  – Cardiac catheterization demonstrates the degree of the stenosis
- Medical management
  – Medications
    · Digoxin and diuretics for signs of heart failure
    · Anticoagulant therapy to prevent thrombus formation around the stenotic valve
    · Prophylactic antibiotics to prevent bacterial endocarditis
  – Surgical repair
    · Balloon angioplasty is being used widely to relieve pulmonic stenosis
    · Valvulotomy may be necessary
- Nursing interventions
  – Explain the heart defect to the child and parents and answer any questions to prepare the child for cardiac catheterization or surgery
  – Monitor vital signs, pulse oximetry, and intake and output to assess renal function and detect changes
  – Assess cardiovascular and respiratory statuses to detect early signs of decompensation
  – Take the child's apical pulse for 1 minute before giving digoxin and withhold the drug to prevent toxicity if the child's heart rate is below 100 beats/minute
  – Monitor fluid status, enforcing fluid restrictions as appropriate to prevent fluid overload
  – Weigh the child daily to determine fluid overload or deficit
  – Weigh soiled diapers to monitor fluid output
  – Organize physical care and anticipate the need to reduce the child's oxygen demands
  – Give the child high-calorie foods that are easy to ingest and digest
  – Raise the head of the bed to ease respiratory status

Complications of pulmonic stenosis

- Bacterial endocarditis
- Heart failure

Managing pulmonic stenosis

- Digoxin and diuretics for heart failure
- Anticoagulant to prevent thrombus formation
- Prophylactic antibiotics to prevent bacterial endocarditis
- Balloon angioplasty to relieve pulmonic stenosis
- Valvulotomy

CONGENITAL HEART DEFECTS — MIXED DEFECTS

● **Characteristics**
- Defects that cause mixed blood flow — oxygenated and deoxygenated blood mix in the heart or great vessels
- Includes transposition of the great vessels, truncus arteriosus, and hypoplastic left heart syndrome

● **Transposition of the great vessels**
- Definition
  - The aorta rises from the right ventricle, and the pulmonary artery from the left ventricle, producing two noncommunicating circulatory systems (see *A look at transposition of the great vessels*)
- Causes
  - Unknown
- Pathophysiology
  - The transposed pulmonary artery carries oxygenated blood back to the lungs, rather than to the left side of the heart
  - The transposed aorta returns unoxygenated blood to the systemic circulation rather than to the lungs
  - Communication between the pulmonary and systemic circulation is necessary for survival; the presence of other congenital defects, such as ASD or VSD, is necessary to sustain life
- Complications
  - Bacterial endocarditis

A look at transposition of the great vessels

This illustration shows transposition of the great vessels, in which the aorta arises from the right ventricle, and the pulmonary artery arises from the left ventricle.

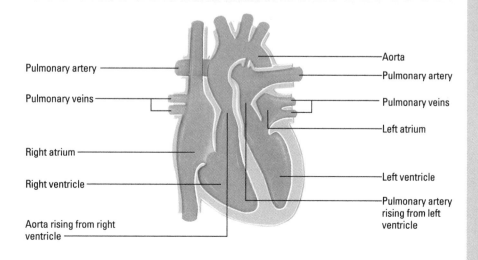

Pulmonary artery

Pulmonary veins

Right atrium

Right ventricle

Aorta rising from right ventricle

Aorta

Pulmonary artery

Pulmonary veins

Left atrium

Left ventricle

Pulmonary artery rising from left ventricle

Characteristics of mixed defects

- Cause mix of oxygenated and deoxygenated blood in heart or great vessels
- Includes transposition of the great vessels, truncus arteriosus, and hypoplastic left heart syndrome

Key facts about transposition of the great vessels

- Aorta rises from right ventricle; pulmonary artery, from left ventricle, producing two noncommunicating circulatory systems
- Unknown cause
- Transposed pulmonary artery carries oxygenated blood back to left side of heart
- Transposed aorta returns unoxygenated blood to systemic circulation rather than to lungs

Key signs of transposition of the great vessels

- Cyanosis and tachypnea (worsen with crying)
- Gallop rhythm
- Tachycardia
- Dyspnea
- Hepatomegaly
- Cardiomegaly
- Murmurs
- Fatigue
- Clubbing

Test findings with transposition of the great vessels

- Oblong appearance of the heart on chest X-ray
- Increased pulmonary vascular markings
- Right axis deviation and right ventricular hypertrophy
- Reversed position of the aorta and pulmonary artery
- Decreased oxygen saturation in left ventricular blood and aortic blood
- Increased right atrial, right ventricular, and pulmonary artery oxygen saturation
- Right ventricular systolic pressure equal to systemic pressure

Managing transposition of the great vessels

- Prostaglandin E to maintain patency of the ductus arteriosus
- Prophylactic antibiotics to prevent bacterial endocarditis
- Atrial balloon septostomy to enlarge patent foramen ovale, improving oxygenation
- Corrective surgery to redirect blood flow

– Death
- Assessment findings
    – Cyanosis from birth and tachypnea (worsen with crying)
    – Gallop rhythm
    – Tachycardia
    – Dyspnea
    – Hepatomegaly
    – Cardiomegaly
    – Murmurs of ASD, VSD, or PDA, loud S_2
    – Diminished exercise tolerance
    – Fatigue
    – Clubbing
- Diagnostic test findings
    – Chest X-ray
        · Right atrial and ventricular enlargement cause a characteristic oblong appearance to heart
        · Increased pulmonary vascular markings
    – ECG
        · May indicate right axis deviation and right ventricular hypertrophy
    – Echocardiography
        · Demonstrates the reversed position of the aorta and pulmonary artery
        · Detects other cardiac defects
    – Cardiac catheterization
        · Decreased oxygen saturation in left ventricular blood and aortic blood
        · Increased right atrial, right ventricular, and pulmonary artery oxygen saturation
        · Right ventricular systolic pressure equal to systemic pressure
        · Dye injection reveals transposed vessels and the presence of any other cardiac defects
- Medical management
    – Medications
        · Prostaglandin E to maintain patency of the ductus arteriosus
        · Prophylactic antibiotics to prevent bacterial endocarditis
    – Atrial balloon septostomy done during cardiac catheterization to enlarge the patent foramen ovale, which improves oxygenation by allowing greater mixing of the pulmonary and systemic circulations
    – Corrective surgery to redirect blood flow by switching the position of the major blood vessels
- Nursing interventions
    – Explain the heart defect to the child and parents and answer any questions to prepare the child for cardiac catheterization or surgery

– Monitor vital signs, pulse oximetry, and intake and output to assess renal function and detect changes

– Assess cardiovascular and respiratory statuses to detect early signs of decompensation

– Monitor fluid status, enforcing fluid restrictions as appropriate to prevent fluid overload

– Weigh the child daily to determine fluid overload or deficit

– Weigh soiled diapers to monitor fluid output

– Organize physical care and anticipate the need to reduce the child's oxygen demands

– Give the child high-calorie foods that are easy to ingest and digest

– Encourage parents to help their child assume new activity levels and independence

● **Truncus arteriosus**

• Definition

– Failure of the common great vessel to divide into the pulmonary artery and aorta, resulting in one major vessel (or "trunk") arising from the left and right ventricles

– Usually accompanied by a VSD

• Causes

– Unknown

– Possibly caused by rubella or another viral illness during early pregnancy

– A parent who had a congenital heart defect

– A mother with diabetes

– Excessive alcohol consumption during pregnancy

– Down syndrome

• Pathophysiology

– Deoxygenated blood from the right ventricle and oxygenated blood from the left ventricle mix and are ejected through the common vessel to the lungs and systemic circulation

• Complications

– Heart failure

– Cardiomegaly

– Death

– Pulmonary hypertension

• Assessment findings

– Cyanosis

– Signs of heart failure

– Hyperactive precordium

– Bounding pulses

– Typical murmur of VSD

– Poor weight gain

– Poor appetite

Test findings with truncus arteriosus

- Cardiomegaly and increased pulmonary blood flow
- Right or biventricular hypertrophy
- Visualization of defect

Key nursing interventions for truncus arteriosus

- Monitor vital signs, pulse oximetry, intake, and output.
- Assess cardiovascular and respiratory statuses.
- Monitor fluid status.
- Take the child's apical pulse for 1 minute before giving digoxin; withhold the drug to prevent toxicity if the heart rate is below 100 beats/minute.
- Organize physical care and anticipate the need to reduce the child's oxygen demands.
- Encourage parents to help the child assume new activity levels and independence.

Key facts about hypoplastic left heart syndrome

- Underdevelopment of left side of heart
- Causes aortic valve atresia or stenosis, mitral valve atresia or stenosis, diminutive or absent left ventricle, and severe hypoplasia of the ascending aorta and aortic arch
- Unknown cause
- Blood from left atrium travels through patent foramen ovale to right ventricle and pulmonary artery, entering the systemic circulation via the ductus arteriosus
- Without surgery, death occurs in early infancy

- Diagnostic test findings
  - Chest X-ray shows cardiomegaly and increased pulmonary blood flow
  - ECG indicates right or biventricular hypertrophy
  - Echocardiography provides visualization of the defect and a VSD
- Medical management
  - Medications: digoxin and diuretics to control heart failure
  - Surgical repair that involves separating the pulmonary arteries and reconnecting them to the right ventricle by implanting an arterial graft with its valves intact, and closure of the VSD
- Nursing interventions
  - Explain the heart defect to the child and parents and answer any questions to prepare the child for surgery
  - Monitor vital signs, pulse oximetry, and intake and output to assess renal function and detect change
  - Assess cardiovascular and respiratory status to detect early signs of decompensation
  - Monitor fluid status, enforcing fluid restrictions as appropriate to prevent fluid overload
  - Take the child's apical pulse for 1 minute before giving digoxin, and withhold the drug to prevent toxicity if the child's heart rate is below 100 beats/minute
  - Weigh the child daily to determine fluid overload or deficit
  - Weigh soiled diapers to monitor fluid output
  - Organize physical care and anticipate the need to reduce the child's oxygen demands
  - Give the child high-calorie foods that are easy to ingest and digest
  - Encourage the parents to help their child assume new activity levels and independence

- **Hypoplastic left heart syndrome**
  - Definition
    - Underdevelopment of the left side of the heart
    - Defects include:
      - Aortic valve atresia or stenosis
      - Mitral valve atresia or stenosis
      - Diminutive or absent left ventricle
      - Severe hypoplasia of the ascending aorta and aortic arch
  - Causes
    - Unknown
  - Pathophysiology
    - Blood from the left atrium travels through a patent foramen ovale to the right ventricle and pulmonary artery, entering the systemic circulation via the ductus arteriosus

– Patency of the ductus arteriosus, which allows blood flow to the systemic circulation, is necessary to sustain life

- Complications
  – Heart failure
  – Death
- Assessment findings
  – Cyanosis
  – Weak or absent pulses
  – Signs of heart failure, such as tachycardia, sweating, cardiomegaly, tachypnea, cyanosis, and peripheral edema
- Diagnostic test findings
  – Echocardiography provides visualization of the defect
- Medical management
  – Medications
    - Prostaglandin E to maintain patency of the ductus arteriosus
    - Digoxin and diuretics to control heart failure
  – Surgical repair
    - Heart transplantation
    - Norwood procedure: a two-stage procedure that involves re-structuring the heart
    - Without surgery, death occurs in early infancy
- Nursing interventions
  – Explain the heart defect to the child and parents and answer any questions to prepare the child for surgery
  – Monitor vital signs, pulse oximetry, and intake and output to assess renal function and detect change
  – Assess cardiovascular and respiratory status to detect early signs of decompensation
  – Monitor fluid status, enforcing fluid restrictions as appropriate to prevent fluid overload
  – Take the child's apical pulse for 1 minute before giving digoxin, and withhold the drug to prevent toxicity if the child's heart rate is below 100 beats/minute
  – Weigh the child daily to determine fluid overload or deficit
  – Weigh soiled diapers to monitor fluid output
  – Organize physical care and anticipate the need to reduce the child's oxygen demands

CONGENITAL HEART DEFECTS — DEFECTS THAT DECREASE PULMONARY BLOOD FLOW

- **Tricuspid atresia**
  - Definition

Signs and symptoms of hypoplastic left heart syndrome

- Cyanosis
- Weak or absent pulses
- Signs of heart failure

Managing hypoplastic left heart syndrome

- Prostaglandin E to maintain patency of the ductus arteriosus
- Digoxin and diuretics to control heart failure
- Heart transplantation
- Norwood procedure

Key facts about tricuspid atresia

- Failure of tricuspid valve to develop prevents blood from entering right ventricle from right atrium
- Unknown cause
- May be associated with pulmonic stenosis or transposition of the great vessels
- Deoxygenated blood mixes with oxygenated blood then passes to left ventricle and through a VSD to right ventricle, pulmonary artery, and lungs or mixed blood refluxes back through the patent ductus arteriosus to lungs

Signs and symptoms of tricuspid atresia

- Cyanosis
- Tachycardia
- Dyspnea
- Murmur

Key test findings with tricuspid atresia

- Enlarged right atrium and decreased pulmonary blood flow
- Left-axis deviation and absent right ventricular forces
- Visualization of the defect and shunting

Key nursing interventions for tricuspid atresia

- Monitor vital signs, pulse oximetry, and intake and output.
- Assess cardiovascular and respiratory statuses.
- Monitor fluid status, enforcing fluid restrictions as appropriate to prevent fluid overload.
- Organize physical care and anticipate the need to reduce the child's oxygen demands.

– Failure of the tricuspid valve to develop, allowing no blood to enter the right ventricle from the right atrium
- Causes
  – Unknown
  – May be associated with pulmonic stenosis or transposition of the great vessels
- Pathophysiology
  – Deoxygenated blood shunts from the right atrium through an ASD or a patent foramen ovale to the left atrium, where it mixes with oxygenated blood
  – This mixed blood then passes to the left ventricle and through a VSD to the right ventricle, pulmonary artery, and lungs, or mixed blood from the aorta refluxes back through the patent ductus arteriosus to the lungs
- Assessment findings
  – Cyanosis
  – Tachycardia
  – Dyspnea
  – Heart murmur
- Diagnostic test findings
  – Chest X-ray shows an enlarged right atrium and decreased pulmonary blood flow
  – ECG indicates left-axis deviation and absent right ventricular forces
  – Echocardiography provides visualization of the defect and shunting
- Medical management
  – Medications: prostaglandin E to maintain ductal patency
  – Surgical repair
    · Subclavian-to-pulmonary artery shunt to improve blood flow to the lungs
    · Fontan procedure: restructures the right side of the heart
- Nursing interventions
  – Explain the heart defect to the child and parents and answer any questions to prepare the child for surgery
  – Monitor vital signs, pulse oximetry, and intake and output to assess renal function and detect changes
  – Assess cardiovascular and respiratory statuses to detect early signs of decompensation
  – Monitor fluid status, enforcing fluid restrictions as appropriate to prevent fluid overload
  – Weigh the child daily to determine fluid overload or deficit
  – Weigh soiled diapers to monitor fluid output
  – Organize physical care and anticipate the need to reduce the child's oxygen demands

A look at tetralogy of Fallot

This illustration shows the cardiac defects that create tetralogy of Fallot.

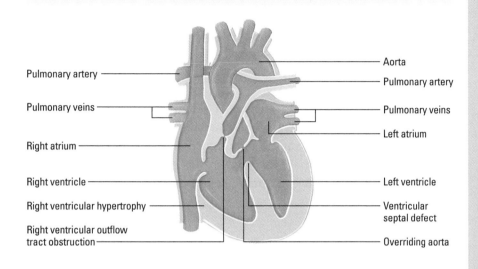

Pulmonary artery

Pulmonary veins

Right atrium

Right ventricle

Right ventricular hypertrophy

Right ventricular outflow tract obstruction

Aorta

Pulmonary artery

Pulmonary veins

Left atrium

Left ventricle

Ventricular septal defect

Overriding aorta

● **Tetralogy of Fallot**
  - Definition
    - Combination of four cardiac defects (see *A look at tetralogy of Fallot*)
      - VSD
      - Right ventricular outflow obstruction
      - Right ventricular hypertrophy
      - Aorta positioned above the VSD (overriding aorta)
  - Causes
    - Unknown
    - May be associated with fetal alcohol syndrome
  - Pathophysiology
    - Unoxygenated venous blood entering the right side of the heart may pass through the VSD to the left ventricle, bypassing the lungs, or it may enter the pulmonary artery, depending on the extent of the pulmonic stenosis
  - Complications
    - Hypercyanotic spells (tet spells)
    - Right ventricular dysfunction
    - Bacterial endocarditis
    - Polycythemia
    - Death
  - Assessment findings
    - Cyanosis
    - Hypercyanotic or "blue" spells (tet spells)

Key signs and symptoms of tetralogy of Fallot

- Cyanosis
- Tet spells
- Clubbing of digits
- Increased dyspnea on exertion
- Growth retardation
- Difficulty eating
- Loud systolic murmur along left sternal border
- Thrill at left sternal border
- Right ventricular impulse and prominent inferior sternum

Key nursing interventions for tetralogy of Fallot

- Monitor vital signs, pulse oximetry, and intake and output.
- Assess cardiovascular and respiratory statuses.
- Monitor fluid status, enforcing fluid restrictions as appropriate to prevent fluid overload.
- Don't interfere when the child is squatting if he appears comfortable; infants may be more comfortable in a knee-chest position.
- Teach parents to recognize serious hypoxic spells.
- If the child has undergone the Blalock-Taussig procedure, don't use the arm on the operative side for measuring blood pressure, inserting I.V. lines, or drawing blood samples.
- Organize physical care and anticipate the need to reduce the child's oxygen demands.
- Encourage parents to help their child assume new activity levels and independence.

– Clubbing of digits
– Diminished exercise tolerance and increased dyspnea on exertion
– Growth retardation
– Difficulty eating
– Squatting to reduce shortness of breath
– Loud systolic murmur heard best along the left sternal border
– Thrill at left sternal border
– Right ventricular impulse and prominent inferior sternum
- Diagnostic test findings
  – Chest X-ray demonstrates a boot-shaped cardiac silhouette and decreased pulmonary vascular markings
  – ECG shows right ventricular hypertrophy, right axis deviation and, possibly, right atrial hypertrophy
  – Echocardiography and cardiac catheterization provide visualization of the defects
- Medical management
  – Knee-chest position and oxygen and morphine administration to improve oxygenation during tet spells
  – Medications
    · Propranolol (Inderal) to prevent tet spells
    · Prophylactic antibiotics to prevent bacterial endocarditis
  – Surgical repair
    · Palliative surgery to reduce hypoxia during tet spells (Blalock-Taussig procedure — joins the subclavian artery to the pulmonary artery)
    · Complete surgical closure to relieve pulmonary stenosis and close the VSD, directing left ventricular outflow to the aorta (Brock procedure); requires cardiopulmonary bypass with hypothermia to decrease oxygen utilization during surgery
- Nursing interventions
  – Explain the heart defect to the child and parents and answer any questions to prepare the child for surgery
  – Monitor vital signs, pulse oximetry, and intake and output to assess renal function and detect changes
  – Assess cardiovascular and respiratory statuses to detect early signs of decompensation
  – Monitor fluid status, enforcing fluid restrictions as appropriate to prevent fluid overload
  – Weigh the child daily to determine fluid overload or deficit
  – Weigh soiled diapers to monitor fluid output
  – Provide adequate nutrition to prevent sequelae of polycythemia
  – Don't interfere when the child is squatting if he appears comfortable; infants may be more comfortable when placed in a knee-chest position

- Teach parents to recognize serious hypoxic spells (which can cause dramatically increased cyanosis; deep, sighing respirations; and loss of consciousness); tell them to report such spells immediately because emergency treatment may be necessary
- If the child has undergone the Blalock-Taussig procedure, don't use the arm on the operative side for measuring blood pressure, inserting I.V. lines, or drawing blood samples because blood perfusion on this side diminishes greatly until collateral circulation develops
- Organize physical care and anticipate the need to reduce the child's oxygen demands
- Give the child high-calorie foods that are easy to ingest and digest
- Encourage parents to help their child assume new activity levels and independence

RHEUMATIC FEVER

● Definition
- A systemic inflammatory disease of childhood, usually recurrent
- Follows a group A streptococcal infection; with an untreated strep infection, 1% to 5% of patients develop rheumatic fever

● Causes
- Altered host resistance to streptococcal infections
- Familial
- Malnutrition
- Crowded living conditions

● Pathophysiology
- Hypersensitivity reaction to a group A beta-hemolytic streptococcal infection in which antibodies manufactured to combat streptococci react and produce characteristic lesions at specific tissue sites, especially in the heart and joints
- Results in antigen-antibody complexes that ultimately destroy heart tissue
- Rheumatic heart disease refers to cardiac manifestations of rheumatic fever
  - Pancarditis (myocarditis, pericarditis, and endocarditis) during the early acute phase
  - Chronic valvular disease later

● Complications
- Valvular disease

● Assessment findings
- The Jones criteria for assessing major rheumatic fever:
  - Carditis
  - Chorea

- Erythema marginatum (temporary, disk-shaped, nonpruritic, red-dened macules that fade in the center, leaving raised margins)
  - Polyarthritis
  - Subcutaneous nodules
- The Jones criteria for assessing minor rheumatic fever:
  - Arthralgia
  - Prolonged PR interval
  - Fever
  - Elevated acute phase reactants (erythrocyte sedimentation rate and C-reactive protein)
- To complete the Jones criteria, evidence of a preceding group A streptococcal infection must also exist

● **Diagnostic test findings**
- Antistreptolysin-O titer is elevated
- Positive throat culture or rapid strep antigen test for group A streptococci
- Erythrocyte sedimentation rate is increased
- ECG shows prolonged PR interval
- Echocardiography helps evaluate valvular damage, chamber size, and ventricular function
- Cardiac catheterization evaluates valvular damage and left ventricular function in severe cardiac dysfunction

● **Medical management**
- Medications
  - Analgesic: anti-inflammatory for arthritis pain
  - Antibiotic: penicillin to prevent damage from future attacks (taken until age 20 or for 5 years after the attack, whichever is longer)
- Strict bed rest for about 5 weeks during the acute phase with active carditis, followed by a progressive increase in physical activity, depending on clinical and laboratory findings and the response to treatment
- Valvular surgery for damaged valves

● **Nursing interventions**
- Monitor vital signs and intake and output to detect fluid volume over-load or deficit
- Institute safety measures for chorea; maintain a calm environment, re-duce stimulation, avoid the use of forks or glass, and assist in walking to prevent injury
- Encourage bed rest as ordered; assist in arranging for home schooling and diversified activities as needed
- Provide appropriate passive stimulation to maintain growth and de-velopment
- Provide emotional support for long-term convalescence to help relieve anxiety
- Note a history of and monitor for penicillin allergy

• Promote good dental hygiene to prevent gingival infection; make sure the child and his family understand the need to comply with prolonged antibiotic therapy and follow-up care and the need for additional antibiotics during dental surgery or procedures

NCLEX CHECKS

It's never too soon to begin your NCLEX preparation. Now that you've reviewed this chapter, carefully read each of the following questions and choose the best answer. Then compare your responses to the correct answers.

1. An infant with a VSD is receiving digoxin (Lanoxin). Which intervention by the nurse is most appropriate before digoxin administration?
- ☐ **1.** Take the infant's blood pressure.
- ☐ **2.** Check the infant's respiratory rate for 1 minute.
- ☐ **3.** Check the infant's radial pulse for 1 minute.
- ☐ **4.** Check the infant's apical pulse for 1 minute.

2. An infant is diagnosed with PDA. Which drug may be administered to achieve pharmacologic closure of the defect?
- ☐ **1.** Digoxin (Lanoxin)
- ☐ **2.** Prednisone (Deltasone)
- ☐ **3.** Furosemide (Lasix)
- ☐ **4.** Indomethacin (Indocin)

3. A nurse checks an infant's apical pulse before digoxin (Lanoxin) administration and finds that the pulse rate is 90 beats/minute. Which nursing action is most appropriate?
- ☐ **1.** Withhold the digoxin and notify the physician.
- ☐ **2.** Administer the digoxin and notify the physician.
- ☐ **3.** Administer the digoxin and document the infant's pulse.
- ☐ **4.** Administer one-half of the digoxin dose and notify the physician.

4. Which cardiac defects are associated with tetralogy of Fallot? Select all that apply.
- ☐ **1.** ASD
- ☐ **2.** VSD
- ☐ **3.** Right ventricular hypertrophy
- ☐ **4.** Aortic stenosis
- ☐ **5.** Hypoplastic left heart syndrome
- ☐ **6.** Right ventricular outflow obstruction
- ☐ **7.** Overriding aorta

TOP 6

Items to study for your next test on the cardiovascular system

1. Structures of the heart
2. Structures involved in fetal circulation
3. Nursing interventions for cardiac catheterization
4. Assessment findings in PDA
5. The four defects of tetralogy of Fallot
6. Jones criteria for assessing rheumatic heart fever

5. A child with coarctation of the aorta has faint femoral pulses bilaterally, 1+ peripheral edema, and cyanosis of the lower extremities extending from midcalf to the toes. Which action should the nurse take?

☐ **1.** Call the physician immediately.

☐ **2.** Obtain a pulse oximetry of the lower extremities.

☐ **3.** Document your findings.

☐ **4.** Call the physician and obtain an order for Doppler studies of the lower extremities.

6. A nurse is caring for a child with AV canal defect. Upon entering the room, the nurse sees the mother lying in bed with the child, who is lying flat and drinking from a bottle. Which intervention should be implemented?

☐ **1.** Immediately raise the child into an upright position.

☐ **2.** Explain to the mother that the child should be in an upright position and should take frequent breaks when eating to ease his breathing.

☐ **3.** Take the bottle from the mother and demonstrate how to hold the child while feeding.

☐ **4.** Inform the mother she shouldn't be lying with her child in bed for safety reasons.

7. A pediatric cardiologist has just informed the parents of a neonate with transposition of the great vessels that he needs a cardiac catheterization. The father asks the nurse, "Why is he going to enlarge a hole in my son's heart? Isn't that going to cause more problems?" Which statement by the nurse is appropriate?

☐ **1.** "I'll have the pediatrician answer your questions."

☐ **2.** "You must have misunderstood; they won't enlarge a hole in your son's heart."

☐ **3.** "I'll have a cardiac nurse explain the procedure to you."

☐ **4.** "The physician will enlarge a 'hole' that's already open in your son's heart. Enlarging it will allow for more oxygenated blood to flow throughout your son's body."

8. A neonate is admitted with a medical diagnosis of tetralogy of Fallot. The mother yells for a nurse and states, "He's having another one of his spells." The nurse notices the client is cyanotic, dyspneic, and is in a fetal position. Which action should the nurse take?

☐ **1.** Administer oxygen and morphine as ordered.

☐ **2.** Raise the head of the bed and increase the oxygen by 2 L.

☐ **3.** Call the pediatrician immediately.

☐ **4.** Call a code.

9. A nurse is caring for a neonate who presents to the neonatal intensive care unit with cyanosis, tachycardia, dyspnea, and a heart murmur. The physician suspects tricuspid atresia. Which diagnostic procedure should the nurse anticipate will be ordered?

☐ **1.** Arterial blood gas (ABG) analysis
☐ **2.** Pulmonary function tests
☐ **3.** ECG
☐ **4.** Cardiac catheterization

10. A child who had rheumatic fever now has a complication of mild mitral valve prolapse. What information should be included in the child's discharge instructions?

☐ **1.** Report bruising and bleeding to the physician.
☐ **2.** Increase intake of fruits and vegetables.
☐ **3.** Encourage exercise.
☐ **4.** Comply with antibiotic therapy during dental surgeries or procedures.

ANSWERS AND RATIONALES

1. CORRECT ANSWER: 4
Before administering digoxin, the nurse should check the infant's apical pulse for 1 minute. Checking the radial pulse may be inaccurate. Checking the blood pressure and respiratory rate isn't necessary before digoxin administration because the medication doesn't affect these parameters.

2. CORRECT ANSWER: 4
Indomethacin is administered to an infant with PDA in hopes of closing the defect. Digoxin and furosemide may be used to treat the symptoms associated with PDA, but they don't achieve closure. Prednisone isn't used to treat PDA.

3. CORRECT ANSWER: 1
The nurse should withhold the digoxin and notify the physician because an apical pulse below 100 beats/minute in an infant is considered bradycardic. The nurse should also document her findings and interventions in the medical record. Administering the drug to an infant who is already bradycardic could further decrease his heart rate and compromise his status.

4. CORRECT ANSWER: 2, 3, 6, 7
VSD, right ventricular hypertrophy, right ventricular outflow obstruction, and an overriding aorta are four cardiac defects associated with tetralogy of Fallot. ASD, aortic stenosis, and hypoplastic left-sided heart failure are other congenital heart defects.

5. CORRECT ANSWER: 3

These findings are typical for a medical diagnosis of coarctation of the aorta and the nurse should document her findings. Pulse oximetry and Doppler studies of the lower extremities can confirm cyanosis, which the nurse has already detected.

6. CORRECT ANSWER: 2

The mother needs education regarding why the child should be raised to an upright position with frequent breaks to help him breath easier. The nurse may demonstrate how to feed the child but the mother requires education regarding frequent breaks so the child may breathe easier. The mother should be allowed to lie in the bed with the child and provide comfort.

7. CORRECT ANSWER: 4

A nurse's role is to be informed of procedures and to explain them to the parents and child. The pediatrician and cardiac nurse shouldn't be called to answer the parent's questions unless the parent has specific medical questions beyond the nurse's ability to answer.

8. CORRECT ANSWER: 1

The medical treatment for tetralogy of Fallot requires oxygenation, morphine, and a knee-to-chest position to ease respiratory cyanosis during these spells. Raising the head of the bed and providing oxygen aren't necessary because the child is already in a fetal position. Calling the pediatrician and a code aren't appropriate interventions at this time since the oxygen and morphine measures haven't been implemented.

9. CORRECT ANSWER: 3

The ECG indicates left-axis deviation and absent right ventricular forces. ABG analysis will validate the hypoxemia which is already known. Pulmonary function tests aren't required since the defect is cardiac in nature. A cardiac catheterization isn't necessary because an ECG will provide the diagnostic information.

10. CORRECT ANSWER: 4

The child with a history of rheumatic fever that has caused valvular damage must be placed on antibiotic therapy for dental procedures and surgeries to prevent carditis. There's no reason to report bruising or bleeding to the physician. Promoting good nutrition is important for all disorders. The child should be on bed rest for 5 weeks during the acute phase.

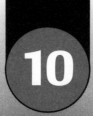

10

Altered gastrointestinal functioning

PRETEST

1. Which condition is suspected when an infant fails to pass meconium in the first 24 hours after birth?

- ☐ 1. Necrotizing enterocolitis
- ☐ 2. Hirschsprung's disease
- ☐ 3. Celiac disease
- ☐ 4. Meckel's diverticulum

CORRECT ANSWER: 2

2. A 6-month-old infant has colicky pain and is passing stools that appear "red and currant jellylike." The nurse should suspect which condition?

- ☐ 1. Intussusception
- ☐ 2. Pyloric stenosis
- ☐ 3. Cystic fibrosis
- ☐ 4. Helicobacter gastritis

CORRECT ANSWER: 1

3. Due to immature liver development, infants are more prone to:

- ☐ 1. hyperglycemia.
- ☐ 2. hypernatremia.
- ☐ 3. hypoglycemia.
- ☐ 4. hyponatremia.

CORRECT ANSWER: 3

4. Which conditions would a nurse expect to see when celiac disease is present?

☐ 1. Hypocalcemia and hyperalbuminemia

☐ 2. Hypocalcemia and hypoalbuminemia

☐ 3. Hypercalcemia and hypoalbuminemia

☐ 4. Hypercalcemia and hyperalbuminemia

CORRECT ANSWER: 2

5. What's the term used to describe cleft palate repair surgery?

☐ 1. Jejunostomy

☐ 2. Fundoplication

☐ 3. Cheiloplasty

☐ 4. Staphylorrhaphy

CORRECT ANSWER: 4

LEARNING OBJECTIVES

After studying this chapter, you should be able to:

● Describe acquired and congenital GI problems that alter nutrition and hydration.

● Assess and plan care for a child with vomiting and diarrhea.

● Plan feeding interventions for children with GI disorders that interfere with proper nutrition and hydration.

CHAPTER OVERVIEW

Acquired and congenital conditions of the GI tract can result in altered GI functioning. A thorough assessment is necessary for prompt treatment. Interventions are geared toward controlling and correcting the problem, promoting adequate nutrition and normal function, and preventing complications.

KEY CONCEPTS

● **Structures and functions**

(See *Characteristics of the pediatric GI system,* page 264.)

- Mouth
  - Teeth begin digestion by chewing food into smaller pieces
  - Salivary glands
    - Provide saliva to moisten the mouth
    - Lubricate food to ease swallowing
    - Begin food breakdown using the enzyme ptyalin
- Esophagus
  - Upper esophageal sphincter relaxes, allowing food to pass into the esophagus
  - Lower esophageal sphincter contractions (called *peristalsis*) push the food gradually down the esophagus and through the lower esophageal sphincter into the stomach
- Stomach
  - Three parts
    - Fundus—the enlarged portion above and to the left of the esophageal opening in the stomach
    - Body—the middle portion of the stomach
    - Pylorus—the lower portion, lying near the junction of the stomach and duodenum
  - Lining secretes gastric juices
  - Churning motion breaks food into tiny particles
  - Limited amounts of water, alcohol, and some drugs are absorbed
  - Liquid portion (chyme) enters the duodenum in small amounts through the pyloric opening
- Small intestine
  - Three segments
    - Duodenum—the beginning portion; the shortest segment
    - Jejunum—the middle portion
    - Ileum—the last portion
  - Where most digestion takes place

Functions of the esophageal sphincters

- Upper sphincter: allows food to pass into the esophagus
- Lower sphincter: pushes food down into the stomach

Functions of the stomach

- Secretes gastric juices
- Churns food to break it into tiny particles

Three parts of the stomach

1. Fundus – top portion
2. Body – middle portion
3. Pylorus – lower portion

Three segments of the small intestine

1. Duodenum
2. Jejunum
3. Ileum

Functions of the small intestines

- Digestion (aided by enzymes in lining)
- Absorption for distribution throughout the body

Functions of the liver

- Stores and filters blood
- Processes sugars, fats, proteins, and vitamins
- Detoxifies drugs, alcohol, and other substances
- Secretes bile

Key facts about bile

- Clear, yellowish fluid
- Neutralizes stomach acids
- Aids emulsification and absorption of fats and fat-soluble vitamins

Four segments of the large intestine

1. Cecum
2. Colon
3. Rectum
4. Anal canal

Characteristics of the pediatric GI system

Here are some characteristics of the pediatric GI system:

- Peristalsis occurs within 2½ to 3 hours in the neonate and extends to 3 to 6 hours in older infants and children.
- The stomach capacity of the neonate is 30 to 60 ml, which gradually increases to 200 to 350 ml by age 12 months and 1,500 ml in the adolescent.
- Up until age 4 to 8 weeks, the neonatal abdomen is larger than the chest and the musculature is poorly developed.
- The sucking and extrusion reflex (a reflex that protects the infant from food substances his system is too immature to digest) persists until age 3 to 4 months.

- Saliva production begins at age 4 months and aids in the process of digestion.
- Spit-ups are frequent in the neonate because of the immature muscle tone of the lower esophageal sphincter and the low volume capacity of the stomach.
- Increased myelination of nerves to the anal sphincter allows for physiologic control of bowel function, usually at about age 2.
- The liver's slow development of glycogen storage capacity makes the infant prone to hypoglycemia.
- From ages 1 to 3, the composition of intestinal flora becomes more adultlike and stomach acidity increases, reducing the number of GI infections.

- Vast array of enzymes from the lining aid in digestion
- Surface area is increased by millions of villi in the mucous membrane lining
- Digested food is absorbed through the walls and into the blood for distribution throughout the body
- Pancreas
  - Large gland located behind the stomach
  - Secretes digestive enzymes, bicarbonate, and hormones into the duodenum
- Liver
  - Stores and filters blood
  - Processes sugars, fats, proteins, and vitamins
  - Detoxifies drugs, alcohol, and other substances
  - Secretes bile
    - A clear, yellowish fluid
    - Neutralizes stomach acids
    - Aids the small intestine to emulsify and absorb fats and fat-soluble vitamins
- Gallbladder
  - Located beneath the liver
  - Stores bile produced by the liver
- Large intestine
  - Four parts

- Cecum—a saclike structure that makes up the first few inches of the large intestine
- Colon—includes the ascending, transverse, descending, and sigmoid colon; the middle part of the large intestine
- Rectum—the last few inches of the large intestine
- Anal canal—where the large intestine ends
 – Larger in diameter than the small intestine
 – Absorbs water and sodium from the digestive material before passing it on for elimination
 – Rectal distention by feces stimulates the defecation reflex which, when assisted by voluntary sphincter relaxation, permits defecation

DIAGNOSTIC TESTS

● **Barium or meglumine diatrizoate (Gastrografin) swallow**
- Purpose
 – Primarily used to examine the esophagus
 – Gastrografin and barium facilitate imaging through X-rays, but gastrografin is less toxic if it escapes from the GI tract
- Nursing interventions
 – Explain the procedure to the child and his parents
 – Maintain the child on a nothing-by-mouth status beginning at midnight before the test
 – Tell the child that he must hold still during the X-ray
 – After the test
 - Monitor bowel movements for excretion of barium
 - Monitor GI function

● **Upper GI imaging**
- Purpose
 – Upper GI series
 - Swallowed barium moves into the esophagus, stomach, and duodenum to reveal abnormalities
 - Barium outlines stomach walls and delineates ulcer craters and filling defects
 – Small-bowel series
 - An extension of the upper GI series
 - Visualizes barium flowing through the small intestine to the ileocecal valve
- Nursing interventions
 – Explain the procedure to the child and his parents
 – Tell the child that he must hold still during the X-ray
 – Make sure the lead apron is properly placed around the genital area

---

Quick guide to diagnostic tests for GI functioning

- **Barium or gastrografin swallow** – used to examine the esophagus
- **Upper GI imaging** – allows visualization of the GI tract from the esophagus to the ileocecal valve
- **Barium enema (lower GI series)** – allows visualization of the colon
- **Stool specimen** – used to test for occult blood as well as for ova, parasites, and fat
- **Fiber-optic testing** – allows visualization of the GI tract from the esophagus to the rectum
- **ERCP** – allows examination of the pancreatic ducts and hepatobiliary tree
- **GI intubation** – allows diagnosis and treatment of GI tract disorders

Two parts of upper GI imaging

1. Upper GI series – barium outlines stomach walls and delineates ulcer craters and filling defects
2. Small bowel series – barium outlines the small intestine to the ileocecal valve

Preparing a patient for a barium enema

- Explain the procedure to the child and his parents.
- Have the child follow a liquid diet for 24 hours before the test, if applicable.
- Tell the child that X-rays will be taken on a test table and that he must hold still.
- Cover the genital area with a lead apron during X-ray.

Types of fiber-optic testing

- Esophagogastroduodenoscopy: the insertion of a fiber-optic scope to allow direct visual inspection of the esophagus, stomach, and duodenum
- Proctosigmoidoscopy: direct inspection of the rectum and distal sigmoid colon
- Colonoscopy: direct inspection of the descending, transverse, and ascending colon

– After the test
  · Monitor bowel movements for excretion of barium
  · Monitor GI function

● Barium enema (lower GI series)
- Purpose
  – Allows X-ray visualization of the colon
- Nursing interventions
  – Explain the procedure to the child and his parents
  – Usually, the child will follow a liquid diet for 24 hours before the test
  – Bowel preparations are administered before the examination
  – Tell the child that X-rays will be taken on a test table and that he must hold still
  – Cover the genital area with a lead apron during X-ray

● Stool specimen
- Purpose
  – Examined for suspected GI bleeding, infection, or malabsorption
  – Tests include the guaiac test for occult blood and microscopic tests for ova, parasites, and fat
- Nursing interventions
  – Obtain the specimen in the correct container (container may need to be sterile or contain preservative)
  – Be aware that the specimen may need to be transported to the laboratory immediately or placed in the refrigerator

● Fiber-optic testing
- Purpose
  – Esophagogastroduodenoscopy — a fiber-optic scope is inserted to allow direct visual inspection of the esophagus, stomach, and duodenum
  – Proctosigmoidoscopy — the rectum and distal sigmoid colon are inspected directly
  – Colonoscopy — the descending, transverse, and ascending colon are inspected directly
- Nursing interventions
  – Explain the procedure to the child and his parents
  – Obtain written, informed consent
  – A mild sedative may be administered before the examination
  – The child may be kept on nothing-by-mouth status beginning at midnight before the test
  – The child may be placed on a liquid diet for 24 hours before the examination or require enemas and laxatives until clear

● Endoscopic retrograde cholangiopancreatography (ERCP)
- Purpose

– Contrast media is injected into the duodenal papilla to allow radiographic examination of the pancreatic ducts and hepatobiliary tree

- Nursing interventions
  - Before the procedure
    - Explain the procedure to the child and his parents
    - Obtain written, informed consent
    - Check the child's history for allergies to cholinergics and iodine
    - Administer a sedative and monitor the child for the drug's effect
  - After the procedure
    - Monitor the child's gag reflex (the child remains on nothing-by-mouth status until his gag reflex returns)
    - Protect the child from aspiration of mucus by positioning the child on his side
    - Monitor the child for urine retention

● **GI intubation**

- Purpose
  - To empty the stomach and intestine
  - To aid diagnosis and treatment
  - To decompress obstructed areas
  - To detect and treat GI bleeding
  - To administer medications or feedings
- Nursing interventions
  - Maintain accurate intake and output records
    - Record the amount, color, odor, and consistency of gastric drainage every 4 hours
    - When irrigating the tube, note the amount of normal saline solution instilled and aspirated
  - Check for fluid and electrolyte imbalances
  - Provide good oral and nasal care; make sure the tube is secure but that it isn't causing pressure on the nostrils
  - To support the tube's weight and prevent its accidental removal, anchor the tube to the child's clothing
  - Check tube placement by checking gastric pH
  - After removing the tube from a child with GI bleeding, watch for signs and symptoms of recurrent bleeding
  - Maintain a calm and reassuring manner and provide emotional support because many children panic at the sight of the tube

NURSING DIAGNOSES

● **Probable nursing diagnoses**

- Bowel incontinence
- Constipation
- Delayed growth and development

TOP 3

Interventions after ERCP

1. Monitor the child's gag reflex.
2. Position the child on his side to protect him from aspiration.
3. Monitor the child for urine retention.

Purposes of GI intubation

- To empty the stomach and intestine
- To aid diagnosis and treatment
- To decompress obstructed areas
- To detect and treat GI bleeding
- To administer medications or feedings

Monitoring intake and output during GI intubation

- Record the amount, color, odor, and consistency of gastric drainage every 4 hours.
- When irrigating the tube, note the amount of normal saline solution instilled and aspirated.

Probable nursing diagnoses for a patient with a GI disorder

- Bowel incontinence
- Constipation
- Delayed growth and development
- Diarrhea
- Imbalanced nutrition: Less than body requirements
- Imbalanced nutrition: More than body requirements
- Impaired swallowing
- Risk for infection
- Nausea

Key facts about appendicitis

- Inflammation of the blind sac at the end of the cecum
- Most common major surgical disease
- Results from an obstruction
- Common in school-age children

TOP 3

Assessment findings in appendicitis

1. Abdominal pain and tenderness that ultimately localizes in the lower right quadrant at McBurney's point
2. Rebound tenderness, especially in the right lower quadrant
3. Abdominal distention, rigidity, and guarding

- Diarrhea
- Imbalanced nutrition: Less than body requirements
- Imbalanced nutrition: More than body requirements
- Impaired swallowing
- Risk for infection
- Nausea

● **Possible nursing diagnoses**
- Feeding self-care deficit
- Impaired oral mucous membrane
- Risk for aspiration
- Risk for constipation
- Risk for imbalanced nutrition: More than body requirements

APPENDICITIS

● **Definition**
- Inflammation and obstruction of the blind sac at the end of the cecum
- Most common major surgical disease

● **Causes**
- Results from an obstruction of the appendicial lumen caused by a fecal mass, stricture, or viral infection
- Common in school-age children

● **Pathophysiology**
- Obstruction starts an inflammatory process that can lead to infection, thrombosis, necrosis, and perforation

● **Complications**
- Ischemic bowel
- Gangrene
- Bowel perforation
- Peritonitis

● **Assessment findings**
- Abdominal pain and tenderness that begins as diffuse, then localizes in the lower right quadrant at McBurney's point
- Fever
- Increased white blood cell (WBC) count
- Rebound tenderness, especially in the right lower quadrant
- Decreased bowel sounds, nausea, vomiting, and anorexia
- Abdominal distention, rigidity, and guarding
- Symptoms of peritonitis if a rupture occurs: fever, sudden relief of pain followed by a diffuse pain

● **Diagnostic test findings**
- Elevated WBC count, with increased immature cells

Medical management
- Surgical intervention (appendectomy)
- If peritonitis develops:
  - GI intubation
  - Parenteral replacement of fluids and electrolytes
  - Administration of antibiotics

Nursing interventions
- Position the child preoperatively in a semi-Fowler's or right side-lying position to decrease pain
- Never apply heat to the right lower abdomen; this may cause the appendix to rupture
- Be aware that, postoperatively, the child with a ruptured appendix may have a drain and a nasogastric (NG) tube attached to low intermittent suction
- Resume oral nutrition when bowel sounds reappear
- Administer antibiotics and pain medication

CELIAC DISEASE

Definition
- Characterized by poor food absorption and intolerance of gluten—a protein found in grains, such as wheat, rye, oats, and barley

Causes
- Gluten intolerance
- Immunoglobulin A deficiency
- Genetic

Pathophysiology
- A decrease in the amount and activity of enzymes in the intestinal mucosal cells
- This causes the villi of the proximal small intestine to atrophy and decreases intestinal absorption
- Usually becomes apparent between ages 6 months and 18 months

Complications
- Osteoporosis
- Lymphoma of the small intestine
- Infertility
- Autoimmune liver disease

Assessment findings
- Steatorrhea (fatty stools)
- Chronic diarrhea or constipation or both
- Anorexia
- Generalized malnutrition and failure to thrive
- Coagulation difficulty from the malabsorption of fat-soluble vitamins

Key facts about celiac disease

- Characterized by poor food absorption and intolerance of gluten
- Caused by immunoglobulin A deficiency
- Becomes apparent between ages 6 and 18 months

TOP 3

Assessment findings in celiac disease

1. Abdominal pain and distention
2. Chronic diarrhea
3. Anorexia

Diagnostic test findings associated with celiac disease

- Hypocalcemia
- Hypoalbuminemia
- Decreased hemoglobin level
- Hypothrombinemia
- Positive immunologic assay screen for celiac disease
- High fat content in stool specimen

Managing celiac disease

- Gluten-free diet
- Folate and iron supplements
- Vitamins A and D in water-soluble forms

Celiac disease–friendly foods

- Corn and rice products
- Soy and potato flour
- Breast milk
- Soy-based formula
- Fresh fruits

Key facts about cleft lip and palate

- Failure of the bone and tissue of the upper jaw and palate to fuse completely at the midline
- Usually a congenital defect
- May be part of another chromosomal abnormality
- May be from prenatal exposure to teratogens
- May be partial or complete, unilateral or bilateral

- Abdominal pain and distention
- Irritability
- Anemia
- Clubbed fingers
- Dental enamel defects
- Vomiting
- Rash

● **Diagnostic test findings**
- Hypocalcemia
- Hypoalbuminemia
- Decreased hemoglobin level
- Hypothrombinemia
- Positive immunologic assay screen for celiac disease
- High fat content in stool specimen
- Intestinal tissue changes indicative of celiac disease (revealed by intestinal biopsy)

● **Medical management**
- Diet that's gluten-free but includes corn and rice products, soy and potato flour, breast milk or soy-based formula, and fresh fruits
- Folate supplements
- Iron supplements
- Vitamins A and D in water-soluble forms

● **Nursing interventions**
- Eliminate all gluten from the diet
- Give the child corn and rice products, soy and potato flour, breast milk or soy-based formula, and fresh fruits
- Replace vitamins and calories; give small, frequent meals
- Monitor for steatorrhea — its disappearance is a good indicator that the child's ability to absorb nutrients is improving
- Inform parents that some hair products and skin products have gluten in them

CLEFT LIP AND PALATE

● **Definition**
- Failure of the bone and tissue of the upper jaw and palate to fuse completely at the midline

● **Causes**
- Congenital defects; in some cases inheritance plays a role
- Part of another chromosomal abnormality
- Prenatal exposure to teratogens

Cleft lip and cleft palate

The illustrations below show the four variations of cleft lip and cleft palate.

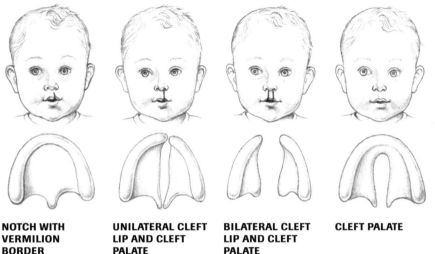

NOTCH WITH VERMILION BORDER

UNILATERAL CLEFT LIP AND CLEFT PALATE

BILATERAL CLEFT LIP AND CLEFT PALATE

CLEFT PALATE

● **Pathophysiology**
  • Defects may be partial or complete, unilateral or bilateral, and may involve just the lip, just the palate, or both (see *Cleft lip and cleft palate*)
  • Defects originate in the second month of pregnancy, when the front and sides of the face and the palatine shelves fuse imperfectly

● **Complications**
  • Speech defects
  • Dental and orthodontic problems
  • Nasal defects
  • Alterations in hearing
  • Shock, guilt, and grief for the parents that may interfere with parent-child bonding
  • Increased risk of aspiration, upper respiratory infections, and otitis media

● **Assessment findings**
  • Abdominal distention from swallowed air
  • Difficulty swallowing
  • Cleft lip
    – Simple notch on the upper lip
    – Complete cleft from the lip edge to the floor of the nostril
    – On either side of the midline but rarely along the midline itself
  • Cleft palate
    – Opening in the palate
    – May be partial or complete

Complications of cleft lip and palate

- Speech defects
- Dental and orthodontic problems
- Nasal defects
- Alterations in hearing
- Possible impaired parent-child bonding
- Increased risk of aspiration, upper respiratory infections, and otitis media

Lip and palate surgeries

- Cheiloplasty — cleft lip repair surgery; typically performed between birth and age 3 months
- Staphylorrhaphy — cleft palate repair surgery; scheduled at about age 18 months

TOP 4

Preoperative interventions for cheiloplasty

1. Feed the infant slowly and in an upright position to decrease the risk of aspiration.
2. Burp the infant often during feeding to eliminate swallowed air and decrease the risk of emesis.
3. Give the infant small, frequent feedings to promote adequate nutrition and to prevent tiring.
4. Feed the infant using a commercially available cleft lip and cleft palate nipple.

● **Diagnostic test findings**
- Prenatal ultrasonography may indicate severe defects

● **Medical management**
- Cheiloplasty (cleft lip repair surgery)
  - Performed between birth and age 3 months
  - Unites the lip and gum edges
    - Provides a route for adequate nutrition and sucking
    - Performed in anticipation of tooth eruption
- Staphylorrhaphy (cleft palate repair surgery)
  - Scheduled at about age 18 months
    - Allows for palate growth
    - Allows for surgery to be done before the infant develops speech patterns
  - Infant must be free from ear and respiratory infections
- Long-term, team-oriented care to address speech defects, dental and orthodontic problems, nasal defects, and possible alterations in hearing
- If cleft lip is detected on sonogram while the infant is in utero, fetal repair may be possible

● **Nursing interventions**
- To help determine an effective feeding method, assess the quality of the child's sucking by determining if the infant can form an airtight seal around a finger or nipple that's placed in his mouth; a specialized nipple can be used for an infant with a cleft lip or palate
- Assess the child's ability to swallow
- Assess for abdominal distension from swallowed air
- Assess respiratory status to detect signs of aspiration
- Monitor vital signs and intake and output to determine fluid volume status
- Preoperative interventions for cheiloplasty
  - Feed the infant slowly and in an upright position to decrease the risk of aspiration
  - Feed the infant using a commercially available cleft lip and cleft palate nipple
  - Burp often during feeding to eliminate swallowed air and decrease the risk of emesis
  - Use gavage feedings if oral feedings are unsuccessful
  - Administer a small amount of water after feedings to prevent formula from accumulating and becoming a medium for bacterial growth
  - Give small, frequent feedings to promote adequate nutrition and prevent tiring of the infant
  - Hold the infant while feeding
  - Promote sucking between meals (sucking is important to speech development)

- Postoperative interventions for cheiloplasty
  - Maintain a patent airway; edema or narrowing of a previously large airway may make the infant appear to be in distress
  - Observe for cyanosis as the infant begins to breathe through his nose to detect signs of respiratory compromise
  - Maintain an intact suture line; keep the infant's hands away from his mouth by using restraints or pinning his sleeves to his shirt
  - Anticipate the infant's needs to prevent crying; don't place him in the prone position
  - Give extra care and support because the infant's emotional needs can't be met by sucking
  - When feeding resumes, use a syringe with tubing to administer foods at the side of the mouth to prevent trauma to the suture line
  - Place the infant on his right side after feedings to prevent aspiration
  - Monitor for pain and administer pain medication as prescribed
- Preoperative interventions for staphylorrhaphy
  - Be aware that the child must be weaned from the bottle or breast before cleft palate surgery; the child must be able to drink from a cup
  - Teach the parents that the child is susceptible to pathogens and otitis media from the altered position of the eustachian tubes
- Postoperative interventions for staphylorrhaphy
  - Position the child on his abdomen or side to maintain a patent airway
  - Assess for signs of altered oxygenation to promote good respiration
  - Keep hard or pointed objects (utensils, straws, frozen dessert sticks) away from the child's mouth to prevent trauma to the suture line
  - Use a cup to feed; don't use a nipple or pacifier, to prevent injury to the suture line
  - Use elbow restraints to keep the child's hands out of his mouth
  - Provide soft toys to prevent injury
  - Start the child on clear liquids and progress to a soft diet
  - Rinse the suture line by giving the child a sip of water after each feeding to prevent infection
  - Distract or hold the child to try to keep his tongue away from the roof of his mouth

DIARRHEA AND GASTROENTERITIS

● Definition
- Diarrhea—increased frequency and amount and decreased consistency of stool
- Gastroenteritis—an inflammation of the lining of the stomach and intestines

Preoperative interventions in staphylorrhaphy

- Make sure that the child has been weaned from the bottle or breast and can drink from a cup.
- Teach the parents that the child is susceptible to pathogens and otitis media.

TOP 5

Postoperative interventions for staphylorrhaphy

1. Position the child on his abdomen or side to maintain a patent airway.
2. Keep hard or pointed objects away from the child's mouth to prevent trauma to the suture line.
3. Use a cup to feed the child to prevent injury to the suture line.
4. Start the child on clear liquids and progress to a soft diet.
5. Rinse the suture line by giving the child a sip of water after each feeding to prevent infection.

Causes of diarrhea and gastroenteritis

- Bacteria
- Amebae
- Parasites
- Viruses
- Toxins
- Medications
- Enzyme deficiencies
- Food allergens

Complications of diarrhea and gastroenteritis

- Metabolic acidosis
- Dehydration

Managing diarrhea and gastroenteritis

- Bed rest
- Nutritional support
- Increased fluid intake
- Antiemetics

TOP 4

Interventions for diarrhea and gastroenteritis

1. Practice enteric precautions and proper hand washing.
2. Initially withhold food and fluids to rest the bowel.
3. Correct dehydration and replace potassium.
4. Restart fluid intake with an electrolyte-balanced solution.

● **Causes**
- Bacteria (responsible for acute food poisoning) such as *Staphylococcus aureus, Salmonella, Shigella, Clostridium botulinum, C. perfringens,* and *Escherichia coli*
- Amebae, especially *Entamoeba histolytica*
- Parasites, such as *Ascaris, Enterobius,* and *Trichinella spiralis*
- Viruses (may be responsible for traveler's diarrhea), such as rotavirus (the most commonly identified viral pathogen), adenoviruses, echoviruses, and coxsackieviruses
- Ingestion of toxins, including plants or toadstools
- Drug reactions (for example, to antibiotics)
- Enzyme deficiencies
- Food allergens

● **Pathophysiology**
- Water in the bowel increases from osmotic pull with electrolyte imbalance
- Peristalsis increases, preventing water from being absorbed
- Can result from anatomic changes or malabsorption

● **Complications**
- Metabolic acidosis
- Dehydration

● **Assessment findings**
- Loose, watery stools
- Abdominal discomfort
- Nausea
- Vomiting
- Fever

● **Diagnostic test findings**
- Stool culture (by direct rectal swab) or blood culture identifies causative bacteria or parasites

● **Medical management**
- Bed rest
- Nutritional support
- Increased fluid intake through the use of I.V. fluids and oral electrolyte replacement fluids with low concentrations of sodium and glucose
- Antiemetics as needed for vomiting and nausea
- Administer rotovirus vaccine

● **Nursing interventions**
- Initially withhold food and oral fluids to rest the bowel
- For the older child:
  – Kaolin and pectin (Kaopectate) to make the stools firmer
  – Paregoric (an opiate) to decrease bowel motility
- Correct dehydration; replace potassium

- Restart oral fluid intake with an electrolyte-balanced solution such as Pedialyte
- Avoid solutions that are high in sodium (broth, milk) because of their osmotic pull
- Practice enteric precautions and proper hand washing
- Measure urine and stool output; use a pediatric plastic urine collector around the urethra to catch urine, if necessary
- Use protective ointments around the anus for prophylactic or therapeutic skin care
- Don't take the child's temperature rectally; use the axillary method

GASTROESOPHAGEAL REFLUX

Definition
- Gastroesophageal reflux (GER) is the return of gastric or duodenal contents into the esophagus from an incompetent or poorly developed esophageal sphincter without associated belching or vomiting

Causes
- Occurs almost immediately after eating
- Typically affects infants but is also seen in young children with spastic cerebral palsy because of decreased muscle tone
- Predisposing factors
  - Prematurity
  - Long-term NG intubation
  - Hiatal hernia with incompetent sphincter
  - Administration of agents that decrease lower esophageal sphincter (LES) pressure

Pathophysiology
- The function of the LES is to prevent gastric contents from backing up into the esophagus
- Normally, the LES creates pressure, closing the lower end of the esophagus, but relaxes after each swallow to allow food into the stomach
- Reflux occurs when LES pressure is deficient or when pressure within the stomach exceeds LES pressure (see *Understanding gastroesophageal reflux*, page 276)

Complications
- Pulmonary symptoms, including nocturnal wheezing, bronchitis, asthma, and cough
- Failure to thrive
- Aspiration pneumonia

Assessment findings
- Irritability
- Vomiting, possibly related to feedings, positioning, and activity level immediately after feedings

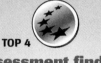

Understanding gastroesophageal reflux

Normally, the lower esophageal sphincter (LES) creates pressure, closing the lower end of the esophagus (as shown below), but relaxes after each swallow to allow food into the stomach.

Reflux occurs when LES pressure is deficient or when pressure within the stomach exceeds LES pressure, allowing the contents of the stomach to pass back up into the esophagus, as shown below.

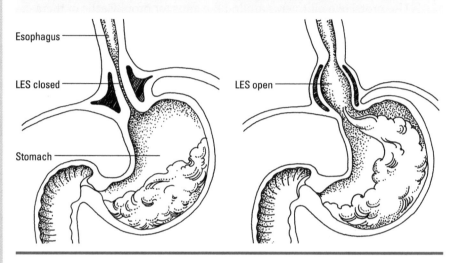

- Esophagitis, indicated by blood in the emesis or stool
- Weight loss
- Aspiration of feedings
- Recurrent pneumonia
- Apnea (many infants may require apnea monitoring)
- Coughing and wheezing

Diagnostic test findings
- 24-hour pH probe study
  - Involves a probe placed in the nose and down to the esophagus
  - The probe is connected to a small data collection device to capture the effects of food, position, and sleeping
- Endoscopy and biopsy allow visualization and confirmation of pathologic changes in the mucosa

Medical management
- Positional therapy is especially useful in infants and children
- Small, frequent feedings of thickened liquids and frequent burping can lessen the chances of regurgitation
- Proton pump inhibitors block production of stomach acid
  - Lansprazole (Prevacid)
  - Omeprasole (Prilosec)
  - Nizatidine (Axid)
- Metoclopramide (Reglan) increases LES tone and stimulates upper GI motility

Managing GER

- Positional therapy
- Small, frequent feedings
- Proton pump inhibitor
- Metoclopramide
- Ranitidine
- Surgery
- Nissen fundoplication procedure
- Placement of a jejunostomy tube

- Ranitidine (Zantac) inhibits gastric acid secretion, lessening the inflammation of the esophagus
- Surgery may be necessary to control severe and refractory symptoms, such as pulmonary aspiration or incompetent LES
- The Nissen fundoplication procedure is a surgical procedure that involves wrapping the stomach fundus around the lower esophagus to increase the pressure necessary for food to enter the esophagus from the stomach
- An alternative for patients requiring long-term, continuous tube feedings is the placement of a jejunostomy tube

● Nursing interventions

- Educate the parents about what causes reflux, how to avoid it, and what symptoms to watch for and report
- To maximize the benefits of medications, administer them 30 minutes before meals
- Provide formula thickened with cereal
- Enlarge the bottle's nipple opening to allow for easier delivery of formula
- Feed the infant in an upright position, burping frequently
- Hold the infant in an upright position for 15 to 30 minutes after feeding
- Give small, frequent feedings
- Prepare for surgery (Nissen's fundoplication) if necessary

HIRSCHSPRUNG'S DISEASE

● Definition

- Absence of parasympathetic ganglionic cells in a segment of the colon (usually at the distal end of the large intestine)
- Lack of nerve innervation causes a lack of, or alteration in, peristalsis in the affected part

● Causes

- Familial, congenital defect
- Commonly coexists with other congenital anomalies, particularly Down syndrome (trisomy 21) and anomalies of the urinary tract

● Pathophysiology

- As a stool enters the affected part, it remains there until additional stool pushes it through
- The affected part of the colon dilates; a mechanical obstruction may result

● Complications

- Severe constipation
- Enterocolitis
  - Severe diarrhea
  - Hypovolemic shock
  - Death

Tips for feeding pediatric patients with GER

- Give small, frequent feedings.
- Provide thickened formula.
- Enlarge the bottle's nipple opening to allow for easier delivery of formula.
- Feed the infant in an upright position, burping frequently.
- Hold the infant upright for 15 to 30 minutes after feeding.

Key facts about Hirschsprung's disease

- Absence of parasympathetic ganglionic cells in a segment of the colon
- Causes lack of, or alteration in, peristalsis
- Commonly coexists with other congenital anomalies

Complications of Hirschsprung's disease

- Severe constipation
- Enterocolitis, possibly resulting in severe diarrhea, hypovolemic shock, and death

TOP 5

Assessment findings in Hirschsprung's disease

1. Failure to pass meconium and stool
2. Liquid or ribbonlike stools
3. Distended abdomen and easily palpable stool masses
4. Signs of dehydration
5. Absence of ganglion cells revealed by rectal biopsy

Surgical treatment for Hirschsprung's disease

- It involves pulling the normal ganglionic segment through to the anus.
- It may be delayed until the infant is at least age 10 months.
- To decompress the colon, a temporary colostomy or ileostomy may be necessary.

Preoperative nursing interventions for Hirschsprung's disease

- Maintain fluid and electrolyte balance.
- Monitor vital signs.
- Administer isotonic enemas.

● **Assessment findings**
- Failure to pass meconium and stool
- Liquid or ribbonlike stools
- Distended abdomen and easily palpable stool masses
- Bile-stained or fecal vomiting
- Irritability and lethargy
- Failure to thrive and weight loss
- Signs of dehydration (pallor, dry mucous membranes, sunken eyes)

● **Diagnostic test findings**
- Rectal biopsy provides definitive diagnosis by showing the absence of ganglion cells
  - Suction aspiration to determine the absence of ganglion cells
  - Full-thickness surgical biopsy under general anesthesia
- Rectal manometry detects failure of the internal anal sphincter to relax and contract
- Abdominal X-rays show distention of the colon

● **Medical management**
- Until surgery is performed, daily colonic lavage to empty the bowel
- Digital examination, performed by a physician, to expand the anus enough to release the impacted stool and provide temporary relief if the megacolon is near the rectum
- Preoperative bowel prep with an antibiotic (neomycin [Mycifradin] or nystatin [Mycostatin])
- Surgical treatment
  - Involves pulling the normal ganglionic segment through to the anus
  - Delayed until the infant is at least age 10 months
  - If total obstruction is present, a temporary colostomy or ileostomy may be necessary to decompress the colon

● **Nursing interventions**
- Preoperative
  - Maintain fluid and electrolyte balance to prevent dehydration and shock
  - Monitor vital signs to prevent sepsis and enterocolitis
  - Administer isotonic enemas (normal saline solution or mineral oil) to evacuate the bowel; don't administer tap water because of the risk of water intoxication
- After colostomy or ileostomy
  - Monitor fluid intake and output (ileostomy is especially likely to cause excessive electrolyte loss)
  - Keep the area around the stoma clean and dry; use colostomy or ileostomy appliances to collect drainage
  - Monitor for return of bowel sounds to begin diet
- After corrective surgery
  - Keep the wound clean and dry to prevent infection

TIME-OUT FOR TEACHING

Teaching about Hirschsprung's disease

Be sure to follow these recommendations when teaching a child and his parents about Hirschsprung's disease:

- Explain Hirschsprung's disease. Make sure the child and his parents understand the necessary diagnostic tests and treatments.
- Before surgery, provide appropriate preoperative teaching to the child and his parents. Reinforce, as necessary, the physician's explanation of the procedure and its possible complications.
- Describe to the child and his parents, as appropriate, the signs of fluid loss and dehydration (decreased urine output, sunken eyes, and poor skin turgor) and enterocolitis (vomiting, diarrhea, fever, lethargy, and sudden, marked abdominal distention).
- Before discharge, if possible, make sure the parents consult an enterostomal therapist for valuable tips on colostomy or ileostomy care.
- Instruct the parents to watch for foods that increase the number of stools and to avoid offering these foods. Reassure them that their child will, in time, probably gain sphincter control and eat a normal diet.
- Warn the child and his parents that complete continence can take years to develop and that constipation may recur.

- Don't use a rectal thermometer or suppositories
- Begin oral feedings when active bowel sounds begin and NG drainage decreases
- Educate the parents on suture line care and the symptoms of the return of constipation (see *Teaching about Hirschsprung's disease*)

INTUSSUSCEPTION

- **Definition**
  - Telescoping or invagination of a bowel segment into itself, the most common site being the ileocecal valve
  - Usually occurs at about age 6 months
  - Occurs in three times more males than females

- **Causes**
  - Unknown in most cases
  - May result from polyps, hyperactive peristalsis, or an abnormal bowel lining
  - May be linked to viral infections because seasonal peaks are noted (spring and summer)

- **Pathophysiology**
  - When a bowel segment invaginates, peristalsis propels it along the bowel, pulling more bowel along with it
  - Invagination causes inflammation and swelling at the affected site
  - Edema eventually causes obstruction and necrosis from occlusion of the blood supply to the bowel

Complications of intussusception

- Bowel obstruction
- Strangulation of the intestine
- Gangrene
- Shock
- Bowel perforation
- Peritonitis
- Death (especially if treatment is delayed for more than 24 hours)

TOP 3

Assessment findings in intussusception

1. Intermittent attacks of colicky pain, causing the child to scream and draw his knees to his chest
2. Passage of red, "currant jellylike" stool containing mucus and blood
3. Distended and tender abdomen with a palpable, sausage-shaped abdominal mass

Indications for surgical management of intussusception

- Failure of hydrostatic reduction
- Recurrent intussusception
- Signs of shock or peritonitis

● Complications

- Bowel obstruction
- Strangulation of the intestine
- Gangrene
- Shock
- Bowel perforation
- Peritonitis
- Death, especially if treatment is delayed for more than 24 hours

● Assessment findings

- Intermittent attacks of colicky pain (screaming, drawing knees to chest, sweating, grunting)
- Emesis containing bile or fecal material
- Passage of red, "currant jellylike" stool containing mucus and blood
- Distended and tender abdomen with a palpable, sausage-shaped abdominal mass

● Diagnostic test findings

- Abdominal X-ray, ultrasound, or computerized tomography shows a soft tissue mass and signs of complete or partial obstruction
- Increased WBC count

● Medical management

- Insertion of an NG tube to decompress the intestine and minimize vomiting
- Hydrostatic reduction
  - Air pressure or solution of barium or water-soluble contrast is introduced to the rectum
  - Force from fluid or air moves invaginated bowel back into its original position
- Surgery
  - Indications
    - Failure of hydrostatic reduction
    - Recurrent intussusception
    - Signs of shock or peritonitis
  - Manual reduction performed first by pulling the intussusception back through the bowel
  - Resection of the affected bowel segment if gangrenous or strangulated

● Nursing interventions

- Prepare for enema (barium or water-soluble contrast) to confirm the condition and reduce the invagination by hydrostatic pressure
- Monitor vital signs; a change in temperature may indicate sepsis
- Monitor intake and output to prevent dehydration
- Monitor NG tube output and replace volume lost, as ordered

- Monitor the child who has undergone hydrostatic reduction for the passage of stools (and barium if used) to determine the need for surgery
- Postoperative interventions
  – Administer antibiotics as ordered to prevent infection
  – Monitor incision site for any signs of infection (inflammation, drainage, or suture separation)
  – Monitor for the return of bowel sounds to allow advancement of the diet
  – Offer emotional support and encouragement to the parents who are usually unprepared for their child's emergency surgery and recovery

PYLORIC STENOSIS

Definition
- Hyperplasia (increased mass) and hypertrophy (increased size) of the circular muscle at the pylorus narrows the pyloric canal (see *Understanding pyloric stenosis*, pages 282)
- Most commonly seen in male infants between ages 1 and 6 months

Causes
- Exact cause unknown
- Not an inherited disorder
- May be associated with malrotation, esophageal atresia, and anorectal abnormalities

Pathophysiology
- Narrowing of passageway between the stomach and the duodenum
- Swelling and inflammation further reduce the size of the lumen and could result in complete obstruction
- Normal emptying of the stomach is prevented

Complications
- Malnutrition
- Dehydration
- Infection
- Metabolic alkalosis
- Failure to thrive

Assessment findings
- Olive-sized bulge below the right costal margin
- Projectile emesis during or shortly after feedings preceded by reverse peristaltic waves (going left to right), but not by nausea
- Child resumes eating after vomiting
- Poor weight gain or weight loss
- Symptoms of malnutrition and dehydration despite the child's apparent adequate intake of food
- Tetany

Postoperative interventions for intussusception

- Administer antibiotics as ordered.
- Monitor incision site.
- Monitor for return of bowel sounds.
- Offer emotional support to parents.

Key facts about pyloric stenosis

- Increased mass and size of the muscle at the pylorus that results in narrowing of the pyloric canal
- Prevents normal emptying of the stomach
- Most commonly seen in males between ages 1 and 6 months
- Unknown cause

Complications of pyloric stenosis

- Malnutrition
- Dehydration
- Infection
- Metabolic alkalosis
- Failure to thrive

TOP 3

Assessment findings in pyloric stenosis

1. Olive-sized bulge below the right costal margin
2. Projectile emesis during or shortly after feedings
3. Hypertrophied sphincter revealed on ultrasound and endoscopy

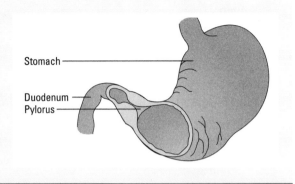

Understanding pyloric stenosis

In pyloric stenosis, hyperplasia (increased mass) and hypertrophy (increased size) of the circular muscle at the pylorus (the lower opening of the stomach leading into the duodenum) prevent the stomach from emptying normally.

Stomach

Duodenum
Pylorus

Care after surgery for pyloric stenosis

- Feed the child small amounts at first.
- Provide a pacifier.
- Position the child on his right side.
- Keep the incision area clean.

Diagnostic test findings
- Arterial blood gas analysis reveals metabolic alkalosis
- Blood chemistry tests reveal hypocalcemia, hypokalemia, and hypochloremia
- Hematest reveals blood in the emesis
- Ultrasound reveals hypertrophied pyloric sphincter
- Endoscopy reveals hypertrophied pyloric sphincter

Medical management
- Nothing-by-mouth status before surgery
- I.V. therapy to correct fluid and electrolyte imbalances
- Insertion of NG tube, kept open for gastric decompression
- Surgical intervention—pyloromyotomy performed by laparoscopy

Nursing interventions
- Weigh the child daily to assess growth
- Monitor vital signs and intake and output to assess renal function and check for signs of dehydration
- Assess for metabolic alkalosis and dehydration from frequent emesis to detect early complications
- Assess abdominal and cardiovascular status to detect early signs of compromise
- Provide small, frequent, thickened feedings with the head of the bed elevated; burp the child frequently to prevent aspiration
- Position the child, preferably on his right side, to prevent the aspiration of vomitus
- Postoperative care
  - Feed the child small amounts of oral electrolyte solution at first, then increase the amount and concentration of food until normal feeding is achieved
  - Provide a pacifier to maintain comfort
  - Position the child on his right side, allowing gravity to help the flow of fluid through the pyloric valve
  - Keep the incision area clean to prevent infection

VOMITING

● **Definition**
- Also known as *emesis*
- The forceful emptying of stomach contents through the mouth
- The body's effort to protect itself from a toxic substance that may be an infectious process or an ingested foreign body
- Nausea
    - The sensation of impending vomiting
    - Associated with excess saliva, pale-colored skin, sweating, and increased heart rate

● **Causes**
- GI disorders, such as spasm of the duodenum, reverse peristalsis from blockage of the pylorus, reflux from an incompetent or lax esophageal sphincter, overdistension of the stomach from increased intake, toxic ingestions, food allergies, and gastroenteritis
- Non-GI disorders, such as increased intracranial pressure or psychogenic problems

● **Pathophysiology**
- Two areas of the medulla in the central nervous system control vomiting
- The chemoreceptor trigger zone, located in the fourth ventricle, can stimulate vomiting
- Vomiting may be a learned behavior in response to a stressful situation such as going to a new school
- A wet burp (spitting up) involves either dribbling of undigested liquids from the mouth and esophagus or their expulsion with the force of a burp

● **Complications**
- Dehydration and electrolyte disturbances
- Malnutrition
- Aspiration
- Mallory-Weiss syndrome (mild to massive, usually painless bleeding resulting from a tear in the mucosa or submucosa of the lower esophagus)

● **Assessment findings**
- Nonprojectile or projectile vomiting (differentiate vomiting from a wet burp or spitting up)
- Accompanying symptoms: fever, nausea, headache, abdominal pain, and constipation or diarrhea
- Characteristics of the vomitus: blood, bile, undigested or digested food, amount, and force
- Metabolic alkalosis from the loss of stomach acids

● **Diagnostic test findings**
- A urinalysis can detect the presence of blood or proteins in the urine

Antiemetic drugs

- Ondansetron – blocks receptors in the chemoreceptor zone
- Metoclopramide – stimulates upper GI peristalsis
- Promethazine – blocks cholinergic receptors in the vomiting center

TOP 6

Items to study for your next test on the gastrointestinal system

1. Characteristics of the pediatric GI system
2. Functions of the liver
3. Key assessment findings for such GI disorders as appendicitis, GER, Hirschsprung's disease, intussusception, and pyloric stenosis
4. Cleft lip and palate surgeries
5. Feeding tips for patients with GER
6. Nursing interventions for the patient with vomiting

due to infection or dehydration

- A basic metabolic panel reveals the levels of electrolytes in the serum
- An abdominal X-ray or ultrasound will reveal structural abnormalities
- Endoscopy involves the insertion of a fiber-optic scope to allow direct visual inspection of the esophagus

● **Medical management**
- The goal is to prevent further episodes of vomiting and to stop the complications from occurring
- Antiemetic drugs include those that block receptors in the chemoreceptor zone (ondansetron [Zofran]), stimulate upper GI peristalsis (metoclopramide [Reglan]), and block cholinergic receptors in the vomiting center (promethazine [Phenergan])

● **Nursing interventions**
- Evaluate feeding methods (amount of burping, air in nipple)
- Prevent aspiration by positioning the child on his side; maintain a patent airway; perform nasotracheal or bulb suctioning, if necessary
- Withhold food and fluids to rest the stomach for 4 to 6 hours; in severe vomiting, I.V. fluids may be needed to prevent dehydration
- If an obstruction isn't the cause, begin administering I.V. fluids or frequent small amounts of clear liquids orally such as ice pops, Pedialyte, or broth
- For older children, administer antiemetic medications (they shouldn't be used in infants)
- Test the emesis for blood
- Record the description and amount of emesis after each vomiting episode
- Raise the head of bed when feeding and shortly thereafter to prevent aspiration
- Provide skin and mouth care after each vomiting episode
- Monitor hydration status, such as daily weight and fluid intake and output
- Monitor bowel status

NCLEX CHECKS

It's never too soon to begin your NCLEX preparation. Now that you've reviewed this chapter, carefully read each of the following questions and choose the best answer. Then compare your responses to the correct answers.

1. A nurse is teaching a parent about her child's diarrhea. The most commonly identified viral pathogen that produces diarrhea is:

☐ **1.** *Giardia.*
☐ **2.** Rotavirus.
☐ **3.** *Salmonella.*
☐ **4.** *Shigella.*

2. Which test provides a definitive diagnosis for Hirschsprung's disease?
- [ ] **1.** Rectal biopsy
- [ ] **2.** Barium enema
- [ ] **3.** Upper GI series
- [ ] **4.** Stool for parasites

3. Which surgical procedure is used to repair a cleft lip?
- [ ] **1.** Rhinoplasty
- [ ] **2.** Herniorrhaphy
- [ ] **3.** Staphylorrhaphy
- [ ] **4.** Cheiloplasty

4. Which signs or symptoms would you expect in an infant with intussusception?
- [ ] **1.** Projectile vomiting containing formula but no bile
- [ ] **2.** Ribbonlike stools
- [ ] **3.** Abdominal distension and pale, watery stools
- [ ] **4.** Severe colicky abdominal pain and a sausage-shaped mass in the right upper quadrant

5. When assessing a child for pyloric stenosis, which assessment finding is most diagnostic?
- [ ] **1.** Projectile vomiting with reverse peristalsis
- [ ] **2.** Spitting up with normal peristalsis
- [ ] **3.** Projectile vomiting with normal peristalsis
- [ ] **4.** Spitting up with reverse peristalsis

6. When explaining to a client and family about what to expect following an upper GI series, which statement by the nurse would be correct?
- [ ] **1.** The client may have diarrhea.
- [ ] **2.** The client may not eat or drink following the examination.
- [ ] **3.** The client may have stools that are chalky colored or gray.
- [ ] **4.** The client may need an enema due to constipation.

7. Which should be the first intervention when caring for a child with severe diarrhea?
- [ ] **1.** Allow the bowel to rest.
- [ ] **2.** Correct any electrolyte imbalance.
- [ ] **3.** Increase oral fluid intake.
- [ ] **4.** Administer bismuth subsalicylate (Kaopectate) as directed.

8. A parent is filling out a menu for his child who was diagnosed with celiac disease. Which food choices by the parent would confirm his understanding of the child's dietary needs?
- [ ] **1.** Chocolate milk and hot dog on a bun
- [ ] **2.** Iced tea and corn tortilla wrap with chicken and cheddar cheese
- [ ] **3.** Fruit juice and grilled cheese on wheat bread
- [ ] **4.** Chocolate milk and a rice cake with peanut butter

9. Which statement best describes the technique to feed an infant with a cleft lip?

☐ **1.** Thicken feedings and enlarge the nipple opening to allow for easier delivery.

☐ **2.** Feed upright and slowly, allowing for frequent breaks.

☐ **3.** Lay the infant on his right side to prevent aspiration.

☐ **4.** Give small, frequent feedings to prevent aspiration.

10. During gastroesophageal reflux, the lower esophageal sphincter (LES) doesn't close or function properly. Identify the location of the LES by placing an "x" over the correct area.

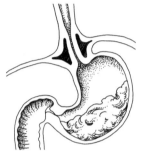

ANSWERS AND RATIONALES

1. CORRECT ANSWER: 2

Rotavirus is the most commonly identified viral pathogen that results in diarrhea. *Salmonella, Giardia,* and *Shigella* are bacterial pathogens.

2. CORRECT ANSWER: 1

Rectal biopsy is the definitive diagnostic test for Hirschsprung's disease. If positive for Hirschsprung's disease, the rectal biopsy shows aganglionic cells in the bowel. A barium enema is the diagnostic test for intussusception. An upper GI series is the diagnostic test for pyloric stenosis. Checking stools for parasites helps diagnose a bacterial infection in the bowel.

3. CORRECT ANSWER: 4

A cleft lip repair is called a cheiloplasty. A herniorrhaphy is repair of a hernia. A rhinoplasty is repair of a deviated nasal septum. Staphylorrhaphy is the procedure used to repair a cleft palate.

4. CORRECT ANSWER: 4

The classic signs of intussusception include an episode of acute, colicky abdominal pain in which the child screams and draws the knees to the chest. The child usually vomits, and you may feel a sausage-shaped mass in the right upper quadrant. Emesis containing milk or formula but no bile is a sign of pyloric stenosis. Ribbonlike stools are characteristic of Hirschsprung's disease. Celiac disease is characterized by abdominal distention and pale, watery stools that have an offensive odor.

5. CORRECT ANSWER: 1

A child with pyloric stenosis usually demonstrates projectile vomiting during or shortly after feedings preceded by reverse peristaltic waves.

6. CORRECT ANSWER: 3

Following an upper GI series, the family and child should be told that stools will be chalky or gray in color because of the barium given during the procedure. A child may become constipated following an upper GI series but the usual treatment is to increase his fluid intake to allow for natural passage of the stool.

7. CORRECT ANSWER: 2

Correcting an electrolyte imbalance is the first intervention that should be made. Diarrhea can cause an acid-base disturbance that leads to shock. Correcting the imbalance with I.V. fluids and electrolytes allows for circulatory volume to be restored. Withholding food and oral fluids is correct but should be done after the imbalance is corrected. Bismuth subsalicylate may be ordered to make stools firmer if the diarrhea occurs in an older child.

8. CORRECT ANSWER: 2

Celiac disease is characterized by poor food absorption and intolerance of gluten, a protein found in grains such as wheat, rye, oats, and barley. All of the foods listed may contain gluten except for iced tea and corn tortilla wrap with chicken and cheddar cheese. Chocolate milk that's commercially prepared contains malt, and processed cheese may contain starch and preservatives not defined as gluten-free.

9. CORRECT ANSWER: 2

Feeding an infant with a cleft lip slowly and in an upright position decreases the risk of aspiration. Thickened feedings with an enlarged nipple is helpful with infants with reflux but doesn't assist with a cleft lip defect. Giving small, frequent feedings is helpful but not the best solution. Laying an infant on the right side wouldn't be helpful with a child with cleft lip but does aid in prevention of aspiration.

10. CORRECT ANSWER:

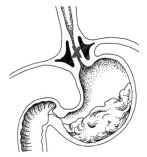

The LES is located at the lower end of the esophagus.

11

Altered genitourinary functioning

PRETEST

1. The most common form of dehydration seen in children is:

☐ 1. hypertonic dehydration.

☐ 2. hypotonic dehydration.

☐ 3. isotonic dehydration.

☐ 4. malignant dehydration.

CORRECT ANSWER: 3

2. The outermost layer of the kidney is called the:

☐ 1. hilum.

☐ 2. cortex.

☐ 3. medulla.

☐ 4. pyramids.

CORRECT ANSWER: 2

3. Which term is used to describe undescended testicles?

☐ 1. Enuresis

☐ 2. Epispadius

☐ 3. Hypospadius

☐ 4. Cryptorchidism

CORRECT ANSWER: 4

4. One cause of isotonic dehydration is:

☐ 1. diarrhea.

☐ 2. fever.

☐ 3. malnutrition.

☐ 4. diabetic ketoacidosis.

CORRECT ANSWER: 1

5. What percentage of an infant's extracellular fluid is exchanged every day?

☐ 1. 10%

☐ 2. 30%

☐ 3. 50%

☐ 4. 70%

CORRECT ANSWER: 3

LEARNING OBJECTIVES

After studying this chapter, you should be able to:

● Describe how a child's fluid and electrolyte status differs from that of an adult.

● Assess and plan care for a dehydrated child.

● Assess and plan care for a child with infected or inflamed renal and urinary systems.

● Discuss two congenital anomalies of the genitourinary tract.

CHAPTER OVERVIEW

Knowing how a child's fluid and electrolyte status differs from that of an adult provides the basis for understanding conditions associated with altered genitourinary function. A thorough assessment is necessary for prompt identification of the problem. Nursing interventions are geared toward controlling and correcting the problem and promoting normal fluid and electrolyte balance and renal function. Intake and output, skin care measures, and medication therapy are crucial components of nursing care.

KEY CONCEPTS

● **Structures**
- Kidneys
  - A pair of organs located retroperitoneally in the lumbar area
  - Right kidney is slightly lower than the left one because the liver is above it
  - Covered by fibrous capsule (renal sinus), perirenal fat, renal fasciae, and pararenal fat (see *Structures of the kidneys*)
  - Anatomy
    - Hilum
      - Located in medial margin of the kidney
      - Indented where blood and lymph vessels enter the kidney and the ureter emerges
    - Cortex
      - Outermost layer of kidney
      - Contains nephrons and glomeruli (networks of minute blood vessels)
    - Medulla
      - Located below the cortex
      - Contains pyramids (cone-shaped structures)
      - Papillae — ends of the pyramids through which formed urine oozes into the minor calyces
      - Minor calyces — converge to form major calyces
      - Major calyces — converge and then narrow into ureter
    - Nephrons
      - The functional units of the kidney
      - Two types
        ·· Cortical — located in the cortex
        ·· Juxtamedullary — located in the medulla
      - The child attains the adult number of nephrons shortly after birth, although these structures continue to mature throughout early childhood
      - Blood flows through the afferent arteriole into the glomerulus and exits through the efferent vessel

---

Quick guide to structures of the genitourinary system

- **Kidneys** — a pair of organs located retroperitoneally in the lumbar area
- **Bladder** — a spherical, hollow, muscular sac that stores formed urine until voiding
- **Ureters** — two ducts that transport urine from the renal pelvis to the urinary bladder
- **Urethra** — a tube that connects the bladder to the external meatus

Tubular components of the nephron

- Bowman's capsule
- Proximal convoluted tubule
- Loop of Henle
- Distal convoluted tubule
- Collecting duct

Structures of the kidneys

This illustration shows the kidneys' structures.

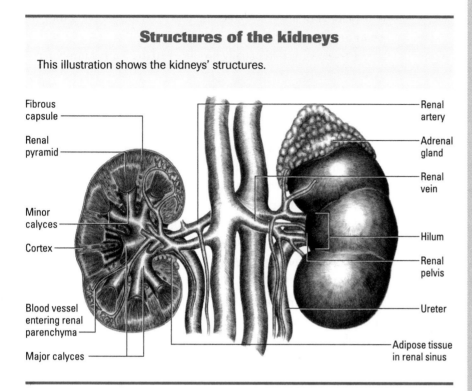

Fibrous capsule

Renal pyramid

Minor calyces

Cortex

Blood vessel entering renal parenchyma

Major calyces

Renal artery

Adrenal gland

Renal vein

Hilum

Renal pelvis

Ureter

Adipose tissue in renal sinus

- Tubular components change filtrate from the glomerulus depending on whether the body needs to reabsorb a substance (such as sodium and water) or excrete a substance (such as urea)
    ·· Bowman's capsule
    ·· Proximal convoluted tubule
    ·· Loop of Henle
    ·· Distal convoluted tubule
    ·· Collecting duct
- Ureters
  - Two ducts—one leading from each kidney
  - Transport urine from renal pelvis to urinary bladder
- Bladder
  - Spherical, hollow muscular sac
  - Storage area for formed urine until voiding (micturition)
  - Located in the abdomen during infancy and drops into pelvis at puberty
  - The number of daily voidings decreases with age (because of increased urine concentration and bladder control)
    • The infant usually produces 5 to 10 ml of urine per hour; the amount of urine voided is measured by weighing the diaper and subtracting dry weight from wet weight (grams equals milliliters)

Key facts about voiding

- An infant usually produces 5 to 10 ml of urine per hour.
- The bladder of a 4-year-old child holds 250 ml.
- A 10-year-old child usually produces 10 to 25 ml of urine per hour.
- An adult usually produces at least 35 ml of urine per hour.
- The number of daily voidings decreases with age.

- The bladder of a 4-year-old child holds 250 ml, allowing the child to stay dry through the night
- The 10-year-old child usually produces 10 to 25 ml of urine per hour
- The adult usually produces at least 35 ml of urine per hour
- Urethra
  - Tube connecting the bladder to the external meatus
  - The child has a short urethra, through which organisms can easily be transmitted into the bladder
  - In males, the urethra travels through the prostate and pelvic floor and exits through the penis
  - In females, the urethra exits in front of the vaginal opening
  - The urethra in a female is shorter and closer to the rectum than in a male, posing a greater risk of contamination by incorrect wiping after a bowel movement

Functions of the kidneys

- Detoxify blood and eliminate wastes
  - Glomerular filtration
    - Process of filtering the blood flowing through the kidneys
    - Blood from afferent vessel passes into glomerulus
    - Glomerular filtrate is formed when substrates (water, electrolytes, and solutes such as glucose) pass through the glomerular membrane into Bowman's capsule
    - Blood pressure drives the glomerular filtration rate (GFR)
    - An infant has a low GFR; however, the rate approaches the adult level by age 2
    - Creatinine clearance is the most accurate measure of glomerular filtration because creatinine is filtered only by the glomerulus and isn't reabsorbed by the tubules
  - Tubular reabsorption and secretion
    - Water, electrolytes, and solutes are reabsorbed or secreted from the filtrate into surrounding peritubular capillaries
    - Transport of filtered substances may be active (requiring the expenditure of energy) or passive (requiring none)
    - Reabsorption of water, sodium, and chloride mainly occurs in the proximal convoluted tubule
    - Inefficient reabsorption of sodium can result in hyponatremia
    - Secretion of potassium excesses and urea occur in the distal convoluted tubule
- Produce erythropoietin
  - Occurs when low oxygen levels are detected in the blood
  - Stimulates bone marrow to produce red blood cells (RBCs) to carry more oxygen
- Regulate blood pressure

Functions of the kidneys

- Detoxify blood and eliminate wastes
- Produce erythropoietin
- Regulate blood pressure
- Maintain fluid and electrolyte balance

– Renin is produced and released when a decrease in blood pressure or blood volume is detected

– Renin acts on a substrate to form angiotensin I, which is converted to angiotensin II

– Angiotensin II increases blood pressure by peripheral vasoconstriction and stimulation of aldosterone secretion

– Aldosterone promotes the reabsorption of sodium and water to correct the fluid deficit

• Maintain fluid and electrolyte balance

– Body water and body weight

• Water is the body's primary fluid

• The amount of water varies with age, sex, and percentage of body fat

• A preterm neonate's weight is 90% water; a full-term neonate's weight is 75% to 80% water

• An infant has a greater percentage of total body water in extracellular fluid (ECF) (42% to 45%) than an adult (20%), which means an infant can't conserve water as well as an adult and has less fluid reserve

• An infant's water turnover rate is two to three times higher than an adult's

  - 50% of an infant's ECF is exchanged every day, compared to only 20% of an adult's

  - An infant is more susceptible than an adult to dehydration

• An infant doesn't concentrate urine at an adult level (average specific gravity is less than 1.010 for an infant; 1.010 to 1.030 for an adult)

• The proportion of body water to body weight decreases with increasing age as body fat increases and solid body structures grow

• The distribution of body water doesn't reach adult levels until late school-age

• The adult percentage of body water (63% for men, 52% for women) is attained by age 3 (after puberty, females have more fat than males)

– Metabolism

• A child's growth depends on, and results in, an increased metabolic rate

• A child's metabolic rate is two to three times higher than that of an adult

• A child produces more metabolic waste

• A child's pulse, respiratory, and peristaltic rates are higher than an adult's

  - A child has a greater proportion of insensible water loss

How the kidneys regulate blood pressure

● They produce renin.
● Renin forms angiotensin I, which is converted to angiotensin II.
● Angiotensin II causes peripheral vasoconstriction and the secretion of aldosterone.
● Aldosterone promotes the reabsorption of sodium and water.

Key facts about an infant's water turnover

● An infant has a greater percentage of total body water in ECF than an adult.
● An infant, who can't conserve water as well as an adult and has less fluid reserve, is more susceptible than an adult to dehydration.
● An infant's water turnover rate is two to three times higher than an adult's.
● Fifty percent of an infant's ECF is exchanged every day.

Key facts about a child's metabolism

● A child's growth depends on an increased metabolic rate, which is two to three times higher than that of an adult.
● A child produces more metabolic waste than an adult.
● A child's pulse, respiratory, and peristaltic rates are higher than an adult's.

- A child needs more water per kilogram of body weight than an adult
– Body surface area
  • A neonate has a greater ratio of body surface area to body weight than an adult
  • The greater ratio of body surface area results in greater fluid loss through the skin

DIAGNOSTIC TESTS

● **Blood tests**
  • Purpose
    – Used to analyze serum levels of chemical substances, such as uric acid, creatinine, blood urea nitrogen (BUN), and electrolytes
  • Nursing interventions
    – Explain the procedure to the parents and child
    – Allow the child to hold a comfort object, such as a stuffed animal or blanket, during the procedure

● **Urinalysis**
  • Purpose
    – Determines urine characteristics such as specific gravity, pH, physical properties (color, clarity, and odor), and detects the presence of RBCs, white blood cells (WBCs), casts, glucose, or bacteria
  • Nursing interventions
    – Explain the importance of cleaning the meatal area thoroughly before collecting for a culture analysis
    – Explain that the culture specimen should be caught midstream in a sterile container
    – Use the clean-catch method to collect urine from a child
    – For an infant, after properly cleaning the skin and genitals, apply a pediatric urine collector to dry skin (powders and creams shouldn't be used)
    – When obtaining a urine specimen from a catheterized child, don't take the sample from the collection bag; aspirate a sample through the collection port in the catheter with a sterile needle and syringe

● **Kidneys-ureters-bladder (KUB) radiography**
  • Purpose
    – To assess the size, shape, position, and possible areas of calcification of the renal organs
  • Nursing interventions
    – Explain the procedure to the parents and child
    – Instruct the child to hold still during the X-ray
    – Shield the genitals of a male child to prevent irradiation of the testes

---

Quick guide to common diagnostic tests for genitourinary disorders

● **Blood tests** – used to analyze serum levels of chemical substances
● **Excretory urography** – allows visualization of the collecting system and ureters
● **KUB radiography** – used to assess renal organs
● **Urinalysis** – used to determine urine characteristics and detect presence of RBCs, WBCs, casts, or bacteria
● **Voiding cystourethrogram** – used to study the bladder and related structures during voiding

Excretory urography

- Purpose
  - Aids in checking renal pelvic structures
  - Contrast media is introduced into the renal pelvis, allowing visualization of the collecting system and ureters
- Nursing interventions
  - Check the child's history for allergies
  - Monitor the child's intake and output
  - Explain the purpose of the test to the parents and child
  - Obtain written, informed consent
  - Maintain the child on nothing-by-mouth status for 8 hours before the test
  - Increase hydration after the procedure

Voiding cystourethrogram

- Purpose
  - Aids in viewing the bladder and related structures during voiding
- Nursing interventions
  - Check the child's history for allergies
  - Monitor the child's intake and output
  - Explain the purpose of the test to the child and his parents
  - Obtain written, informed consent
  - Insert a urinary catheter just before the test
  - After the procedure, remove the urinary catheter and encourage the child to drink lots of fluid to reduce burning on urination and to flush out residual dye

NURSING DIAGNOSES

Probable nursing diagnoses

- Risk for infection
- Acute pain
- Impaired urinary elimination
- Urinary retention

Possible nursing diagnoses

- Total urinary incontinence
- Disturbed body image
- Deficient knowledge (disease process and treatment regimen)

ACUTE GLOMERULONEPHRITIS

Definition

- An autoimmune immune-complex disorder occurring 1 to 2 weeks after a group A beta-hemolytic streptococcal infection

Probable nursing diagnoses for a patient with a genitourinary disorder

- Risk for infection
- Acute pain
- Impaired urinary elimination
- Urinary retention

Key facts about acute glomerulonephritis

- Autoimmune-complex disorder occurring 1 to 2 weeks after a streptococcal infection
- Sometimes follows a skin infection
- Most common in boys ages 3 to 7
- Usually resolves within 2 weeks

Complications of acute glomerulonephritis

- Chronic renal failure
- Heart failure from hypervolemia leads to pulmonary edema

TOP 4

Findings in acute glomerulonephritis

1. Decreased urine output
2. Fatigue, irritability, lethargy, and an anemic appearance
3. Protein, blood, RBCs, and WBCs in the urine
4. Cola-colored urine

- Most common in boys ages 3 to 7
- Usually resolves within 2 weeks

Causes

- Follows a group A beta-hemolytic streptococcal infection of the respiratory tract
- Less commonly, follows a skin infection such as impetigo

Pathophysiology

- Antibodies are made against the toxin of the streptococci
- The antigen-antibody complex becomes entrapped in the glomerular capillary membrane (see *A look at glomerulonephritis*)
- The condition induces inflammatory damage and impedes glomerular function
- The glomerulus loses the ability to be selectively permeable, and allows RBCs and proteins to filter through as the GFR falls
- Streptococcus isn't present in the kidney at any time

Complications

- Chronic renal failure
- Heart failure from hypervolemia leads to pulmonary edema

Assessment findings

- Mild to moderate edema
- Cola-colored (smoky) urine
- Decreased urine output
- Fatigue, irritability, lethargy, and an anemic appearance
- Mild to severe increased blood pressure (hypertension)
- Possibly in children, encephalopathy with seizures and focal neurologic deficits

Diagnostic test findings

- Increased erythrocyte sedimentation rate indicates inflammation
- Increased antistreptolysin-O titer indicates recent streptococcal infection
- Urinalysis reveals the presence of protein, blood, RBCs, and WBCs in the urine
- Elevated creatinine level
- Renal ultrasound may show a slightly enlarged kidney
- Kidney biopsy may reveal the cause of the inflammation

Medical management

- Supportive measures include bed rest, fluid and dietary sodium restrictions, and correction of electrolyte imbalances
- Diuretics such as furosemide (Lasix) to reduce fluid overload
- Antihypertensive drug to treat increased blood pressure
- Antibiotic (penicillin) if a staphylococcal infection is documented

Nursing interventions

- Monitor intake and output and daily weight; watch for signs of acute

A look at glomerulonephritis

The immune complex depositions that occur in glomerulonephritis are shown in the illustration below.

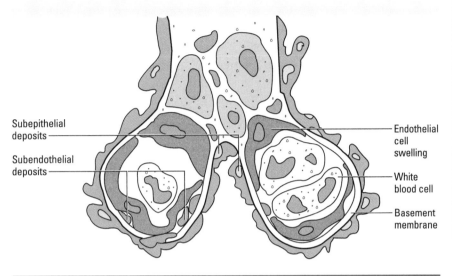

Subepithelial deposits

Subendothelial deposits

Endothelial cell swelling

White blood cell

Basement membrane

renal failure, including decreased (less than 1 mg/kg/hour), or no urine output
- Teach the parents about possible long-term penicillin therapy to prevent further renal damage in a subsequent streptococcal infection
- Institute moderate sodium restrictions for the child with hypertension or edema
- Administer medications to control hypertension
- Bed rest is necessary during the acute phase; aid the patient in gradually resuming normal activities

DEHYDRATION

● **Definition**
- Fluid output exceeds fluid intake
- Expressed as a percentage of body weight lost as water
- Isotonic dehydration
  - A deficiency of fluid and electrolytes in approximately equal proportions
  - Primary form of dehydration in children
  - 15% loss in the infant is considered severe
  - 9% loss in the older child is considered severe
  - Plasma sodium levels remain in the normal value range (130 to 150 mEq/L)
- Hypotonic dehydration

TOP 4

Ways to manage acute glomerulonephritis

1. Bed rest
2. Fluid and dietary sodium restrictions
3. Diuretics to reduce fluid overload
4. Antihypertensive drugs to decrease blood pressure

Types of dehydration

- Isotonic dehydration – fluid and electrolytes are deficient in approximately equal proportions
- Hypotonic dehydration – electrolyte loss is greater than fluid loss and plasma sodium levels are less than the normal value range
- Hypertonic dehydration – fluid loss is greater than electrolyte loss and plasma sodium levels are greater than normal value range

– Electrolyte loss is greater than fluid loss, causing extracellular-to-intracellular movement of water that results in shock
– Plasma sodium levels are less than the normal value range
- Hypertonic dehydration
    – Fluid loss is greater than electrolyte loss, causing intracellular-to-extracellular movement of water that results in neurologic changes, such as confusion, inability to concentrate, and motor tremors
    – Plasma sodium levels are greater than normal value range

● **Causes**
- Isotonic dehydration
    – Burns
    – Diarrhea
    – Excessive diaphoresis
    – Hemorrhage
    – Prolonged nothing-by-mouth status
    – Vomiting
- Hypotonic dehydration
    – Diabetic ketoacidosis
    – Fever
    – Tube feedings
- Hypertonic dehydration
    – Chronic illness
    – Malnutrition

● **Pathophysiology**
- Isotonic dehydration
    – Loss of isotonic fluids from the ECF space
    – No shifting of fluids between ECF and intracellular fluid (ICF)
    – Results in decreased blood volume and shock
- Hypotonic dehydration
    – Losses of sodium and potassium from ECF
    – Water shifts from ECF to ICF
    – Results in decreased blood volume, hyponatremia, and hypokalemia
- Hypertonic dehydration
    – Water loss from ECF greater than electrolyte losses
    – Water shifts from ICF to ECF
    – Results in cellular shrinkage and increased blood volume

● **Complications**
- Blood volume depletion
- Circulatory collapse
- Hypovolemic shock
- Cardiac arrhythmias

● **Assessment findings**
- Decreased urine output

- Concentrated urine
- Sudden weight loss
- Dry skin with poor tissue turgor
- Sunken anterior fontanel in the infant
- Decrease in tears and saliva
- Dry mucous membranes
- Sunken and soft eyeballs
- Thirst
- Pale, cool skin with poor perfusion, cool extremities, decreased body temperature
- Tachycardia, tachypnea, and hypotension
- Lethargy, irritability, and a high-pitched, weak cry

● **Diagnostic test findings**
- Isotonic dehydration
  - Normal sodium plasma level
  - Increased hematocrit and hemoglobin level
  - Increased urine specific gravity
- Hypotonic dehydration
  - Decreased sodium plasma level
  - Increased hematocrit and hemoglobin level
  - Decreased urine specific gravity
- Hypertonic dehydration
  - Increased sodium plasma level
  - Normal or decreased hematocrit and hemoglobin level
  - Increased urine specific gravity

● **Medical management**
- Administration of oral fluids
- I.V. fluids are used when oral intake is insufficient, severe vomiting or severe abdominal distention is present, or circulatory collapse is imminent
  - Isotonic solutions (normal saline solution or lactated Ringer's solution) are the first choice for rapid rehydration and are given as I.V. boluses
  - Maintenance fluids may contain sodium, water, and glucose to replace lost electrolytes; glucose is withheld from patients suffering from diabetic ketoacidosis
  - Potassium is withheld from I.V. fluids until kidney function is adequate
- Begin oral feedings slowly with an oral replacement solution such as Pedialyte and advance as tolerated

● **Nursing interventions**
- Record hourly all stools, vomitus, and urine
  - Note the amount, color, consistency, concentration, time, and relation to meals or stress

– Note the results of specific gravity and other values from urine dipstick tests
- Withhold food and fluids and use I.V. replacement of fluids; provide sucking stimulation to the young infant
- Provide mouth care
- Provide skin care
  – Turn the child every 2 hours
  – Keep the extremities warm
- Carefully measure intake and output
  – Weigh the diapers
  – Record the fluids used to take medications
  – Indicate the fluid lost by diaphoresis, suctioning, or other tubes
- Weigh the child using the same scale at the same time each day, with the child naked or wearing the same type and amount of clothing
- Provide rest
- Monitor for and prevent shock
- Note that an increase in ambient heat or water loss requires greater fluid intake to meet hydration needs

ENURESIS

Definition
- Repeated involuntary urination after age 5
- Usually occurs while the child is asleep (may also occur during the day)
- Primary enuresis — the child has never achieved complete bladder control
- Secondary enuresis — the child has achieved a period of bladder control
- Nocturnal enuresis — occurs when the child is sleeping

Causes
- Stress, such as the birth of a sibling, moving to a new home, or divorce
- Incomplete muscle maturation
- Altered sleep patterns
- Irritable bladder that can't handle large amounts of urine

Pathophysiology
- The child may sleep too soundly to recognize the cues of a full bladder
- A child with enuresis may have a smaller bladder capacity than other children

Complications
- Low self-esteem
- Social withdrawal from peers because of ridicule
- Anger, rejection, and punishment by caregivers

Assessment findings
- Acute urgency to void followed by discomfort and restlessness

- Voiding during sleep, especially at night

● **Diagnostic test findings**
  - Routine physical examination and history determines age of toilet training, onset of enuresis, and frequency of occurrences
  - Functional bladder capacity is determined by having the child hold his urine until the last possible moment and then void into a calibrated container; ability to hold a night's urine is probable when functional bladder capacity reaches 300 ml
  - Urinalysis, urine culture and sensitivity, and blood studies, including BUN and creatinine, to evaluate renal function and possible urinary tract infection (UTI)

● **Medical management**
  - Dry-bed therapy may include the use of an enuresis alarm (an alarm that sounds when the bed pad becomes wet), social motivation, self-correction of accidents, and positive reinforcement
  - Drug therapy may include the use of tricyclic antidepressants, antidiuretics, and antispasmodics

● **Nursing interventions**
  - Be aware that treatment varies with the cause
  - Remind the child to use the toilet every 2 hours
  - Decrease fluids after 5 p.m. except to satisfy the child's thirst
  - Teach bladder-stretching exercises during the day
    - Have the child drink large amounts of fluid
    - Try to have the child keep the bladder enlarged for a while before emptying
  - Provide emotional support to the child and his parents
    - Don't embarrass or punish the child
    - Don't refer to enuresis as an accident

HYPOSPADIAS AND EPISPADIAS

● **Definition**
  - Hypospadias—a congenital anomaly of the penis in which the urethral meatus opens on the ventral surface (underside) of the penis
  - Epispadias—a rare condition in which the urinary meatus opens on the dorsal surface (top side) of the penis
  - Both conditions shorten the distance to the bladder, offering bacteria easier access

● **Causes**
  - Exact cause is unknown
  - Genetic factors most likely contribute to the cause

Dry-bed therapy techniques

- Enuresis alarm
- Social motivation
- Self-correction of accidents
- Positive reinforcement

Key facts about hypospadias and epispadias

- Hypospadias is a congenital anomaly in which the urethral meatus opens on the underside of the penis.
- Epispadias is a rare condition in which the urinary meatus opens on the top side of the penis.
- The cause is unknown.
- Recurrent UTIs are a complication.

Hypospadias and epispadias

The illustrations at right show the placement of the urethral opening in males with hypospadias and epispadias.

HYPOSPADIAS

EPISPADIAS

Assessment findings in hypospadias

- Altered angle of urination
- Urethral opening is located on underside of penis

Assessment findings in epispadias

- The urethral opening is located on the topside of the penis.
- In epispadias with bladder exstrophy, the bladder is exposed and urine seeps onto the abdominal wall.

Pathophysiology

- Hypospadias
  - The urethral opening is on the ventral surface of the penis
  - In severe cases, the urethral opening is located on the perineal or scrotal region
  - Occurs in 1 in 300 live male births
- Epispadias
  - The urethral opening is on the dorsal surface of the penis
  - Less frequent than hypospadias; occurs in 1 in 200,000 live male births (see *Hypospadias and epispadias*)

Complications

- Sexual disability
- Recurrent UTIs

Assessment findings

- Hypospadias
  - Altered angle of urination
  - Normal urination with penis elevated is impossible because of chordee (band of fibrous tissue causing penis curvature)
  - Urethral opening is located on underside of penis
- Epispadias
  - Urethral opening is located on topside of penis
  - With bladder exstrophy
    - Exposed bladder appears bright red and is obvious at birth
    - Urine seeps onto the abdominal wall from abnormal ureteral openings

Diagnostic test findings

- Diagnostic testing isn't necessary because observation confirms abnormal placement of the urethral opening

- **Medical management**
  - Hypospadias
    - Avoid circumcision (the foreskin may be needed later for surgical repair)
    - No treatment is necessary in mild disorder
    - Meatotomy—a surgical procedure performed to extend the urethra into a normal position
    - Surgery to release the chordee
      - Typically performed when the child is 12 to 18 months old
      - If extensive repair is needed, surgery is delayed until age 4
  - Epispadias
    - Surgery typically requires multiple procedures
    - Associated bladder exstrophy is closed preferably within the first few days of life
    - The second phase of surgery involves the lengthening and straightening of the penis and the creation of a more distal urethral opening

- **Nursing interventions**
  - Keep the area clean to prevent bacterial infection
  - Be aware that surgery involving implants or reconstruction may be needed to reduce the chance of UTIs and infertility
  - Encourage the parents to express their feelings and concerns, and provide emotional support

NEPHROTIC SYNDROME (NEPHROSIS)

- **Definition**
  - Nephrotic syndrome is an autoimmune process that occurs 1 week after an immune assault
  - It increases glomerular permeability to protein, especially albumin
  - The condition is common among toddlers

- **Causes**
  - Idiopathic glomerulonephritis (about 75% of cases)
  - Metabolic diseases such as diabetes mellitus
  - Collagen-vascular diseases such as systemic lupus erythematosus
  - Circulatory diseases such as sickle cell anemia
  - Nephrotoxins such as mercury
  - Allergic reactions
  - Infections such as tuberculosis

- **Pathophysiology**
  - Diseases increase glomerular permeability to proteins (especially albumin) leading to decreased serum levels of albumin (hypoalbuminemia)
  - Hypoalbuminemia results in reduced plasma volume as fluids shift from the ECF space to the ICF space

TOP 2

Interventions for hypospadias and epispadias

1. Keep the area clean to prevent bacterial infection.
2. Encourage the parents to express their feelings and concerns, and provide emotional support.

Key facts about nephrotic syndrome

- Autoimmune process that occurs 1 week after an immune assault
- Increases glomerular permeability of protein
- Common among toddlers
- Can be caused by numerous conditions including allergic reactions, toxins, and infections

GO WITH THE FLOW

What happens in nephrotic syndrome

The flowchart below shows the pathophysiology of nephrotic syndrome.

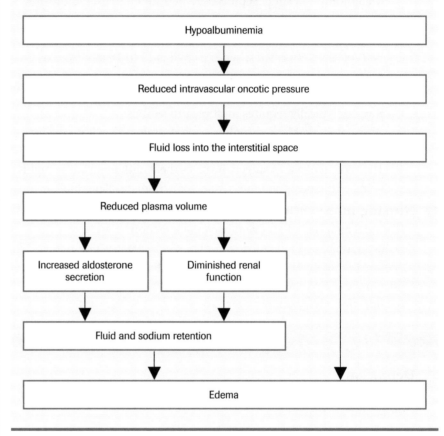

- The final result is edema from salt and water retention (see *What happens in nephrotic syndrome*)

● Complications
- Peritonitis
- End-stage renal failure

● Assessment findings
- Dark, foamy, and frothy urine
- Decreased urine production
- Edema
  - Dependent body edema accompanies weight gain
  - Periorbital edema occurs in the morning
  - Abdominal ascites and increased abdominal girth are evident
  - Scrotal edema occurs

Complications of nephrotic syndrome

- Peritonitis
- End-stage renal failure

– Ankle edema develops by midday
– Diarrhea, anorexia, and malnutrition result from edema of the intestinal mucosa
- Stretched, shiny skin with a waxy pallor
- Fatigue and lethargy

Diagnostic test findings

- Proteinuria
- High urine specific gravity
- Microscopic hematuria; frank bleeding doesn't occur
- Decreased protein and potassium levels revealed through blood analysis
- Kidney biopsy diagnoses the disease and shows a renal lesion

Medical management

- Protein replacement with a high-protein diet
- Diuretics and a low-sodium diet to alleviate edema
- Antibiotics for treatment of underlying infections
- Oral steroid (such as prednisone) therapy to suppress the autoimmune response and to stimulate vascular reabsorption of edema
- Angiotension-converting enzyme (ACE) inhibitors to help reduce protein loss in urine

Nursing interventions

- Provide skin care to edematous skin; don't use adhesive strip bandages, tape, or I.M. injections
- Provide warm soaks to decrease periorbital edema
- Elevate the head of the bed
- Turn the child frequently
- Provide scrotal support and place padding between body parts to prevent irritation
- Test the first void of the day for protein
- Feed small, frequent meals
- Measure intake and output and daily weight
- Prevent contact with persons who have an infection
- Anticipate diuresis in 1 to 3 weeks
  – Maintain bed rest during rapid diuresis
  – Monitor hydration status and vital signs

UNDESCENDED TESTES

Definition

- Also known as *cryptorchidism*
- One or both testes fail to descend into the scrotum, remaining in the abdomen, in the inguinal canal, or at the external ring
- If the testes aren't descended at birth, they may descend on their own in a few weeks

Key facts about undescended testes

- Also known as *cryptorchidism*
- One or both testes fail to descend into the scrotum
- Testes remain in the abdomen, in the inguinal canal, or at the external ring
- May descend on their own a few weeks after birth

Complications of undescended testes

- Sterility
- Trauma to testes
- Testicular cancer

Key facts about orchiopexy

- Surgical correction of undescended testes
- Secures the testes in the scrotum
- Performed if testes don't spontaneously descend by age 1
- Commonly performed before the child reaches age 4

Causes

- Failure of the gubernaculum, a fibromuscular band that connects the testes to the floor of the scrotum, to form
- Testosterone deficiency causing the failure of gonadal differentiation and gonadal descent
- Structural factors, such as ectopic testis or short spermatic cord, that impede gonadal descent
- In preterm neonates, early gestational age
- Rarely, genetic predisposition

Pathophysiology

- The testes descend from the abdomen into the scrotum during the last 2 months of gestation
- Testosterone stimulates the formation of the gubernaculum
- The gubernaculum probably helps pull the testes into the scrotum by shortening as the fetus grows
- Undescended testes may result if testosterone levels are inadequate or if there's a defect in the testes or gubernaculum

Complications

- If the testes remain in the abdominal cavity after age 5, the seminiferous tubules may degenerate because of increased body temperature in the abdomen, resulting in sterility
- Increased risk of trauma to testes, if untreated
- Increased risk of testicular cancer, if untreated

Assessment findings

- Testis on the affected side isn't palpable in the scrotum
- Scrotum appears underdeveloped

Diagnostic test findings

- Expect additional diagnostic tests to check kidney function because the kidneys and the testes arise from the same germ tissue

Medical management

- Surgical correction (orchiopexy)
  - Performed if testes don't spontaneously descend by age 1
  - Secures the testes in the scrotum
  - Commonly performed before the child reaches age 4

Nursing interventions

- Educate the parents on postoperative expectations
  - Explain that one suture passes through the testes and scrotum and attaches to the thigh
  - Instruct them to prevent pulling on the thigh suture postoperatively because the testes could reascend into the abdomen through the inguinal canal if the suture disconnects

URINARY TRACT INFECTION

● **Definition**
  - A microbial invasion of the kidneys, ureters, bladder, or urethra
  - In the neonatal period, UTIs occur most commonly in males, possibly because of the higher incidence of congenital abnormalities
  - By age 4 months, UTIs are more common in females because of the placement and size of the urethra

● **Causes**
  - Incomplete bladder emptying
  - Irritation by bubble baths
  - Poor hygiene
  - Vesicoureteric reflux
  - Urinary tract obstruction

● **Pathophysiology**
  - Bacteria enter the urethra and ascend the urinary tract
  - *Escherichia coli* causes approximately 75% to 90% of all UTIs in females

● **Complications**
  - Vesicoureteric reflux
  - Glomerulonephritis
  - Bacteremia
  - Sepsis
  - Septic shock

● **Assessment findings**
  - Abdominal pain
  - Enuresis
  - Frequent urges to void with pain or burning on urination
  - Hematuria
  - Lethargy or irritability
  - Low-grade fever
  - Poor feeding patterns
  - Cloudy, foul-smelling urine

● **Diagnostic test findings**
  - Clean-catch urine culture yields large amounts of bacteria
  - Increased urine pH

● **Medical management**
  - Forced fluids to flush infection from the urinary tract
  - Antibiotics: co-trimoxazole (Bactrim) or ampicillin (Omnipen) to prevent glomerulonephritis

Locations of UTIs
- Kidneys
- Ureters
- Bladder
- Urethra

Causes of UTIs
- Incomplete bladder emptying
- Irritation by bubble baths
- Poor hygiene
- Vesicoureteric reflux
- Urinary tract obstruction

TOP 5
Findings in UTIs
1. Frequent urges to void with pain or burning on urination
2. Lethargy or irritability
3. Low-grade fever
4. Cloudy, foul-smelling urine
5. Large amounts of bacteria present in clean-catch urine culture

Key nursing interventions for UTIs

- Administer antibiotics as prescribed.
- Force fluids.
- Teach proper toileting hygiene.
- Encourage the child to void every 2 hours.
- Discourage the use of bubble baths.
- Instruct the parents in ways to prevent UTIs.

TOP 7

Items to study for your next test on the genitourinary system

1. Structures and functions of the genitourinary system
2. Pediatric metabolism
3. Proper method for obtaining a urine specimen from an infant or a child
4. Signs and symptoms of dehydration
5. The difference between hypospadias and epispadias
6. Findings in nephrotic syndrome
7. Signs and symptoms of UTIs and key nursing interventions

TIME-OUT FOR TEACHING

Teaching about urinary tract infections

Be sure to include these points in your teaching plan for the parents of a child with a urinary tract infection:
- compliance with medication regimen
- increased need for fluids and suggestions for choices
- proper perineal hygiene
- avoidance of irritants
- signs and symptoms of recurrence.

● **Nursing interventions**
- Administer antibiotic as prescribed; instruct parents to complete the entire course of antibiotics even though the child's symptoms may be gone
- Force fluids to flush the infection from the urinary tract
- Teach proper toileting hygiene (front-to-back wiping)
- Encourage the child to use the toilet every 2 hours
- Discourage the use of bubble baths
- Instruct the parents in measures to prevent future UTIs (see *Teaching about urinary tract infections*)

NCLEX CHECKS

It's never too soon to begin your NCLEX preparation. Now that you've reviewed this chapter, carefully read each of the following questions and choose the best answer. Then compare your responses to the correct answers.

1. Which finding most likely indicates a child has a UTI?
- ☐ **1.** He has clear urine.
- ☐ **2.** He's toilet trained but experiences enuresis.
- ☐ **3.** He drinks a lot of fluids at frequent intervals.
- ☐ **4.** He urinates once in the morning and once in the evening.

2. A nurse is caring for a child with hypospadias. Which description of this condition is most accurate?
- ☐ **1.** Ventral curvature of the penis
- ☐ **2.** Meatal opening located on the dorsal surface of the penis
- ☐ **3.** Narrowing or stenosis of the preputial opening of the foreskin
- ☐ **4.** Urethral opening located behind the glans penis or along the ventral surface of the penile shaft

3. A nurse is examining a 2-year-old with nephrotic syndrome. Which signs or symptoms should she expect to find?

☐ **1.** Hyperalbuminemia
☐ **2.** Hypoalbuminemia
☐ **3.** Hyperlipidemia
☐ **4.** Increased urine production

4. A male neonate is diagnosed with cryptorchidism. When teaching the neonate's parents about the condition, the nurse explains that cryptorchidism is:

☐ **1.** protrusion of abdominal contents into the scrotum.
☐ **2.** narrowing of the preputial opening of the foreskin.
☐ **3.** failure of one or both testes to descend into the scrotum.
☐ **4.** fluid in the scrotum.

5. An 8-year-old girl is diagnosed with a UTI. Which statement indicates that the parent understands your instructions about UTIs?

☐ **1.** "It's OK for my daughter to use bubble bath."
☐ **2.** "She shouldn't drink too much water."
☐ **3.** "She should take the antibiotics until all the pills are used."
☐ **4.** "I should teach her to wipe from back to front."

6. Which is the most common bacteria present in females with UTIs?

☐ **1.** Adenovirus
☐ **2.** *Escherichia coli*
☐ **3.** Klebsiella
☐ **4.** Proteus

7. A 10-year-old was treated for a streptococcal throat infection 2 weeks ago and now has hypertension and cola-colored urine. The nurse should suspect which condition?

☐ **1.** Enuresis
☐ **2.** Nephrotic syndrome
☐ **3.** Glomerulonephritis
☐ **4.** Hypospadias

8. What diagnostic test findings should a nurse expect to find in a child with hypertonic dehydration?

☐ **1.** Increased hematocrit and hemoglobin level
☐ **2.** Decreased sodium plasma
☐ **3.** Normal sodium
☐ **4.** Increased urine specific gravity

9. How many milliliters of urine does a 10-year-old child produce per hour?

☐ **1.** 5 to 10
☐ **2.** 10 to 25
☐ **3.** 35
☐ **4.** 60

10. Place in chronological order the correct sequence for how the kidneys regulate blood pressure.

1. Renin forms angiotensin I.	
2. Aldosterone is secreted.	
3. Sodium and water are reabsorbed.	
4. Kidneys produce renin.	
5. Peripheral vasoconstriction occurs.	
6. Angiotensin II is produced.	

ANSWERS AND RATIONALES

1. CORRECT ANSWER: 2

Suspect a UTI if a toilet-trained child has enuresis (urine incontinence), frequent voiding with urgency, or cloudy, strong-smelling urine. A child who drinks large amounts of fluid at frequent intervals should be tested for diabetes.

2. CORRECT ANSWER: 4

With hypospadias, the urethral opening is located behind the glans penis or along the ventral surface of the penile shaft. A ventral curvature of the penis is called *chordee*. Phimosis is narrowing or stenosis of the preputial opening of the foreskin. Epispadias is diagnosed when the meatal opening is located on the dorsal surface of the penis.

3. CORRECT ANSWER: 2

In nephrotic syndrome, the glomerular membrane becomes permeable to proteins, especially albumin. Excess protein lost in the urine causes serum hypoalbuminemia and proteinuria. This also decreases colloidal osmotic pressure in the capillaries, causing fluid to accumulate in the interstitial spaces (edema). Nephrotic syndrome doesn't cause hyperlipidemia. Nephrotic syndrome causes urine production to decrease.

4. CORRECT ANSWER: 3

Cryptorchidism is the failure of one or both testes to descend through the inguinal canal into the scrotum. Protrusion of the abdominal contents into the scrotum is an inguinal hernia. Phimosis is a narrowing of the preputial opening of the foreskin. Fluid in the scrotum is a hydrocele.

5. CORRECT ANSWER: 3

The child should complete the full course of antibiotics. The parents should notify a health care provider if the child's condition gets worse or can't tolerate the medication. A child with a UTI shouldn't use bubble bath or let the soap float around in the bathtub because bubble bath and soap can cause urethral irritation. Fluid intake should be increased in a patient with a UTI. Girls should learn to wipe from front to back to prevent infection.

6. CORRECT ANSWER: 2
All are bacteria that may cause an infection but *E. coli* causes approximately 75% to 90% of all urinary tract infections in females.

7. CORRECT ANSWER: 3
Glomerulonephritis usually begins 7 to 21 days after group A beta-hemolytic streptococcal infection of either the throat or skin. It presents with mild to moderate edema and cola-colored urine. Enuresis is involuntary urination after the age of 5 that doesn't produce a particular color urine. Nephrotic syndrome produces dark, foamy, and frothy urine. Hypospadias is the placement of urethral opening on the dorsal surface of the penis and doesn't produce a colored urine.

8. CORRECT ANSWER: 4
There's an increased urine specific gravity, normal, or decreased hematocrit and hemoglobin, and an increased sodium plasma level in hypertonic dehydration. Increased hematocrit and hemoglobin are found in hypotonic and isotonic dehydration. In hypotonic dehydration, the sodium plasma level is decreased. In isotonic dehydration, the sodium plasma level is normal.

9. CORRECT ANSWER: 2
A 10-year-old child usually produces 10 to 25 ml of urine per hour. An infant usually produces 5 to 10 ml of urine per hour. An adult usually produces 35 ml of urine per hour. An output of 60 ml of urine per hour would be considered increased urination in an adult.

10. CORRECT ANSWER:

| 4. Kidneys produce renin. |
| 1. Renin forms angiotensin I. |
| 6. Angiotensin II is produced. |
| 5. Peripheral vasoconstriction occurs. |
| 2. Aldosterone is secreted. |
| 3. Sodium and water are reabsorbed. |

The kidneys produce renin. Renin forms angiotensin I which is converted to angiotensin II. Angiotensin II causes peripheral vasoconstriction and the secretion of aldosterone. Aldosterone promotes the reabsorption of sodium and water.

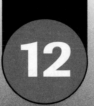

Altered musculoskeletal functioning

12

PRETEST

1. What's the name of the sheath of connective tissue that binds muscle fibers together?

☐ 1. Myosin
☐ 2. Sarcoplasm
☐ 3. Perimysium
☐ 4. Endomysium

CORRECT ANSWER: 3

2. What's the function of ligaments?

☐ 1. Protect internal tissue and organs
☐ 2. Bind bones to other bones
☐ 3. Cushion and absorb shock
☐ 4. Prevent transmission to the bone

CORRECT ANSWER: 2

3. Which type of osteogenesis perfecta is characterized by fractures that are present at birth and occur frequently during childhood?

- ☐ 1. Type I
- ☐ 2. Type II
- ☐ 3. Type III
- ☐ 4. Type IV

CORRECT ANSWER: 3

4. Which type of scoliosis can occur after polio?

- ☐ 1. Paralytic
- ☐ 2. Congenital
- ☐ 3. Idiopathic
- ☐ 4. Nonstructural

CORRECT ANSWER: 1

5. Legg-Calvé Perthes disease occurs in five stages. Which stage is considered the residual stage?

- ☐ 1. Reabsorption
- ☐ 2. Growth arrest
- ☐ 3. Reossification
- ☐ 4. Healed stage

CORRECT ANSWER: 4

LEARNING OBJECTIVES

After studying this chapter, you should be able to:

- ● Determine the nursing interventions necessary for the child with common pediatric musculoskeletal disorders.
- ● Assess and plan care for the child with a musculoskeletal defect.
- ● Describe how musculoskeletal development from birth through adolescence predisposes the child to various orthopedic conditions.

Structures of the musculoskeletal system

- Skeletal muscles
- Tendons
- Ligaments
- Bones
- Cartilage
- Joints
- Bursae

Types of muscle fibers

- Endomysium – sheath of fibrous connective tissue that surrounds the exterior of the fiber
- Sarcolemma – plasma membrane of cell that lies beneath the endomysium and above the nuclei
- Sarcoplasm – cytoplasm contained within the sarcolemma
- Myofibrils – tiny, threadlike structures that make up the bulk of the fiber
- Myosin (thick filaments) and actin (thin filaments) – fine fibers within the myofibrils

Functions of the skeletal muscles

- Maintain posture
- Produce voluntary and reflex movements
- Generate body heat
- Permit several types of movement

CHAPTER OVERVIEW

Musculoskeletal development from birth through adolescence predisposes a child to various orthopedic conditions. A thorough assessment of body part function, bone and tissue quality, bone alignment, and muscle response is crucial to the child's care. The various orthopedic conditions require different treatments. Nursing interventions are focused on maintaining optimal function and adaptation and assisting with, correcting, or controlling the problem, ultimately enhancing the child's level of functioning.

KEY CONCEPTS

- **Structures and functions**
  - Skeletal muscles
    - Attached to bone
      - Directly—the epimysium of the muscle fuses to the periosteum, the fibrous membrane covering the bone
      - Indirectly—the epimysium extends past the muscle as a tendon, or aponeurosis, and attaches to the bone
    - Consist of striated tissue
    - Composed of large, long cell groups called muscle fibers (see *Muscle structure up close*)
      - Endomysium—a sheath of fibrous connective tissue that surrounds the exterior of the fiber
      - Sarcolemma—the plasma membrane of the cell that lies beneath the endomysium and just above the cells' nuclei
      - Sarcoplasm—the muscle cell's cytoplasm, which is contained within the sarcolemma
      - Myofibrils—tiny, threadlike structures that run the fiber's length and make up the bulk of the fiber
      - Myosin (thick filaments) and actin (thin filaments)
        - Finer fibers within the myofibrils
        - Contained within compartments called sarcomeres
    - Develop when existing muscle fibers hypertrophy
      - Strength and size differ among individuals
    - Contract when stimulated by impulses
      - During contraction, the muscle shortens, pulling on the bones to which it's attached
      - Force is applied to the tendon
      - One bone is pulled toward, moved away from, or rotated around a second bone, depending on the type of muscle that has contracted
      - Most movement involves groups of muscles
    - Maintain posture
    - Generate body heat

Muscle structure up close

Skeletal muscle contains cell groups called *muscle fibers.* The illustration below shows the muscle and its fibers.

IN A BIND
The *perimysium* — a sheath of connective tissue — binds muscle fibers together into a fasciculus. The *epimysium* binds the fasciculi (bundles of muscle fibers) together; beyond the muscle, it becomes a tendon.

MUSCLE FIBERS ARE SURROUNDED
A sarcolemma (plasma membrane) surrounds each muscle fiber. Tiny myofibrils within the muscle fibers contain even finer fibers called myosin (thick filaments) and actin (thin filaments).

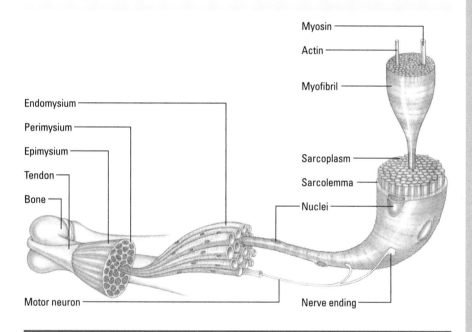

Types of skeletal muscle movement

- Flexion — bending
- Adduction — moving toward a body axis
- Abduction — moving away from a body axis
- Circumduction — circular movement

- Produce voluntary and reflex movements
- Permit several types of movement
  - Flexors permit bending (flexion)
  - Adductor muscles permit movement toward a body axis (adduction)
  - Abductor muscles permit movement away from a body axis (abduction)
  - Circumductor muscles allow a circular movement (circumduction)
- Tendons
  - Bands of fibrous connective tissue
  - Attach muscles to the periosteum, the fibrous covering of the bone
  - Enable bones to move when skeletal muscles contract
- Ligaments

Key facts about ligaments

- Dense, strong, flexible bands of fibrous connective tissue
- Bind bones to other bones
- Hold organs in place
- Limit or promote movement
- Provide stability

Functions of the bones

- Protect internal tissues and organs
- Stabilize and support the body
- Provide a surface for muscle, ligament, and tendon attachment
- Move through "lever" action when contracted
- Produce red blood cells in the bone marrow
- Store mineral salts

– Dense, strong, flexible bands of fibrous connective tissue
– Bind bones to other bones
– Hold organs in place
– Either limit or promote movement
– Provide stability

- Bones
  – The human skeleton contains 206 bones
    - 80 bones form the axial skeleton, which lies along the central line, or axis, of the body
      - Facial and cranial bones
      - Hyoid bone
      - Vertebrae
      - Ribs and sternum
    - 126 bones form the appendicular skeleton relating to the limbs, or appendages of the body
      - Clavicle
      - Scapula
      - Humerus, radius, ulna, carpals, metacarpals, and phalanges
      - Pelvic bone
      - Femur, patella, fibula, tibia, tarsals, metatarsals, and phalanges
  – Classified by shape
    - Long
    - Short
    - Flat
    - Irregular
    - Sesamoid
    - Wormian or sutural
  – Perform various anatomic (mechanical) and physiologic functions
    - Protect internal tissues and organs
    - Stabilize and support the body
    - Provide a surface for muscle, ligament, and tendon attachment
    - Move through "lever" action when contracted
    - Produce red blood cells in the bone marrow (a process called *hematopoiesis*)
    - Store mineral salts
  – Formation
    - At 3 months in utero, the fetal skeleton is composed of cartilage
    - At 6 months, fetal cartilage has transformed into bony skeleton
    - After birth, some bones ossify or harden
      - Carpals
      - Tarsals
  – Remodeling
    - The continuous process whereby bone is created and destroyed (see *Bone growth and remodeling*)

Bone growth and remodeling

The ossification of cartilage into bone, or *osteogenesis,* begins at about the 9th week of fetal development. The diaphyses of long bones are formed by birth, and the epiphyses begin to ossify about that time. Below are the stages of growth and remodeling of the epiphyses of a long bone.

CREATION OF AN OSSIFICATION CENTER

At about the 9th month, an ossification center develops in the epiphysis. Some cartilage cells enlarge and stimulate ossification of surrounding cells. The enlarged cells die, leaving small cavities. New cartilage continues to develop.

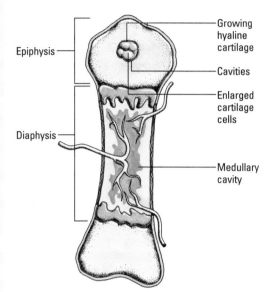

Epiphysis

Diaphysis

Growing hyaline cartilage

Cavities

Enlarged cartilage cells

Medullary cavity

OSTEOBLASTS FORM BONE

Osteoblasts begin to form bone on the remaining cartilage, creating the trabeculae network of cancellous bone. Cartilage continues to form on the outer surfaces of the epiphysis and along the upper surface of the epiphyseal plate.

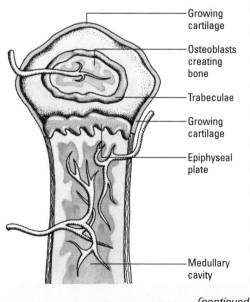

Growing cartilage

Osteoblasts creating bone

Trabeculae

Growing cartilage

Epiphyseal plate

Medullary cavity

(continued)

Key facts about bone remodeling

- It's a continuous process whereby bone is created and destroyed.
- It's performed by osteocytes.
- Osteoblasts deposit new bone.
- Osteoclasts increase long bone diameter.

Bone growth and remodeling *(continued)*

BONE GROWTH

Cartilage is replaced by compact bone near the outer surfaces of the epiphysis. Only cartilage cells on the upper surface of the diaphyseal plate continue to multiply rapidly, pushing the epiphysis away from the diaphysis. This new cartilage ossifies, creating trabeculae on the medullary side of the epiphyseal plate.

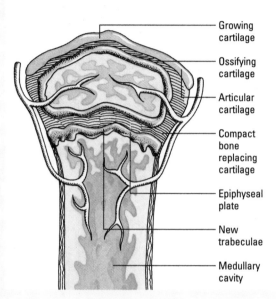

- Growing cartilage
- Ossifying cartilage
- Articular cartilage
- Compact bone replacing cartilage
- Epiphyseal plate
- New trabeculae
- Medullary cavity

REMODELING

Osteoclasts produce enzymes and acids that reduce trabeculae created by the epiphyseal plate, thus enlarging the medullary cavity. In the epiphysis, osteoclasts reduce bone, making its calcium available for new osteoblasts that give the epiphysis its adult shape and proportion. In young adults, the epiphyseal plate completely ossifies (closes) and becomes the epiphyseal line; longitudinal growth of bone then ceases.

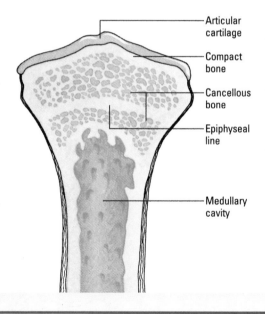

- Articular cartilage
- Compact bone
- Cancellous bone
- Epiphyseal line
- Medullary cavity

• Performed by the osteocytes
  - Osteoblasts
    ·· Deposit new bone
  - Osteoclasts
    ·· Increase long bone diameter

··Promote longitudinal bone growth by reabsorbing the previously deposited bone

- Cartilage
  - Dense connective tissue
  - Consists of fibers embedded in a strong, gel-like substance
  - Has the flexibility of firm plastic
  - Has no blood supply or innervation
  - Supports and shapes various structures
  - Cushions and absorbs shock, preventing direct transmission to the bone
- Joints (articulations)
  - Points of contact between two bones that hold the bones together
  - Allow flexibility and movement
  - Structural classifications
    - Fibrous
      - The articular surfaces of two bones are bound closely by fibrous connective tissue
      - Little movement is possible
    - Cartilaginous
      - Cartilage connects one bone to another
      - Allow some movement
    - Synovial
      - Contiguous bony surfaces are separated by a viscous, lubricating fluid, the synovia, and by the cartilage
      - Freely movable
  - Functional classifications
    - Synarthrosis — immovable
    - Amphiarthrosis — slightly movable
    - Diarthrosis — freely movable
- Bursae
  - Small synovial fluid sacs
  - Located at friction points around joints between tendons, ligaments, and bones
  - Act as cushions and decrease stress on adjacent structures

DIAGNOSTIC TESTS

● Arthroscopy
- Purpose
  - To perform a visual examination of the interior of a joint with a fiber-optic endoscope
- Nursing interventions
  - Explain the procedure to the parents and the child
  - Obtain written, informed consent

Key facts about cartilage

- Dense connective tissue
- Consists of fibers embedded in strong, gel-like substance
- Has the flexibility of firm plastic
- No blood supply or innervation
- Supports and shapes various structures
- Cushions and absorbs shock, preventing direct transmission to the bone

Functions of joints

- Points of contact between bones
- Allow flexibility
- Allow movement
- May be fibrous, cartilaginous, or synovial

Functional classifications of joints

- Synarthrosis – immovable
- Amphiarthrosis – slightly movable
- Diarthrosis – freely movable

Functions of bursae

- Act as cushions around joints
- Decrease stress on adjacent structures

Quick guide to common diagnostic tests for musculoskeletal problems

- **Arthroscopy** – uses a fiber-optic endoscope to visualize the interior of a joint
- **CT scan** – identifies injuries to the soft tissue, ligaments, tendons, and muscles
- **Magnetic resonance imaging** – allows cross-sectional imaging of bones and joints and visual assessment of certain muscle and soft-tissue injuries
- **Myelography** – allows detection of abnormalities of the spinal canal and cord through use of serial X-rays
- **X-rays** – help measure bone density and identify joint disruption; calcifications; and bone deformities, fractures, and destruction

Preprocedure myelography interventions

- Explain the procedure to the parents and the child.
- Obtain written, informed consent.
- Check for allergies to the contrast medium.
- If metrizamide is used, discontinue phenothiazines 48 hours before the test.

– Tell the child and his parents that he may need to fast after midnight before the procedure
– Note allergies because local anesthesia is used
– Tell the child he may feel a thumping sensation as the cannula is inserted in the joint capsule

● **Computed tomography (CT) scan**
- Purpose
  – To identify injuries to the soft tissue, ligaments, tendons, and muscles
- Nursing interventions
  – Explain the procedure to the parents and the child
  – Obtain written, informed consent
  – Tell the child to hold still during the procedure
  – Tell the child that he'll be placed in a tubelike circle and pictures will be taken

● **Magnetic resonance imaging (MRI)**
- Purpose
  – Using a strong magnetic field and radio waves, allows cross-sectional imaging of bones and joints and visual assessment of certain muscle and soft-tissue injuries
- Nursing interventions
  – Note if the child has any metal implants, which would be a contraindication for the procedure
  – Explain the procedure to the parents and child
  – Instruct the child to hold still during the procedure; sedation may be necessary

● **Myelography**
- Purpose
  – An invasive procedure that involves injection of a radiopaque contrast medium and serial X-rays used to evaluate abnormalities of the spinal canal and cord
- Nursing interventions
  – Before the procedure
    · Explain the procedure to the parents and the child
    · Obtain written, informed consent
    · Check for allergies to the contrast medium
    · If metrizamide (Amipaque) is used as the contrast medium, discontinue phenothiazines 48 hours before the test
  – During the procedure
    · When the contrast medium is injected, tell the child that he may experience a burning sensation, warmth, headache, salty taste, nausea, and vomiting
  – After the procedure
    · Have the child sit in his room or lie in bed with his head elevated 60 degrees

- Make sure he doesn't lie flat for at least 8 hours
- Encourage the child to drink extra fluids
- Check that the child voids within 8 hours

● **X-rays**
  - Purpose
    – To help identify joint disruption, calcifications, and bone deformities, fractures, and destruction
    – To help measure bone density
  - Nursing interventions
    – Explain the test to the parents and child
    – Tell the child he must hold still during the X-ray
    – Cover the genital area with a lead apron

NURSING DIAGNOSES

● **Probable nursing diagnoses**
  - Delayed growth and development
  - Impaired physical mobility
  - Risk for peripheral neurovascular dysfunction
  - Impaired walking
  - Disturbed body image
  - Acute pain
  - Activity intolerance
  - Risk for injury

● **Possible nursing diagnoses**
  - Risk for impaired skin integrity
  - Impaired gas exchange
  - Chronic pain
  - Ineffective role performance
  - Fatigue
  - Compromised family coping
  - Powerlessness
  - Dressing or grooming self-care deficit
  - Ineffective breathing pattern
  - Bathing or hygiene self-care deficit
  - Anxiety
  - Fear

CLUBFOOT

● **Definition**
  - A congenital disorder in which the foot and ankle are twisted and can't be manipulated into the correct position

Probable nursing diagnoses for a patient with a musculoskeletal disorder

- Delayed growth and development
- Impaired physical mobility
- Risk for peripheral neurovascular dysfunction
- Impaired walking
- Disturbed body image
- Acute pain
- Activity intolerance
- Risk for injury

Key facts about clubfoot

- Congenital disorder in which the foot and ankle are twisted
- Abnormal development of the foot during fetal growth leads to abnormal muscles and joints and contracture of soft tissue
- Deformity usually obvious at birth
- Unilateral type is more common

- Also known as *talipes*
- Unilateral clubfoot is more common than bilateral

● **Causes**
- Arrested development during the 9th and 10th weeks of embryonic life, when the feet are formed
- Deformed talus and shortened Achilles tendon
- Possible genetic predisposition

● **Pathophysiology**
- Abnormal development of the foot during fetal growth leads to abnormal muscles and joints and contracture of soft tissue
- Apparent clubfoot
  – Results when a fetus maintains a position that gives his feet a clubfoot appearance at birth; it can usually be corrected manually
  – Another form of apparent clubfoot is inversion of the feet, resulting from the denervation type of progressive muscular atrophy and progressive muscular dystrophy

● **Complications**
- Delayed growth and development
- Impaired mobility
- Physical injury

● **Assessment findings**
- Deformity usually obvious at birth (see *Recognizing clubfoot*)
- Inability to correct deformity manually (distinguishes true clubfoot from apparent clubfoot)

● **Diagnostic test findings**
- X-rays show superimposition of the talus and calcaneus and a ladder-like appearance of the metatarsals

● **Medical management**
- Correcting the deformity
  – A series of casts to gradually stretch and realign the angle of the foot and, after cast removal, application of Denis Browne splint at night until age 1
  – Surgical correction
    · Can improve clubfoot with good function but can't correct it
    · The affected calf muscle will remain slightly underdeveloped
  – Correction usually occurs in sequential order (correcting all three deformities at once results in a misshapen, rocker-bottomed foot)
    · Forefoot adduction
    · Varus (inversion)
    · Equinus (plantar flexion)
- Maintaining the correction until the foot gains normal muscle balance
- Observing the foot closely for several years to prevent the deformity from recurring

Complications of clubfoot

- Delayed growth and development
- Impaired mobility
- Physical injury

Correction sequence for clubfoot

- Forefoot adduction
- Varus (inversion)
- Equinus (plantar flexion)

Recognizing clubfoot

Clubfoot (talipes) may have various names, depending on the orientation of the deformity, as shown in these illustrations.

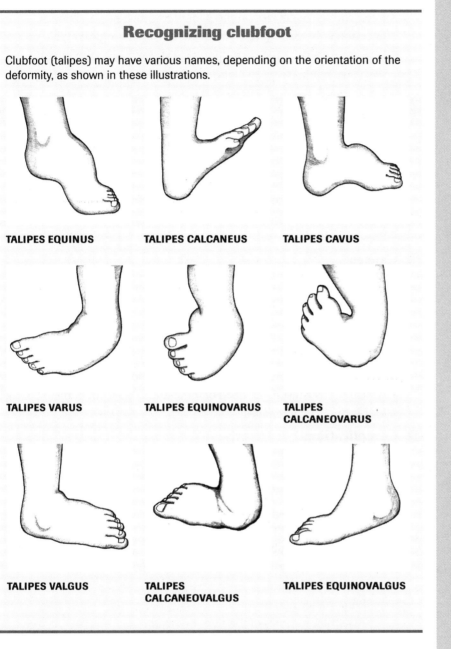

TALIPES EQUINUS

TALIPES CALCANEUS

TALIPES CAVUS

TALIPES VARUS

TALIPES EQUINOVARUS

TALIPES CALCANEOVARUS

TALIPES VALGUS

TALIPES CALCANEOVALGUS

TALIPES EQUINOVALGUS

Types of clubfoot

- Talipes equinus
- Talipes calcaneus
- Talipes cavus
- Talipes varus
- Talipes equinovarus
- Talipes calcaneovarus
- Talipes valgus
- Talipes calcaneovalgus
- Talipes equinovalgus

● Nursing interventions
- For the patient with a cast
  - Assess neurovascular status to ensure circulation to the foot
  - Use a blow-dryer on the cool setting to provide relief of itching
  - Discuss the importance of placing nothing inside the cast
- Ensure that shoes fit correctly to promote comfort and prevent skin breakdown
- Prepare the patient for surgery, if necessary, to maintain and promote healing process and decrease anxiety

Key nursing interventions for clubfoot

- Assess neurovascular status to ensure circulation to the foot.
- Ensure that shoes fit correctly.
- Prepare the patient for surgery, if necessary.
- Keep corrective devices on the patient as much as possible.
- Perform passive ROM exercises.

- Keep corrective devices on the patient as much as possible
- Encourage the patient to walk as exercise after surgical repair
- Perform passive range-of-motion (ROM) exercises; don't use excessive force when trying to manipulate the foot

DEVELOPMENTAL DYSPLASIA OF THE HIP

● Definition
- An abnormal development of the hip socket
- The disorder can affect one or both hips
- Occurs in varying degrees of dislocation, from partial (subluxation) to complete (see *Complete dysplasia of the hip*)
- Present at birth

● Causes
- Breech birth
- Position of fetus in utero
- Genetic predisposition
- Laxity of the ligaments

● Pathophysiology
- The head of the femur is still cartilaginous and the acetabulum (socket) is shallow; as a result, the head of the femur comes out of the hip socket
- More common in females

● Complications
- Delayed growth and development
- Impaired mobility
- Impaired skin integrity
- If corrective treatment isn't begun until after age 2
  - Degenerative hip changes
  - Abnormal acetabular development
  - Lordosis (abnormally increased concave curvature of the lumbar and cervical spine)
  - Joint malformation
  - Avascular necrosis of the femoral head

● Assessment findings
- On the affected side, an increased number of folds on the posterior thigh when the child is in a supine position with knees bent
- Appearance of a shortened limb on the affected side
- Restricted abduction of the hips
- Barlow's sign
  - A click is felt when the infant is placed supine with abducted hips flexed 90 degrees, knees fully flexed, and the hip adducted to midline
- Ortolani's click

Complete dysplasia of the hip

In complete dislocation, the femoral head is totally displaced outside the acetabulum, as shown at right (see arrow).

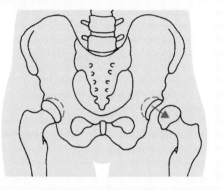

TOP 5

Assessment findings in developmental dysplasia of the hip

1. Increased number of folds on posterior thigh when the child is in a supine position with knees bent
2. Shortened limb
3. Barlow's sign
4. Ortolani's click
5. Positive Trendelenburg's test

- The infant is placed on his back, with hip flexed and in adduction; the hip is then abducted while the examiner presses the femur downward to dislocate the hip
- A click or jerk (produced by the femoral head moving over the acetabular rim) indicates subluxation in a neonate younger than 1 month; the sign indicates subluxation or complete dislocation in an older infant
- Positive Trendelenburg's test
  - When the child stands on the affected leg, the opposite pelvis dips to maintain erect posture

● Diagnostic test findings
- Sonography and MRI may be used to assess reduction
- Ultrasonography shows the involved cartilage and acetabulum
- X-rays
  - Show the location of the femur head and shallow acetabulum
  - Can also be used to monitor progression of the disorder

● Medical management
- Infants younger than age 3 months
  - Gentle manipulation to reduce the dislocation, followed by splint-brace or harness to hold the hips in a flexed and abducted position to maintain the reduction
  - Splint brace or harness worn continuously for 2 to 3 months, then a night splint for another month to tighten and stabilize the joint capsule in correct alignment
- Infants older than age 3 months
  - Bilateral skin traction (in infants) or skeletal traction (in children who have started walking)
  - Bryant's traction or divarication traction (both extremities placed in traction, even if only one is affected, to help maintain immobi-

Managing developmental dysplasia of the hip

- In infants younger than age 3 months — gentle manipulation and splint brace or harness
- In infants older than age 3 months — bilateral skin traction, skeletal traction, closed reduction under general anesthesia and a spica cast, or open reduction and osteotomy and a spica cast
- In children ages 2 to 5 — skeletal traction and subcutaneous adductor tenotomy

lization) for children younger than 3 years and weighing less than 35 lb (16 kg) for 2 to 3 weeks
- Gentle closed reduction under general anesthesia, followed by a spica cast (the legs are abducted with a bar between them) for 3 months if traction fails
- If hip isn't reducible, open reduction and pelvic or femoral osteotomy to correct bony deformity, followed by immobilization in a spica cast for 6 to 8 weeks
• In children ages 2 to 5
- Treatment is difficult; if begun after age 5, rarely restores satisfactory hip function
- Skeletal traction and subcutaneous adductor tenotomy (surgical cutting of the tendon)

● **Nursing interventions**
• Assess circulation before application of cast or traction; after application, have the child wiggle toes to detect signs of impaired circulation; the nurse should be able to place one finger between the child's skin and cast
• Give reassurance that early, prompt treatment will probably result in complete correction to decrease anxiety
• Assure the parents that the child will adjust to restricted movement and return to normal sleeping, eating, and play in a few days
• Inspect the skin and provide skin care, especially around bony prominences, to detect cast complications and prevent skin breakdown
• Be aware that the goal of treatment is to enlarge and deepen the socket by pressure

DUCHENNE'S MUSCULAR DYSTROPHY

● **Definition**
• Also known as *pseudohypertrophic dystrophy*
• A genetic disorder marked by muscular deterioration that progresses throughout childhood
- Onset is insidious
- Onset occurs between ages 3 and 5

● **Causes**
• Sex-linked recessive trait

● **Pathophysiology**
• Occurs only in males because of a defect in the X chromosome
• A lack of production of dystrophin results in breakdown of muscle fibers
• Muscle fibers are replaced with fatty deposits and collagen in muscles
• Weakness results

Key nursing interventions in developmental dysplasia of the hip

• Assess circulation.
• Give reassurance that early treatment will probably result in correction.
• Assure the parents that the child will adjust to restricted movement.
• Provide skin care.

Key facts about Duchenne's muscular dystrophy

• Also known as *pseudohypertrophic dystrophy*
• Genetic disorder
• Marked by muscular deterioration that causes weakness
• Occurs only in males because of a defect in the X chromosome

Complications

- Death in the late teens to early 20s
  - Cardiac failure
  - Respiratory failure
- Impaired mobility
- Intellectual retardation is possible

Assessment findings

- Begins with pelvic girdle weakness, indicated by waddling gait and falling
- Cardiac or pulmonary failure
- Decreased ability to perform self-care activities
- Delayed motor development
- Eventual contractures and muscle hypertrophy
- Gowers' sign (use of hands to push self up from floor) when rising from a sitting or supine position
- Toe-walking

Diagnostic test findings

- Electromyography typically demonstrates short, weak bursts of electrical activity in affected muscles
- Muscle biopsy shows variations in the size of muscle fibers and, in later stages, shows fat and connective tissue deposits, with no dystrophin

Medical management

- Gene therapy (under investigation to prevent muscle degeneration)
- High-fiber, high-protein, low-calorie diet
- Physical therapy
- Surgery to correct contractures (for mobility purposes only)
- Use of devices such as splints, braces, trapeze bars, overhead slings, and a wheelchair to help preserve mobility

Nursing interventions

- Perform ROM exercises to promote joint mobility
- Provide emotional support to the child and parents to decrease anxiety and promote coping mechanisms
- Initiate genetic counseling to inform the child and family about passing the disorder on to future children
- If respiratory involvement occurs, encourage coughing, deep-breathing exercises, and diaphragmatic breathing to maintain a patent airway and mobilize secretions to prevent complications associated with retained secretions
- Encourage use of a footboard or high-topped sneakers and a foot cradle to increase comfort and prevent footdrop
- Encourage adequate fluid intake, increase dietary fiber, and obtain an order for a stool softener to prevent constipation from inactivity

---

Complications of Duchenne's muscular dystrophy

- Death in late teens to early 20s, resulting from cardiac or respiratory failure
- Impaired mobility
- Possible intellectual retardation

TOP 2

Assessment findings in Duchenne's muscular dystrophy

1. Pelvic girdle weakness
2. Gowers' sign

Managing Duchenne's muscular dystrophy

- Gene therapy
- Diet
- Physical therapy
- Surgery
- Use of assistive devices

Key facts about fractures

- They're a discontinuation of continuity of the bone.
- There are two types of causes: trauma-related or pathological.
- They may cause muscle, nerve, and other soft-tissue damage.

Factors affecting prognosis of arm and leg fractures

- Extent of disablement or deformity
- Amount of vascular and tissue damage
- Adequacy of reduction and immobilization
- Health
- Nutritional status

The five Ps of assessing fractures

1. Pain and point tenderness
2. Pallor
3. Pulse loss
4. Paresthesia
5. Paralysis

FRACTURES, ARM AND LEG

- **Definition**
  - A discontinuation of the continuity of the tissue of the bone in the arm or leg

- **Causes**
  - Trauma
    - Fall
    - Sport-related injury
    - Child abuse (suspected in the case of multiple or repeated episodes of fractures)
    - Motor vehicle accidents
    - Repetitive force on a bone (stress fracture)
  - Pathological
    - Bone tumors
    - Metabolic disease

- **Pathophysiology**
  - Commonly cause substantial muscle, nerve, and other soft-tissue damage
  - Prognosis varies
    - Extent of disablement or deformity
    - The amount of vascular and tissue damage
    - Adequacy of reduction and immobilization
    - Health
    - Nutritional status
  - Children's bones usually heal rapidly and without deformity

- **Complications**
  - Permanent deformity and dysfunction if bones fail to heal (nonunion) or heal improperly (malunion)
  - Aseptic necrosis of bone segments from impaired circulation
  - Hypovolemic shock as a result of blood vessel damage (this is especially likely to develop in patients with a fractured femur)
  - Muscle contractures
  - Renal calculi from decalcification (due to prolonged immobility)
  - Fat embolism
  - Compartment syndrome

- **Assessment findings**
  - The "five Ps"
    - Pain and point tenderness
    - Pallor
    - Pulse loss
    - Paresthesia
    - Paralysis
  - Deformity

- Swelling
- Discoloration
- Crepitus
- Loss of limb function
- Arterial compromise or nerve damage
  – Numbness and tingling
  – Mottled cyanosis
  – Cool skin at the end of the extremity
  – Loss of pulse distal to the injury
- Open fractures
  – Skin wound

● **Diagnostic test findings**
- X-rays confirm a diagnosis of fracture

● **Medical management**
- Splinting the limb above and below the suspected fracture
- Applying a cold pack
- Elevating the limb to reduce edema and pain
- Severe fractures that cause blood loss
  – Apply direct pressure to control bleeding
  – Administer fluid replacement as soon as possible to prevent or treat hypovolemic shock
- Reduction
  – Restores displaced bone segments to their normal position
  – After reduction, the fractured arm or leg must be immobilized by a splint, cast, or with traction
  – Closed reduction
    · Manual manipulation facilitates the muscle stretching necessary to realign the bone
    · X-rays determine the outcome of an attempt at closed reduction
  – Open reduction
    · Used when closed reduction is impossible
    · Reduces and immobilizes the fracture
      - Rods
      - Plates
      - Screws
    · Casting
  – Traction
    · Uses a series of weights and pulleys
    · Used when a splint or cast fails to maintain the reduction
    · Skin traction
      - Adhesives, moleskin, elastic bandages, and sheepskin coverings are used to attach traction devices to the child's skin
      - Traction pulls indirectly on the skeleton by pulling on the skin

Signs and symptoms of arterial compromise or nerve damage

- Numbness and tingling
- Mottled cyanosis
- Cool skin at the end of the extremity
- Loss of pulse distal to the injury

TOP 3

Ways to manage a fracture

1. Splint the limb above and below the suspected fracture.
2. Apply a cold pack.
3. Elevate the limb to reduce edema and pain.

Three types of fracture reduction

1. Closed
2. Open
3. Traction

Managing open fractures

- Tetanus prophylaxis
- Prophylactic antibiotics
- Surgery to repair soft-tissue damage
- Thorough debridement of the wound

Signs of shock

- Rapid pulse
- Decreased blood pressure
- Pallor
- Cool, clammy skin

Nursing interventions for long-term immobilization

- Reposition the child often.
- Assist with active ROM exercises.
- Encourage deep breathing and coughing.

Signs and symptoms of impaired circulation

- Skin coldness
- Numbness
- Tingling
- Discoloration

- Skeletal traction
  - Pulls directly on the skeleton via pins or wires
  - A pin or wire inserted through the bone distal to the fracture and attached to a weight allows for prolonged traction
- Open fractures
  - Tetanus prophylaxis
  - Prophylactic antibiotics
  - Surgery to repair soft-tissue damage
  - Thorough debridement of the wound

● **Nursing interventions**
- Watch for signs of shock in the child with a severe open fracture of a large bone such as the femur
- Monitor vital signs, and be especially alert for rapid pulse, decreased blood pressure, pallor, and cool, clammy skin—all of which may indicate the child is in shock
- Administer I.V. fluids as ordered
- Offer reassurance to the child, who may be frightened and in pain
- Ease pain with analgesics as needed
- Help the child and parents set realistic goals for recovery
- When a fracture requires long-term immobilization with traction
  - Reposition the child often to increase comfort and prevent pressure ulcers
  - Assist with active ROM exercises to prevent muscle atrophy
  - Encourage deep breathing and coughing to avoid hypostatic pneumonia
- Urge adequate fluid intake to prevent urinary stasis and constipation
- Watch for signs of renal calculi (flank pain, nausea, and vomiting)
- Provide good cast care
  - Support the cast with pillows
  - Observe for skin irritation near cast edges
  - Check for foul odors or discharge
  - Tell the child to report signs and symptoms of impaired circulation
    - Skin coldness
    - Numbness
    - Tingling
    - Discoloration
  - Warn the child not to get the cast wet
  - Instruct the child not to insert foreign objects under the cast (see *Teaching about cast care*)
- Encourage the child to start moving around as soon as he's able
  - Help him to walk
  - Demonstrate how to use crutches properly
- After cast removal, refer the child to a physical therapist to restore limb mobility

TIME-OUT FOR TEACHING

Teaching about cast care

Be sure to include these points in your teaching plan for the parents of a child with a cast:
- mechanism of bone healing and necessity for casting
- cast care, including air exposure, elevation, and moving
- measures to protect the cast
- measures for skin care
- methods to relieve itching and irritation
- measures to keep cast dry
- ways to test for sensation, movement, and circulation
- measures to cope with swelling
- monitoring for wound drainage
- exercises for the casted extremity.

HERNIA

Definition
- Protrusion of an organ through the abnormal musculature caused by muscle weakness
- Inguinal hernias are most common

Causes
- Congenital abnormality
- Failure of structures to close after birth
- Obesity
- Muscle weakness
- Surgery
- Illness

Pathophysiology
- Umbilical hernia
  - A weakness in the umbilical area, where umbilical blood vessels traveled
  - Failure of the umbilical muscles to close at birth results in protrusion of the omentum and intestine through the naval
- Inguinal canal hernia
  - A weakness in the area where the testes descended from the abdomen to the scrotum
  - Failure of the proximal portion of the inguinal canal to atrophy results in protrusion
- Irreducible hernia—a protrusion that won't return to its normal position

Complications
- Ischemic tissue
- Sepsis

Key facts about hernia
- It's a protrusion of an organ through the abnormal musculature caused by muscle weakness.
- Inguinal hernias are most common.
- Causes include congenital abnormalities, obesity, muscle weakness, surgery, and illness.

Types of hernias
- Umbilical hernia – a protrusion of the omentum and intestine through the naval that's caused by failure of the umbilical muscles to close at birth
- Inguinal canal hernia – a protrusion in the area where the testes descend from the abdomen to the scrotum that's caused by the failure of the proximal portion of the inguinal canal to atrophy
- Irreducible hernia – a protrusion that won't return to its normal position

● **Assessment findings**
  • Lump appears over the herniated area when the child strains, coughs, or cries
  • The lump disappears when the patient is relaxed or supine
  • Usually, no pain

● **Diagnostic test findings**
  • Diagnostic tests aren't usually necessary
  • Hernias are generally visible or palpable
  • They're more obvious in the infant who is crying, coughing, or straining causing increased abdominal pressure

● **Medical management**
  • If the hernia doesn't resolve, surgical intervention (herniorrhaphy) may be required
  • Herniorrhaphy returns the contents of the herniated sac into the abdominal cavity and closes the opening

● **Nursing interventions**
  • Observe for the signs and symptoms of incarceration
    – Pain
    – Irritability
    – Intestinal obstruction caused by the loop of the bowel becoming occluded so that solids can't pass
  • Tell the parents that home measures such as belly bands and abdominal binders aren't effective
  • Remember that the abdominal muscles commonly strengthen as the child grows, and the hernia may resolve without treatment
  • Repair done based on child's age, weight, and severity of hernia

LEGG-CALVÉ-PERTHES DISEASE

● **Definition**
  • Ischemic necrosis leading to eventual flattening of the head of the femur due to vascular compromise
  • Typically unilateral; occurs bilaterally in 20% of patients
  • Occurs most frequently in boys ages 4 to 8 and tends to run in families

● **Causes**
  • Unknown
  • Theories
    – Venous obstruction with secondary intraepiphyseal thrombosis
    – Trauma to retinacular vessels
    – Vascular irregularities (congenital or developmental)
    – Vascular occlusion secondary to increased intracapsular pressure from acute transient synovitis

---

Signs of an incarcerated hernia

• Pain
• Irritability
• Intestinal obstruction

Key facts about Legg-Calvé-Perthes disease

• Ischemic necrosis of bone
• Causes vascular compromise that eventually leads to flattening of the head of the femur
• Typically unilateral (can be bilateral)
• Occurs more commonly in boys and tends to run in families

– Increased blood viscosity resulting in stasis and decreased blood flow

● **Pathophysiology**
- Occurs in five stages
  - Growth arrest
    - Avascular phase
    - May last 6 to 12 months
  - Subchondral fracture
    - Radiographic visualization of the fracture varies with the age of the child at clinical onset and the extent of epiphyseal involvement
    - May last 3 to 8½ months
  - Reabsorption (fragmentation or necrosis)
    - The necrotic bone beneath the subchondral fracture is gradually and irregularly absorbed
    - Lasts 6 to 12 months
  - Reossification (healing stage)
    - Ossification of the primary bone begins irregularly in the subchondral area and progresses centrally
    - Takes 6 to 24 months
  - Healed stage (residual stage)
    - Complete ossification of the epiphysis of the femoral head
    - Occurs with or without residual deformity
- Usually runs its course in 3 to 4 years but may lead to premature osteoarthritis later in life from misalignment of the acetabulum and flattening of the femoral head

● **Complications**
- Impaired mobility
- Premature osteoarthritis

● **Assessment findings**
- Persistent thigh pain or limp that becomes progressively severe
- Mild pain in the hip, thigh, or knee that's aggravated by activity and relieved by rest
- Muscle spasms
- Atrophy of muscles in the upper thigh
- Slight shortening of the leg
- Severely restricted abduction and internal rotation of the hip

● **Diagnostic test findings**
- Anterior-posterior X-ray and MRI enhance diagnosis of necrosis and visualization of articular surface

● **Medical management**
- Containment of the femoral head within the acetabulum to protect it from further stress and damage

Five stages of Legg-Calvé-Perthes disease

1. Growth arrest
2. Subchondral fracture
3. Reabsorption
4. Reossification
5. Healed stage

Complications of Legg-Calvé-Perthes disease

● Impaired mobility
● Premature osteoarthritis

TOP 2
Assessment findings in Legg-Calvé-Perthes disease

1. Mild pain in the hip, thigh, or knee during activity
2. Muscle spasms

Managing Legg-Calvé-Perthes disease

- Containment of the femoral head within the acetabulum
- Bedrest for 1 to 2 weeks
- Reduced weight bearing by means of bed rest and then application of hip abduction splint, cast, or weight bearing while a splint, cast, or brace holds the leg in abduction
- Braces for 6 to 18 months
- For a young child in early stage of disease, osteotomy and subtrochanteric derotation
- Postoperative spica cast for approximately 2 months

Avoiding cast complications

- Report dusky, cool, or numb toes immediately.
- Follow a consistent plan of skin care to prevent skin breakdown; never use oils or powders under the cast because they increase skin breakdown and soften the cast.
- Check under the cast daily for odors to detect skin breakdown or wound problems.
- Report persistent soreness.

Ways to relieve itching under a cast

- Use a hair-dryer to blow in cool air.
- Get an order for an antipruritic.
- Advise the patient and his parents never to insert objects under the cast.

- Bedrest for 1 to 2 weeks
- Reduced weight bearing by means of bed rest in bilateral splint counterpoised traction, then application of hip abduction splint, cast, or weight bearing while a splint, cast, or brace holds the leg in abduction
- Braces for 6 to 18 months
- For a young child in the early stages of the disease, osteotomy and subtrochanteric derotation provide maximum confinement of the epiphysis within the acetabulum to allow return of the femoral head to normal shape and full range of motion
- Postoperative spica cast for approximately 2 months
- Analgesics

● **Nursing interventions**
- Monitor intake and output
  - Maintain sufficient fluid balance
  - Provide a diet sufficient for growth without causing excessive weight gain, which might necessitate cast change and loss of the corrective position
- Provide good cast care; turn the child every 2 to 3 hours to expose the cast to air
- Watch for complications
  - Check toes for color, temperature, swelling, sensation, and motion; report dusky, cool, or numb toes immediately
  - Check the skin under the cast with a flashlight every 4 hours while the patient is awake
  - Follow a consistent plan of skin care to prevent skin breakdown; never use oils or powders under the cast because they increase skin breakdown and soften the cast
  - Check under the cast daily for odors, particularly after surgery, to detect skin breakdown or wound problems
  - Report persistent soreness
- Administer analgesics as ordered
- Relieve itching by using a hair-dryer (set on cool) at the cast edges; this also decreases dampness from perspiration
  - If itching becomes excessive, get an order for an antipruritic
  - Never insert an object under the cast to scratch
- Provide continuous emotional support
  - Explain all procedures and the need for bed rest, casts, or braces to the child; encourage him to verbalize his fears and anxiety
  - Encourage parents to participate in their child's care; teach them proper cast care and how to recognize signs of skin breakdown
  - Offer tips for easiest home management of the bedridden child
  - Tell parents what special supplies are needed
    - Pajamas and trousers that are a size larger than the child's regular size (open the side seam, and attach Velcro fasteners to close it)

- Bedpan
- Adhesive tape
- Moleskin
- Possibly, a hospital bed
- When cast is removed, debride dry, scaly skin gradually by applying lotion after bathing
- Stress the need for follow-up care to monitor rehabilitation
- Stress home tutoring and socialization to promote normal mental and emotional growth and development

OSTEOGENESIS IMPERFECTA

Definition
- Brittle bones
- A hereditary disease of bones and connective tissue

Causes
- Autosomal dominant
  - Type I
  - Type IV
- Autosomal recessive
  - Type II
  - Type III
- Defective osteoblastic activity and a defect of mesenchymal collagen (embryonic connective tissue) and its derivatives (sclerae, bones, and ligaments)

Pathophysiology
- The reticulum fails to differentiate into mature collagen or causes abnormal collagen development
  - Immature bones
  - Coarse bone formation
  - Cortical bone thinning
- Results in pathologic fractures and impaired healing

Complications
- Fractures
- Pain
- Impaired mobility
- Death (intrauterine or early infancy)
- Scoliosis

Assessment findings
- Type I
  - Fractures that occur from minimal trauma; the number of fractures may spontaneously decrease in adolescence
  - Blue, purple, or gray tint to sclera

– Yellow or grayish blue teeth from opalescent dentin
  • Children with dental abnormalities are shorter and have more fractures at birth, more frequent fractures, and more severe skeletal deformities than children with normal teeth
– Bowing of the lower limbs

• Type II
  – Intrauterine fractures due to extreme bone fragility, heart failure, pulmonary hypertension, or respiratory failure
  – Intrauterine or early infant death

• Type III
  – Fractures are usually present at birth and occur frequently during childhood
    • Progressive skeletal deformity
    • Impaired mobility
  – Poor growth rate
    • Below the third percentile in height for specific age
  – Normal or light blue sclerae

• Type IV
  – Osteoporosis (increased bone fragility)
  – Sclerae
    • Light blue at birth
    • Normal in adolescents
  – Bowed limbs
  – Short stature
  – Fractures (the number may decrease spontaneously at puberty)
  – Possible skull deformity

● **Diagnostic test findings**
• Collagen biochemical studies of cultured skin fibroblasts confirm the diagnosis
• Ultrasound identifies mutation
  – Limb shortening
  – In utero fractures
  – Polyhydramnios
• X-rays reveal old fractures and skeletal deformities
• Skull X-rays show wide sutures with small, irregularly shaped islands of bone (wormian bones) between them

● **Medical management**
• Prevent deformities
  – Traction
  – Immobilization
  – Both
• Aid normal development and rehabilitation
• Dental care

Key findings in osteogenesis imperfecta

• Limb shortening
• In utero fractures
• Polyhydramnios
• Old fractures and skeletal deformities
• Wide sutures with small, irregularly shaped islands of bone between them
• Blue sclerae

Nursing interventions

- Check the child's circulatory, motor, and sensory abilities
- Encourage him to walk when possible (these children develop a fear of walking)
- Promote preventive dental care and repair of dental caries
- Provide gentle handling in all child-care activities
- Provide a padded and soft environment
- Teach preventive measures
  - Avoid contact sports
  - Avoid strenuous activities
  - Wear knee pads, helmets, or other protective devices when engaging in sports
  - Diet management—encourage a diet high in calcium and vitamins D and C
  - Maintain a healthy weight

SCOLIOSIS

Definition

- A lateral curvature of the spine that may occur in the thoracic, lumbar, or thoracolumbar spinal segment
- Most common in females and identified at puberty and throughout adolescence
- Types
  - Nonstructural, functional, or postural scoliosis—a nonprogressive C curvature caused by another condition
  - Structural or progressive scoliosis—a progressive S curvature

Causes

- Nonstructural, functional, or postural scoliosis
  - Poor posture
  - Discrepancy in leg lengths
  - Poor vision
  - Paraspinal inflammation
  - Acute disk disease
- Structural or progressive scoliosis
  - Deformity of the vertebral bodies
  - Rib changes
  - Neuromuscular changes; muscle weakness or paralysis

Pathophysiology

- Nonstructural scoliosis
  - The pelvic tilt caused by unequal leg lengths, poor posture, paraspinal inflammation, acute disk disease, or head tilt associated with poor vision leads to a spinal deviation
  - There is little change in the shape of the vertebrae

TOP 5

Ways to prevent fractures in children with osteogenesis imperfecta

1. Provide gentle handling in all child-care activities.
2. Provide a padded and soft environment.
3. Tell the child to avoid contact sports.
4. Suggest that the child avoid strenuous activities.
5. Tell the child to wear knee pads, helmets, and other protective devices when engaging in sports.

Key facts about scoliosis

- Lateral curvature of the spine
- May occur in the thoracic, lumbar, or thoracolumbar spinal segment
- Most common in females

Types of scoliosis

- Nonstructural, functional, or postural – a nonprogressive C curvature caused by another condition
- Structural or progressive – a progressive S curvature caused by deformity of the vertebral bodies or rib changes

Three classifications of idiopathic scoliosis

- Infantile
- Juvenile
- Adolescent

Key findings in nonstructural scoliosis

- C-shaped curvature of the spine
- Curve of spine disappears when the child bends at the waist

Key findings in structural scoliosis

- S-shaped curvature of the spine
- Curve fails to straighten when the child bends at the waist
- Asymmetrical hips, ribs, shoulders, and shoulder blades

- Structural scoliosis
  - Congenital—usually related to a congenital defect, such as wedge vertebrae, fused ribs or vertebrae, or hemivertebrae; may result from trauma to zygote or embryo
  - Paralytic or musculoskeletal—develops several months after asymmetrical paralysis of the trunk muscles due to polio, cerebral palsy, or muscular dystrophy
  - Idiopathic—the most common form; may be transmitted as an autosomal dominant or multifactorial trait
    - Appears in previously straight spine during the growing years
    - Brain stem dysfunction, possibly due to a lesion of the posterior columns or the inner ear, may be the cause
    - Three classifications
      - Infantile—affects mostly male infants between birth and age 3 and causes left thoracic and right lumbar curves
      - Juvenile—affects both sexes between ages 4 and 10 and causes varying types of curvature
      - Adolescent—generally affects girls between ages 10 and achievement of skeletal maturity and causes varying types of curvature
- Scoliosis stops progressing when bone growth stops

● **Complications**
- Impaired growth and development
- Body image disturbances
- Impaired mobility
- Debilitating back pain
- Severe deformity
- With thoracic curve exceeding 60 degrees: possible reduced pulmonary function
- With thoracic curve exceeding 80 degrees: increased risk of cor pulmonale in middle age

● **Assessment findings**
- Nonstructural scoliosis
  - A C-shaped curvature of the spine
  - The curve of the spine disappears when the child bends at the waist to touch the toes
- Structural scoliosis
  - A curve in the thoracic segment of the spine, with convexity to the right, and compensatory curves (S curves) in the cervical segment above and the lumbar segment below, both with a convexity to the left
  - The spinal curve fails to straighten when the child bends forward with the knees straight and the arms hanging down toward the feet
  - The hips, ribs, shoulders, and shoulder blades are asymmetrical

- Backache
- Fatigue
- Dyspnea

● **Diagnostic test findings**
- X-rays of the spine reveal curvature
- A scoliometer measures the degree of spine curvature

● **Medical management**
- Nonstructural scoliosis
  – Corrective lenses if the problem is associated with poor vision that results in a head tilt
  – Postural exercises
  – Shoe lifts
- Structural scoliosis
  – Electrical stimulation for mild to moderate curvatures
  – Harrington, Luque, or Cotrel-Dubousset rods for curves greater than 40 degrees (to realign the spine or when curves fail to respond to orthotic treatment)
  – Possible prolonged bracing (Milwaukee or Boston brace)
    · Worn over a T-shirt for 23 hours per day
    · Brace adjustments every 3 months
  – Skin traction or halo femoral traction
  – Spinal fusion with bone from the iliac crest

● **Nursing interventions**
- After spinal fusion and the insertion of rods
  – Monitor vital signs and intake and output to prevent fluid volume deficit
  – Turn the child only by logrolling to prevent injury
  – Maintain correct body alignment to promote joint mobility and prevent injury
  – Keep the bed in a flat position to prevent injury and complications
  – Help the child adjust to the increase in height and altered self-perception to promote self-esteem and decrease anxiety
- Teach the child to perform stretching exercises for the spine
- Help the child to maintain self-esteem
- Teach the child and parents about the brace
  – How to apply it and how long to wear it
  – How to prevent skin breakdown
    · Keep the skin beneath the brace clean and dry
    · Wear a tight fitting T-shirt under the brace

Managing nonstructural scoliosis

- Corrective lenses (if scoliosis is associated with poor vision)
- Postural exercises
- Shoe lifts

Managing structural scoliosis

- Electrical stimulation
- Harrington, Luque, or Cotrel-Dubousset rods for curves greater than 40 degrees
- Prolonged bracing
- Skin traction or halo femoral traction
- Spinal fusion with bone from the iliac crest

TOP 3

Postoperative interventions for structural scoliosis

1. Monitor vital signs and intake and output.
2. Turn the child by logrolling.
3. Maintain the bed in a flat position.

TOP 7

Items to study for your next test on the musculoskeletal system

1. Functions of muscles and bones
2. Bone growth and remodeling
3. Assessment findings in developmental dysplasia of the hip
4. Principles of skin traction and skeletal traction
5. Proper method for cast care
6. The difference between structural and nonstructural scoliosis
7. Management of scoliosis

NCLEX CHECKS

It's never too soon to begin your NCLEX preparation. Now that you've reviewed this chapter, carefully read each of the following questions and choose the best answer. Then compare your responses to the correct answers.

1. A nurse is assessing a neonate in the nursery. She performs Ortolani's test to rule out which defect?

- ☐ **1.** Neural tube defects
- ☐ **2.** Congenital clubfoot
- ☐ **3.** Development dysplasia of the hip
- ☐ **4.** Osteogenesis imperfecta

2. A 13-year-old with structural scoliosis had surgery to insert Harrington rods. Which postoperative position is best for this adolescent?

- ☐ **1.** Flat in bed
- ☐ **2.** Side-lying position
- ☐ **3.** Semi-Fowler's position
- ☐ **4.** High Fowler's position

3. A 13-year-old has been diagnosed with structural scoliosis and is fitted with a Milwaukee brace. How long should she wear the brace?

- ☐ **1.** 8 hours per day
- ☐ **2.** 12 hours per day
- ☐ **3.** 23 hours per day
- ☐ **4.** 24 hours per day

4. A child who is wearing a cast to correct clubfoot develops an itch under the cast. What should the nurse do to help relieve the itch?

- ☐ **1.** Use sterile applicators to relieve the itch.
- ☐ **2.** Apply water under the cast.
- ☐ **3.** Apply cool air under the cast with a blow-dryer.
- ☐ **4.** Apply hydrocortisone cream.

5. A nurse is developing a dietary teaching plan for a child with Duchenne's muscular dystrophy. What type of diet should the child follow? Select all that apply.

- ☐ **1.** Low-calorie
- ☐ **2.** High-calorie
- ☐ **3.** Low-protein
- ☐ **4.** High-protein
- ☐ **5.** Low-fiber
- ☐ **6.** High-fiber

6. Which classifications of the function of joints describes an immovable joint?

☐ **1.** Amphiarthrosis
☐ **2.** Diarthrosis
☐ **3.** Synarthrosis
☐ **4.** Synovial

7. Which assessment finding confirms a diagnosis of Duchenne's muscular dystrophy?

☐ **1.** Ortolani's sign
☐ **2.** Trendelenburg sign
☐ **3.** Barlow's sign
☐ **4.** Gowers' sign

8. Which is the highest priority nursing diagnosis for a child with a musculoskeletal disorder?

☐ **1.** *Impaired physical mobility*
☐ **2.** *Impaired walking*
☐ **3.** *Disturbed body image*
☐ **4.** *Risk for peripheral neurovascular dysfunction*

9. A nurse is caring for a child with a broken wrist that has just been placed in a cast. Why would the nurse elevate the arm?

☐ **1.** To promote healing
☐ **2.** To prevent edema
☐ **3.** To discourage infection
☐ **4.** To ensure proper bone alignment

10. Which common therapy for children with Legg-Calvé-Perthes disease should a nurse describe to the parents?

☐ **1.** Surgery with supporting rods
☐ **2.** Passive range-of-motion exercises
☐ **3.** A nonweight-bearing period
☐ **4.** Exercise to increase muscle strength of the knee joint

ANSWERS AND RATIONALES

1. CORRECT ANSWER: 3
Ortolani's test is performed to determine whether the neonate has developmental dysplasia of the hip. Neural tube defects are diagnosed by X-ray, magnetic resonance imaging, or computed tomography scan (if not visible externally). Clubfoot, a twisting of the foot, is visually diagnosed. Osteogenesis imperfecta, or bone fragility, is marked by bone fractures, blue sclerae, progressive bone deformities, and hypoplastic teeth.

2. CORRECT ANSWER: 1
After placement of Harrington rods, the client must remain flat in bed. In addition, the nurse should tape the latch of a manual bed or unplug an elec-

tric bed to prevent the head or foot of the bed from being raised. Other positions would be detrimental to the success of surgery because they wouldn't maintain the spine in a straight position.

3. CORRECT ANSWER: 3

A Milwaukee brace should be worn 23 hours per day. The brace may be removed for 1 hour per day for bathing and hygiene purposes. Periods of 8 hours and 12 hours are too short to provide the necessary support. A period of 24 hours per day doesn't allow for bathing or for skin integrity checks.

4. CORRECT ANSWER: 3

Itching underneath a cast can be relieved by directing a blow-dryer on the cool setting toward the itchy area. The nurse shouldn't put anything inside the cast because this can cause further skin irritation. Water would wet the cast and wouldn't help relieve the itch. Hydrocortisone cream can ball up and be irritating, and it would be difficult to apply inside the cast.

5. CORRECT ANSWER: 1, 4, 6

A child with muscular dystrophy is prone to constipation and obesity. He should follow a diet that's low in calories, high in protein, and high in fiber. Adequate fluid intake should also be encouraged.

6. CORRECT ANSWER: 3

Synarthrosis is a term that describes the function of an immovable joint. Amphiarthrosis is a joint that's slightly movable. Diarthrosis is a joint that's freely movable. Synovial describes a joint structure, not its function.

7. CORRECT ANSWER: 4

Gowers' sign (the use of hands to push up from the floor when rising from a sitting or supine position) is an assessment finding used to diagnose Duchenne's muscular dystrophy. Ortolani's, Trendelenburg, and Barlow's signs are used to diagnose developmental dysplasia of the hip, not Duchenne's muscular dystrophy.

8. CORRECT ANSWER: 4

Risk for peripheral neurovascular dysfunction is the highest priority nursing diagnosis for a child with a musculoskeletal disorder. The other nursing diagnoses are important, but the neurovascular considerations must be the priority to maintain future function of the affected body part.

9. CORRECT ANSWER: 2

After placing an extremity in a cast, the extremity should remain elevated to decrease edema to the dependent parts. Elevating the arm won't promote healing, discourage infection, or ensure proper bone alignment.

10. CORRECT ANSWER: 3

The only management of this disorder is reduced weight bearing and bed rest for 1 to 2 weeks, followed by a brace and decreased activity for up to 18 months.

13

Altered endocrine and metabolic functioning

1. Which endocrine gland serves as a storage area for hormones produced by the hypothalamus?

- ☐ 1. Thymus
- ☐ 2. Parathyroid
- ☐ 3. Adrenal
- ☐ 4. Posterior pituitary

CORRECT ANSWER: 4

2. Which cells produce somatostatin?

- ☐ 1. Alpha
- ☐ 2. Delta
- ☐ 3. Beta
- ☐ 4. Acinar

CORRECT ANSWER: 2

3. Which disorder can be a complication of Cushing's syndrome?

☐ 1. Menstrual disturbances

☐ 2. Nocturia

☐ 3. Polyuria

☐ 4. Peripheral neuropathy

CORRECT ANSWER: 1

4. One sign or symptom of hyperglycemia is:

☐ 1. diaphoresis.

☐ 2. tachycardia.

☐ 3. fruity breath odor.

☐ 4. palpitations.

CORRECT ANSWER: 3

5. Which inborn error of metabolism causes amino acids to degrade?

☐ 1. Phenylketonuria

☐ 2. Maple syrup urine disease

☐ 3. Galactosemia

☐ 4. Hypothyroidism

CORRECT ANSWER: 2

LEARNING OBJECTIVES

After studying this chapter, you should be able to:

● Assess and plan care for the child with diabetes mellitus.

● Assess the alterations in growth and development from the hyposecretion of thyroid hormones.

● Assess and plan care for the child with an inborn error of metabolism.

CHAPTER OVERVIEW

Altered endocrine function involves a hyposecretion or hypersecretion of hormones, which affect the body's metabolic processes and function. Nursing care involves measures to support hormonal secretion (such as hormonal replacement) or curtail secretion (such as through radiation therapy). Inborn errors of metabolism involve a biochemical alteration that affects metabolism.

KEY CONCEPTS

- **Structures and functions**
  - Glands—specialized cell clusters or organs
    - Pituitary gland
      - The hypophysis or master gland
      - Rests in the sella turcica, a depression in the sphenoid bone at the base of the brain
      - Pea-size
      - Anterior pituitary (adenohypophysis)
        - The larger region of the pituitary gland
        - Produces seven hormones
          - ·· Growth hormone (GH), or somatotropin
          - ·· Thyroid-stimulating hormone (TSH), or thyrotropin
          - ·· Corticotropin (ACTH)
          - ·· Follicle-stimulating hormone (FSH)
          - ·· Luteinizing hormone (LH)
          - ·· Prolactin
          - ·· Melanocyte-stimulating hormone
      - Posterior pituitary (neurohypophysis)
        - Makes up about 25% of the gland
        - Serves as a storage area for hormones produced by the hypothalamus
          - ·· Antidiuretic hormone (ADH), or vasopressin
          - ·· Oxytocin
    - Thyroid gland
      - Lies directly below the larynx, partially in front of the trachea
      - Two lateral lobes
        - One on either side of the trachea
        - Joined by a narrow tissue bridge called the isthmus, which gives the gland its butterfly shape
        - Lobes function as one unit to produce hormones
          - ·· Thyroid hormones (triiodothyronine [T_3] and thyroxine [T_4])
          - ·· Calcitonin
    - Parathyroid glands
      - Two glands that work together as a single gland

Quick guide to endocrine glands

- **Adrenal glands** – produce mineralocorticoids, glucocorticoids, some sex hormones, and catecholamines
- **Anterior pituitary gland** – produces GH, TSH, FSH, corticotropin, LH, prolactin, and melanoctye-stimulating hormone
- **Gonads** – produce estrogen and progesterone in females and testosterone in males
- **Pancreas** – consists of acinar cells that regulate exocrine function and various islet cells that produce glucagon, insulin, and somatostatin
- **Parathyroid glands** – produce PTH
- **Pineal gland** – produces melatonin
- **Posterior pituitary gland** – stores hormones produced by the hypothalamus (such as ADH and oxytocin)
- **Thymus** – produces T cells and peptide hormones
- **Thyroid gland** – produces thyroid hormones and calcitonin

- The body's smallest known endocrine glands
- Embedded on the posterior surface of the thyroid, one in each corner
- Produce parathyroid hormone (PTH)

– Adrenal glands
  - Two almond-shaped glands
  - Lie on top of each kidney
  - Contain two distinct structures
    - Adrenal cortex
      - The large outer layer that forms the bulk of the adrenal gland
      - Has three zones, or cell layers, that produce mineralocorticoids, glucocorticoids, and some sex hormones
    - Adrenal medulla
      - The inner layer
      - Functions as part of the sympathetic nervous system
      - Produces two catecholamines that play an important role in the autonomic nervous system: epinephrine and norepinephrine

– Pancreas
  - A triangular organ
  - Nestled in the curve of the duodenum
  - Stretches horizontally behind the stomach and extends to the spleen
  - Performs endocrine and exocrine functions
  - Cells that make up the pancreas
    - Acinar cells
      - Make up most of the gland
      - Regulate pancreatic exocrine function
    - Islets of Langerhans (islet cells)
      - Exist in clusters and are scattered among the acinar cells
      - Alpha cells produce glucagon, which raises the blood glucose level by triggering the breakdown of glycogen to glucose
      - Beta cells produce insulin, which lowers the blood glucose level by stimulating the conversion of glucose to glycogen
      - Delta cells produce somatostatin, which inhibits the release of GH, corticotropin, and certain other hormones

– Thymus
  - Located below the sternum
  - Contains lymphatic tissue
  - Reaches maximal size at puberty and then starts to atrophy
  - Produces T cells that are important in cell-mediated immunity
  - Produces peptide hormones that promote the growth of peripheral lymphoid tissue

Key facts about the pancreas

- Triangular organ that's nestled in the curve of the duodenum
- Performs endocrine and exocrine functions
- Made up of acinar cells and islets of Langerhans (islet cells)

Key facts about the islets of Langerhans

- They exist in clusters.
- Alpha cells produce glucagon.
- Beta cells produce insulin.
- Delta cells produce somatostatin.

– Pineal gland
  - Tiny gland
  - Lies at the back of the third ventricle of the brain
  - Produces melatonin, which may play a role in the neuroendocrine reproductive axis as well as other widespread actions
– Gonads
  - Ovaries (in females)
    - Paired, oval glands
    - Located on either side of the uterus
    - Produce ova (eggs)
    - Produce estrogen and progesterone, which promote the development and maintenance of female sex characteristics, regulate the menstrual cycle, maintain the uterus for pregnancy, and prepare the mammary glands for lactation
  - Testes (in males)
    - Paired structures
    - Lie in the extra-abdominal pouch (scrotum)
    - Produce spermatozoa
    - Produce the male hormone testosterone, which stimulates and maintains male sex characteristics
- Hormones
  – Chemical substances secreted by glands in response to stimulation
  – Trigger or regulate the activity of an organ or a group of cells
  – Classified by their molecular structure
    - Polypeptides
      - Protein compounds
      - Made of many amino acids that are connected by peptide bonds
      - Types
        ·· Anterior pituitary hormones (GH, TSH FSH, LH, and prolactin)
        ·· Posterior pituitary hormones (ADH and oxytocin)
        ·· PTH
        ·· Pancreatic hormones (insulin and glucagon)
    - Steroids
      - Derived from cholesterol
      - Adrenocortical hormones secreted by the adrenal cortex
        ·· Aldosterone
        ·· Cortisol
      - Sex hormones secreted by the gonads
        ·· Estrogen and progesterone (in females)
        ·· Testosterone (in males)
    - Amines
      - Derived from tyrosine, an essential amino acid found in most proteins

Functions of estrogen and progesterone

- Promote the development and maintenance of female sex characteristics
- Regulate the menstrual cycle
- Maintain the uterus for pregnancy
- Prepare the mammary glands for lactation

Key facts about hormones

- They're released by the glands and then bind to specific receptors.
- They have varying release patterns.
- They may have different effects at different target sites.
- They trigger or regulate the activity of an organ or a group of cells.
- They're classified as polypeptides, steroids, or amines, depending on their molecular structure.

Key facts about steroids

- Derived from cholesterol
- Adrenocortical hormones (aldosterone and cortisol) secreted by the adrenal cortex
- Sex hormones (estrogen, progesterone, and testosterone) secreted by the gonads

Target cells

A hormone acts only on cells that have receptors specific to that hormone. The sensitivity of a target cell depends on how many receptors it has for a particular hormone (the more receptor sites, the more sensitive the target cell).

- Types
  - ·· Thyroid hormones (T_4 and T_3)
  - ·· Catecholamines (epinephrine, norepinephrine, and dopamine)
- Hormone release patterns vary greatly
- When hormones reach their target site, they bind to a specific receptor
- After binding, each hormone produces unique physiologic changes, depending on the target site and its specific action at that site
- One hormone may have different effects at different target sites
- Regulation
  - A feedback mechanism involving hormones, blood chemicals and metabolites, and the nervous system that regulates hormone production and secretion
  - For normal function, each gland must contain enough appropriately programmed secretory cells to release active hormone on demand
  - Secretory cells are stimulated and inhibited to actively control the rate and duration of hormone release
- Receptors
  - Protein molecules
  - Trigger specific physiologic changes in a target cell in response to hormonal stimulation
  - Located in target cells (see *Target cells*)
  - May be found on the cell membrane or within the cell

Key facts about receptors

- Protein molecules that trigger specific changes in a target cell
- Respond to hormonal stimulation
- May be found on the target cell membrane or within the target cell

DIAGNOSTIC TESTS

● **Endocrine function study**
  • Purpose
    – Focuses on measuring the level or effect of a hormone such as the effect of insulin on blood glucose levels
  • Nursing interventions
    – Explain the test to the child and his parents
    – Check with the laboratory and consult facility protocol to determine specific actions before the test (for example, nothing-by-mouth for blood glucose test)

● **Radioimmunoassay**
  • Purpose
    – Used to measure minute quantities of hormones
  • Nursing interventions
    – Explain the test to the child and his parents

NURSING DIAGNOSES

● **Probable nursing diagnoses**
  • Delayed growth and development
  • Imbalanced nutrition: Less than body requirements
  • Activity intolerance
  • Excess fluid volume
  • Impaired skin integrity
  • Risk for infection
  • Imbalanced nutrition: More than body requirements

● **Possible nursing diagnoses**
  • Interrupted family process
  • Deficient knowledge (treatment regimen)
  • Disturbed body image
  • Risk for deficient fluid volume
  • Disturbed thought processes
  • Ineffective coping
  • Risk for injury
  • Sexual dysfunction
  • Deficient fluid volume
  • Disturbed sensory perception: Visual
  • Impaired oral mucous membrane
  • Impaired physical mobility
  • Chronic pain
  • Hypothermia
  • Situational low self-esteem
  • Ineffective tissue perfusion: Cardiopulmonary

Diagnostic tests for endocrine problems

● Endocrine function study – measures the level or effect of a hormone
● Radioimmunoassay – measures minute quantities of hormones

Probable nursing diagnoses for a patient with an endocrine or a metabolic disorder

● Delayed growth and development
● Imbalanced nutrition: Less than body requirements
● Activity intolerance
● Excess fluid volume
● Impaired skin integrity
● Risk for infection
● Imbalanced nutrition: More than body requirements

- Constipation
- Decreased cardiac output

CUSHING'S SYNDROME

Definition
- Clinical manifestation of glucocorticoid excess, particularly cortisol
- May also reflect excess secretion of mineralocorticoids and androgens

Causes
- Pituitary microadenoma
- Excess production of corticotropin
- Corticotropin-producing tumor in other organs
- Administration of synthetic glucocorticoids or corticotropin over long periods (common cause in older children)
- Cortisol-secreting adrenal tumor (most common cause in infants and young children)

Pathophysiology
- A loss of normal feedback inhibition by cortisol occurs
- Elevated levels of cortisol don't suppress hypothalamic and anterior pituitary secretion of corticotropin-releasing hormone and corticotropin
- The result is excessive levels of circulating cortisol

Complications
- Osteoporosis and pathologic fractures
- Peptic ulcer
- Dyslipidemia
- Impaired glucose tolerance
- Diabetes mellitus
- Frequent infections
- Slow wound healing
- Suppressed inflammatory response
- Hypertension
- Ischemic heart disease; heart failure
- Menstrual disturbances
- Psychiatric problems ranging from mood swings to frank psychosis

Assessment findings
- Fatigue
- Obesity
- Muscle weakness and wasting
- Sleep disturbances
- Water retention
- Amenorrhea or impotence
- Irritability, emotional instability

- Symptoms resembling those of hyperglycemia
- Thin hair
- Moon-shaped face
- Hirsutism
- A buffalo-humplike back
- Thin extremities
- Petechiae, ecchymoses, and purplish striae
- Delayed wound healing
- Swollen ankles
- Hypertension
- Acne

● **Diagnostic test findings**
- Elevated salivary free cortisol level
- Decreased corticotropin levels in adrenal disease and increased in excess pituitary or ectopic secretion of corticotropin
- Blood chemistry possibly showing hypernatremia, hypokalemia, hypocalcemia, and elevated blood glucose level
- Elevated urinary free cortisol level
- Elevated plasma cortisol level
- Ultrasonography, computed tomography (CT) scan, and magnetic resonance imaging may show the location of a pituitary or adrenal tumor
- A low-dose dexamethasone suppression test shows failure of plasma cortisol levels to be suppressed

● **Medical management**
- Restore hormone balance and reverse Cushing's syndrome
- Management approaches (may be used in combination with each other)
  – Radiation
  – Removal of excess glucocorticoids by reducing exogenous steriods
  – Drug therapy
    · Aminoglutethimide
    · Antifungal agents
    · Antihypertensives
    · Diuretics
    · Potassium supplements
    · Antineoplastic, antihormone agents
    · Cortisol therapy (during and after surgery)
  – Surgery
    · Possible hypophysectomy (removal of pituitary gland or tumor)
    · Bilateral adrenalectomy
    · Excision of nonendocrine, corticotropin-producing tumor, followed by drug therapy
    · Glucocorticoid administration on the morning of surgery can help prevent acute adrenal insufficiency during surgery

TOP 8

Findings in Cushing's syndrome

1. Obesity
2. Moon-shaped face
3. Thin extremities
4. Acne
5. Hypertension
6. Elevated urinary free cortisol level
7. Elevated plasma cortisol level
8. Failure of plasma cortisol levels to be suppressed (revealed by a low-dose dexamethasone suppression test)

Managing Cushing's syndrome

- Radiation
- Drug therapy
- Surgery
- Combination of radiation, drugs, and surgery

Medications used to treat Cushing's syndrome

- Aminoglutethimide
- Antifungal agents
- Antihypertensives
- Diuretics
- Cortisol therapy (during and after surgery)
- Potassium supplements
- Antineoplastic, antihormone agents

• Cortisol therapy is essential during and after surgery to help the child tolerate the physiologic stress caused by removal of the pituitary or adrenal glands

Nursing interventions
- Administer medications as ordered
- Monitor fluids and electrolytes
- Restrict sodium and water intake
- Evaluate for hyperglycemia
- Consult a nutritionist
- Use protective measures to reduce the risk of infection
- Use meticulous hand-washing technique
- Schedule adequate rest periods
- Institute safety precautions
- Provide meticulous skin care
- Encourage verbalization of feelings by the child and the parents
- Offer emotional support
- Help to develop effective coping strategies
- After hypophysectomy using the transsphenoidal approach
  - Keep the head of the bed elevated at least 30 degrees
  - Maintain nasal packing
  - Provide frequent mouth care
  - Avoid activities that increase intracranial pressure (ICP)
  - Monitor for cerebral fluid leaks
- After bilateral adrenalectomy or hypophysectomy, assess the child for:
  - Changes in neurologic and behavioral status
  - Severe nausea, vomiting, and diarrhea
  - Bowel sounds
  - Adrenal hypofunction
  - Increased ICP
  - Transient diabetes insipidus
  - Hemorrhage
  - Shock

DIABETES MELLITUS

Definition
- A chronic disease of absolute or relative insulin deficiency or resistance
- Type 1 diabetes mellitus is the most common childhood endocrine disorder
- The incidence of type 2 diabetes mellitus in childhood is rising because of the increase of childhood obesity and sedentary lifestyles

Causes
- Genetic factors

What to assess for after bilateral adrenalectomy or hypophysectomy

- Changes in neurologic and behavioral status
- Severe nausea, vomiting, and diarrhea
- Bowel sounds
- Adrenal hypofunction
- Increased ICP
- Transient diabetes insipidus
- Hemorrhage
- Shock

Key facts about diabetes mellitus

- It's a chronic disease of absolute or relative insulin deficiency or resistance.
- There are two types: type 1 and type 2.
- Type 1 diabetes mellitus is the most common childhood endocrine disorder.
- The incidence of type 2 diabetes mellitus in childhood is rising because of the increase of childhood obesity and sedentary lifestyles.
- It's characterized by disturbances in carbohydrate, protein, and fat metabolism.

- Autoimmune factors (type 1)
- Viral infection

Pathophysiology

- Characterized by disturbances in carbohydrate, protein, and fat metabolism
- Insulin
  - Allows glucose transport into the cells for use as energy or storage as glycogen
  - Stimulates protein synthesis and free fatty acid storage in adipose tissues
  - Deficiency compromises the body tissues' access to essential nutrients for fuel and storage
- Two primary forms
  - Type 1, characterized by absolute insulin insufficiency
  - Type 2, characterized by insulin resistance with varying degrees of insulin secretory defects

Complications

- Hypoglycemia (insulin reaction)
- Ketoacidosis
- Hyperosmolar, hyperglycemic syndrome
- Cardiovascular disease
- Peripheral vascular disease
- Retinopathy, blindness
- Nephropathy, renal failure
- Diabetic dermopathy
- Peripheral neuropathy
- Autonomic neuropathy
- Amputation
- Impaired resistance to infection
- Cognitive depression
- Poor wound healing

Assessment findings

- Polyuria
- Polydipsia
- Polyphagia
- Nocturia
- Weight loss and hunger
- Weakness and fatigue
- Dehydration
  - Dry mucous membranes
  - Poor skin turgor
- Vision changes
  - Retinopathy or cataract formation

Types of diabetes mellitus

- Type 1 — absolute insulin insufficiency
- Type 2 — insulin resistance with varying degrees of insulin secretory defects

Key complications of diabetes mellitus

- Hypoglycemia
- Ketoacidosis
- Cardiovascular disease
- Peripheral neuropathy
- Poor wound healing

TOP 3

Assessment findings in diabetes mellitus

1. Polyuria
2. Polydipsia
3. Polyphagia

– Can lead to blindness
- Frequent skin and urinary tract infections
- Acanthosis nigricons (a velvety hyperpigmented thickening of the skin around the nape of the neck that's mostly seen in type 2 diabetes)
- Skin changes
  – Dry, itchy skin (especially on the hands and feet)
  – Cool temperature
- Numbness or pain in the hands or feet
- Postprandial feeling of nausea or fullness
- Nocturnal diarrhea
- Decreased peripheral pulses
- Diminished deep tendon reflexes
- Orthostatic hypotension
- Characteristic "fruity" breath odor in ketoacidosis
- Possible hypovolemia and shock in ketoacidosis and hyperosmolar hyperglycemic state
- Type 1 specific
  – Rapidly developing symptoms
  – Muscle wasting and loss of subcutaneous fat
  – Honeymoon period
    · A one-time remission of the symptoms, which occurs shortly after insulin treatment is started
    · A last-ditch effort by pancreas to produce insulin
  – The child can be insulin-free for up to 1 year but may need oral hypoglycemics
  – Symptoms of hyperglycemia will reappear, and the child will be insulin-dependent for life
- Type 2 specific
  – Hypertension
  – Vague, long-standing symptoms that develop gradually
  – Severe viral infection
  – Other endocrine diseases
  – Recent stress or trauma
  – Use of drugs that increase blood glucose levels
  – Obesity, particularly in the abdominal area
  – Acanthosis nigricans

● **Diagnostic test findings**
- Fasting plasma glucose level greater than or equal to 126 mg/dl on at least two occasions
- Random blood glucose level greater than or equal to 200 mg/dl
- Two-hour postprandial blood glucose level greater than or equal to 200 mg/dl
- Glycosylated hemoglobin increased

Findings in type 1 diabetes mellitus

- Rapidly developing symptoms
- Muscle wasting and loss of subcutaneous fat
- Honeymoon period
- Reappearing symptoms
- Insulin-dependent for life

Findings in type 2 diabetes mellitus

- Vague, long-standing symptoms
- Severe viral infection
- Other endocrine diseases
- Recent stress or trauma
- Use of drugs that increase blood glucose levels
- Obesity, particularly in the abdominal area

- Urinalysis possibly showing acetone or glucose
- Ophthalmologic examination may show diabetic retinopathy

Medical management

- Glycemic control to prevent complications
    - Exogenous insulin (type 1)
        - Regular (Humulin R)
            - Onset: 30 to 60 minutes
            - Peaks in 2 to 3 hours
        - NPH (Humulin N)
            - Onset: 1 to 1½ hours
            - Peaks in 4 to 12 hours (8 hours average)
        - Lente (Humulin L)
            - Onset: 1 to 2½ hours
            - Peaks in 7 to 15 hours
        - Ultralente (Humulin U Ultralente)
            - Onset: 4 to 8 hours
            - Peaks in 10 to 30 hours
        - Lispro (Humalog)
            - Onset: less than 15 minutes
            - Peaks in 30 to 90 minutes
    - The most common insulin regimen for children consists of a combination of rapid-acting (regular) and intermediate-acting (NPH or Lente) insulins mixed in one syringe and administered twice daily, before breakfast and before dinner
    - Oral antidiabetic drugs (type 2); insulin may be required
    - Insulin pump; gives insulin on a more regular basis
- Surgery
    - Kidney transplantation
    - Pancreas transplantation
    - Islet cell transplantation
- Diet
    - Modest caloric restriction for weight loss or maintenance
    - Counting carbs to give the exact amount of regular insulin
    - About 1 unit of regular insulin per 30 g of carbohydrates
    - Follow American Diabetes Association recommendations to reach target glucose, glycosylated hemoglobin, lipid, and blood pressure levels
- Regular aerobic exercise

Nursing interventions

- Administer medications as ordered
- Monitor for hypoglycemia (insulin shock)
    - Can result from increased insulin use, excessive exercise, or failure to eat
    - Recognize signs and symptoms

TOP 3

Ways to manage diabetes

1. Glycemic control with insulin or oral antidiabetic drugs
2. Diet
3. Regular aerobic exercise

Types of exogenous insulin commonly used in children

- Rapid acting (Regular) — clear, short-acting; onset of 30 minutes; peaks in 2 to 3 hours
- Intermediate acting (NPH or Lente) — cloudy; onset of 1 to 2½ hours; peaks in 4 to 15 hours

Signs and symptoms of hypoglycemia

- Behavior changes (belligerence, confusion, slurred speech)
- Diaphoresis
- Palpitations
- Tachycardia
- Tremors

Signs and symptoms of hyperglycemia

- Abdominal cramping
- Dry, flushed skin
- Fatigue
- Fruity breath odor
- Headache
- Mental status changes
- Nausea
- Thin appearance and possible malnourishment
- Vomiting
- Weakness

- Behavior changes (belligerence, confusion, slurred speech)
- Diaphoresis
- Palpitations
- Tachycardia
- Tremors
  - If hypoglycemia occurs, give rapidly absorbed carbohydrates such as orange juice or, if the child is unconscious, glucagon or I.V. dextrose as ordered
- Monitor for hyperglycemia
  - Recognize signs and symptoms
    - Abdominal cramping
    - Dry, flushed skin
    - Fatigue
    - Fruity breath odor
    - Headache
    - Mental status changes
    - Nausea
    - Thin appearance and possible malnourishment
    - Vomiting
    - Weakness
  - Administer I.V. fluids and insulin replacement for hyperglycemic crisis as ordered
- If it can't be determined whether a stuporous diabetic is suffering from hypoglycemia or hyperglycemia, treat for hypoglycemia
- Provide meticulous skin care, especially to the feet and legs
- Treat all injuries, cuts, and blisters immediately
- Avoid constricting hose, slippers, or bed linens
- Encourage adequate fluid intake
- Consult a nutritionist
- Encourage verbalization of feelings
- Offer emotional support
- Help to develop effective coping strategies
- Provide patient teaching
  - The disorder, diagnostic studies, and treatment
  - Insulin (see *Insulin-dependent diabetes mellitus*)
    - When giving a combination of clear and cloudy insulins, draw up clear insulin first to prevent contamination
    - To prevent air bubbles, don't shake the vial; intermediate forms are suspensions and should be gently rotated
    - Administer insulin as ordered (commonly twice daily; however, more injections per day may be ordered), 30 minutes before breakfast and 30 minutes before dinner; know that both injections will include a combination of fast-acting and intermediate-acting insulin

TIME-OUT FOR TEACHING

Insulin-dependent diabetes mellitus

Be sure to include these points in your teaching plan for the parents of a child with insulin-dependent diabetes mellitus:
- insulin dosage, frequency, administration, and storage
- subcutaneous injection technique
- site selection and rotation
- signs and symptoms of hyperglycemia and hypoglycemia
- fingerstick blood glucose measurement
- diet therapy
- compliance with laboratory tests and follow-up
- factors associated with altering insulin requirements
- possible complications.

- Insulin dosages vary; the dosage for one day is based on blood glucose levels of the previous day, with two-thirds of the daily dose usually given in the morning injection and one-third in the evening injection
- Watch for hypoglycemic reactions during the peak action times for fast-acting and intermediate-acting insulins
- Rotate injection sites to prevent lipodystrophy
- Teach maintenance of insulin pump
- Make sure the child eats when the insulin peaks, such as a midafternoon and bedtime snack
- Keep in mind that insulin requirements may be altered with illness, stress, growth, food intake, and exercise; blood glucose measurements are the best way to determine insulin adjustments
- Instruct parents in all aspects of insulin therapy
  - When to notify the physician
  - Appropriate exercise plan
  - Self-monitoring of glucose
  - Signs and symptoms of hyperglycemia, hypoglycemia, infection, and diabetic neuropathy
  - Foot care
  - Safety precautions

HYPOTHYROIDISM

● Definition
- Deficiency of thyroid hormone secretion (T_3 and T_4) during fetal development or early infancy (see *Understanding thyroid gland hormones, page 358*)

Understanding thyroid gland hormones

- The thyroid gland secretes the iodinated hormones thyroxine and triiodothyronine.
- Thyroid hormones, necessary for normal growth and development, act on many tissues to increase metabolic activity and protein synthesis.
- Deficiency of thyroid hormones causes varying degrees of hypothyroidism, from a mild, clinically insignificant form to life-threatening myxedema coma.

- If left untreated, results in congenital hypothyroidism (or infantile cretinism)
- Cretinism is three times more common in girls than in boys
- Early diagnosis and treatment allow the best prognosis
  - Infants treated before age 3 months usually grow and develop normally
  - Athyroid children who remain untreated beyond age 3 months and children with acquired hypothyroidism who remain untreated beyond age 2 years suffer irreversible mental retardation; their skeletal abnormalities are reversible with treatment

Causes
- Defective embryonic development (most common cause), causing congenital absence or underdevelopment of the thyroid gland
- Inherited autosomal recessive defect in the synthesis of thyroxine (next most common cause)
- Antithyroid drugs taken during pregnancy, causing cretinism in infants
- Chronic autoimmune thyroiditis (cretinism after age 2 years)
- Iodine deficiency during pregnancy

Pathophysiology
- Hypothyroidism in infants and children is related to decreased thyroid hormone production or secretion
- Loss of functional thyroid tissue can be caused by an autoimmune process
- Defective thyroid synthesis may be related to congenital defects, with thyroid dysgenesis (defective development) the most common
- Hypothyroidism may also be related to decreased TSH secretion or resistance to TSH

Complications
- Skeletal malformations and irreversible mental retardation (for hypothyroid infants not treated by age 3 months; early treatment helps prevent retardation)
- Learning disabilities
- Accelerated or delayed sexual maturation
- Myxedema coma

Causes of hypothyroidism

- Defective embryonic development
- Inherited autosomal recessive defect
- Antithyroid drugs taken during pregnancy
- Chronic autoimmune thyroiditis
- Iodine deficiency during pregnancy

Complications of hypothyroidism

- Skeletal malformations and irreversible mental retardation
- Learning disabilities
- Accelerated or delayed sexual maturation

● Assessment findings

A child may be asymptomatic until age 6 months for acquired hypothyroidism

- General
  - Delayed dentition
  - Lethargy or, in infants, excessive sleeping
  - Enlarged, dry tongue
  - Hypotonia
  - Legs shorter in relation to trunk size
  - Cognitive impairment (develops as the disorder progresses)
  - Short stature with the persistence of infant proportions
  - Short, thick neck
- Associated with slow basal metabolic rate
  - Cool body and skin temperature
  - Dry, scaly skin
  - Easy weight gain
  - Slow pulse
- Untreated hypothyroidism in infants
  - Hoarse cry
  - Persistent jaundice
  - Respiratory difficulties
- Untreated hypothyroidism in older children
  - Bone and muscle dystrophy
  - Cognitive impairment
  - Stunted growth (dwarfism)

● Diagnostic test findings

- Elevated TSH level associated with low T_3 and T_4 levels point to cretinism (because early detection and treatment can minimize the effects of cretinism, many states require measurement of infant thyroid hormone levels at birth)
- Thyroid ultrasound and radioactive iodine uptake tests show decreased uptake levels and confirm the absence of thyroid tissue in athyroid children
- Increased gonadotropin levels accompany sexual precocity in older children and may coexist with hypothyroidism
- Electrocardiogram shows bradycardia and flat or inverted T waves in untreated infants
- Hip, knee, and thigh X-rays reveal absence of the femoral or tibial epiphyseal line and delayed skeletal development that's markedly inappropriate for the child's chronological age
- Low T_4 and normal TSH levels suggest hypothyroidism secondary to hypothalamic or pituitary disease (rare)

TOP 6

Findings in hypothyroidism

1. Lethargy
2. Hypotonia
3. Short, thick neck
4. Cool body and skin temperature
5. Dry, scaly skin
6. Elevated TSH level with low T_3 and T_4 levels

Medications for hypothyroidism

- Synthetic levothyroxine
- Synthetic liothyronine
- Supplemental vitamin D

Key interventions for hypothyroidism

- Administer medications as ordered.
- Provide adequate rest periods.
- If the infant's tongue is unusually large, position him on his side and observe him frequently to prevent airway obstruction.
- Monitor blood pressure and pulse rate.

Signs of thyroid hormone replacement medication toxicity

- Hypertension
- Tachycardia
- Fever
- Irritability
- Sweating

● **Medical management**
- Medication
  - Long-term thyroid hormone replacement therapy
    · Synthetic levothyroxine
    · Synthetic liothyronine
  - Supplemental vitamin D to prevent rickets resulting from rapid bone growth
- Surgery for the underlying cause such as pituitary tumor
- Routine monitoring of T_4 and TSH levels
- Periodic evaluation of growth to ensure thyroid replacement is adequate

● **Nursing interventions**
- Administer medications as ordered
- Provide adequate rest periods
- Apply antiembolism stockings
- Encourage coughing and deep-breathing exercises
- Maintain fluid restrictions and a low-salt diet
- Reorient the patient as needed
- Offer support and encouragement
- Provide meticulous skin and mucous membrane care
- If the infant's tongue is unusually large, position him on his side and observe him frequently to prevent airway obstruction
- Check rectal temperature every 2 to 4 hours; keep the patient warm as needed
- Encourage the patient to express his feelings
- Help to develop effective coping for the child and the parents
- Discuss the importance of the child wearing a medical identification bracelet
- During early management of infantile hypothyroidism, monitor blood pressure and pulse rate; report hypertension and tachycardia immediately (normal infant heart rate is approximately 120 beats/minute); these signs, as well as fever, irritability, and sweating, indicate the dose of thyroid hormone replacement medication is too high
- Adolescent girls require future-oriented counseling that stresses the importance of adequate thyroid hormone replacement during pregnancy

INBORN ERRORS OF METABOLISM

● **Definition**
- Multiple conditions, most of them autosomal recessive, resulting from altered biochemistry
- Enzyme abnormalities result in accumulation of a reactant that may have toxic effects

● **Causes**
  - Genetic
● **Pathophysiology**
  - An absence or deficiency of a substance essential to metabolism on a cellular level
    – Phenylketonuria (PKU)
      · Results from a defect that prevents conversion of phenylalanine to tyrosine
      · Dietary phenylalanine builds up, resulting in brain damage and mental retardation
    – Galactosemia
      · A deficiency in galactose enzymes
      · Galactose fails to be converted into glucose; it builds up in the bloodstream and spills into the urine
      · Results in liver failure, renal tubular problems, and cataracts
    – Maple syrup urine disease (MSUD)
      · A deficiency of decarboxylase that degrades some amino acids
      · Results in altered tonicity and seizures
      · If untreated, this disease can be fatal
● **Complications**
  - Developmental delays
  - Coma
  - Seizures
  - Death
● **Assessment findings**
  - General
    – Lethargy
    – Persistent vomiting
    – Respiratory difficulty
    – Hypothermia
    – Coma
    – Seizures
    – Jaundice
    – Hepatomegaly
    – Coarse facial features
    – Macroglossia
    – Diarrhea
    – Abnormal odor
    – Abnormal hair
  - PKU
    – Athetosis (movement disorder)
    – Brain damage
    – Urine has a musty odor

Quick guide to inborn errors of metabolism

- **PKU** – phenylalanine can't convert to tyrosine, which causes phenylalanine to build up in the body
- **Galactosemia** – galactose doesn't convert to glucose, causing it to build up in the bloodstream and spill into the urine
- **MSUD** – a deficiency of de-carboxylase causes amino acids to degrade

Complications of inborn errors of metabolism

- Developmental delays
- Coma
- Seizures
- Death

Assessment findings for inborn errors of metabolism

- Lethargy
- Persistent vomiting
- Respiratory difficulty
- Hypothermia
- Coma
- Seizures
- Jaundice
- Hepatomegaly
- Coarse facial features
- Macroglossia
- Diarrhea
- Abnormal odor
- Abnormal hair

– Seizures
- Galactosemia
  – Lethargy, hypotonia
  – Diarrhea
  – Vomiting
  – Jaundice
  – Development of bilateral cataracts
- MSUD
  – Urine has the odor of maple syrup
  – Feeding difficulties
  – Loss of Moro reflex
  – Irregular respirations
  – Seizures

● **Diagnostic test findings**
- PKU
  – Genetic screening is positive for the disorder
  – The Guthrie blood test reveals serum phenylalanine levels greater than 4 mg/dl (most states require screening for PKU at birth)
- Galactosemia
  – Genetic screening is positive for the disorder
  – Increased blood levels of galactose
  – Decreased UDP galactose transferase activity in erythrocytes
- MSUD
  – Genetic screening is positive for the disorder

● **Medical management**
- PKU
  – Eliminate dietary phenylalanine
    · An enzymatic hydrolysate of casein, such as Lofenalac powder or Pregestimil powder, is substituted for milk in the diets of affected infants
    · Dietary restrictions should probably continue throughout life
      - Avoid foods highest in phenylalanine, including meats, eggs, and milk
      - Foods low in phenylalanine include orange juice, bananas, potatoes, lettuce, spinach, and peas
  – This special diet calls for careful monitoring; because the body doesn't make phenylalanine; overzealous dietary restriction can induce phenylalanine deficiency, producing lethargy, anorexia, anemia, rashes, and diarrhea
- Galactosemia
  – Eliminate dietary galactose (generally available as lactose) (see *Diet for galactosemia*)
  – As the child grows, a balanced, galactose-free diet must be maintained

---

Diagnostic findings for inborn errors of metabolism

- PKU – Genetic screening is positive for the disorder; Guthrie blood test reveals serum phenylalanine levels greater than 4 mg/dl.
- Galactosemia – Blood levels of galactose are increased; UDP galactose transferase activity in erythrocytes is decreased.

Managing inborn errors of metabolism

- PKU – eliminate dietary phenylalanine
- Galactosemia – eliminate dietary galactose (generally available as lactose)
- MSUD – restrict branched-chain amino acids, such as leucine, isoleucine, and valine, and provide a diet high in thiamine

Diet for galactosemia

A patient with galactosemia must follow a lactose-free diet. He may eat these foods:
- fish and animal products (except brains and mussels)
- fresh fruits and vegetables (except peas and lima beans)
- bread and rolls made from cracked wheat.

He should avoid these foods:
- dairy products
- such snacks as puddings, cookies, cakes, and pies
- food coloring
- instant potatoes
- canned and frozen foods (if lactose is listed as an ingredient).

- MSUD
  - Restrict branched-chain amino acids, such as leucine, isoleucine, and valine, and provide a diet high in thiamine
  - If necessary, peritoneal dialysis, hemodialysis, or both

● **Nursing interventions**
- Test urine specimens and blood samples after the first 24 hours of feeding
- Check diapers for color, amount, and odor of urine
- For neonates discharged within 24 hours of birth, ensure home visits by a nurse to obtain blood samples for testing and provide rapid test results; refer for abnormal test results

PRECOCIOUS PUBERTY

● **Definition**
- In females, the onset of pubertal changes before age 8 (the mean age for menarche is 13)
  - Breast development
  - Pubic and axillary hair development
  - Menarche
- In males, manifestation of sexual development before age 9

● **Causes**
- Unknown
- In girls, precocious puberty generally occurs as an isolated event
- Familial (in boys)

● **Pathophysiology**
- More common in girls than boys
- True precocious puberty
  - Early activation of the hypothalamic-pituitary-gonadal system
    - Premature maturation and development of the gonads and premature secretion of sex hormones
      - Premature development of secondary sex characteristics

- Occasional production of mature sperm or ova
  – Constitutional or functional idiopathic precocious puberty
    • Early development and activation of the endocrine glands without corresponding abnormality
  – Pathologic
    • Central nervous system (CNS) disorders resulting from tumors, trauma, infection, or lesions
      ·· Hypothalamic tumors
      ·· Intracranial tumors
      ·· Hydrocephaly
      ·· Degenerative encephalopathy
      ·· Tuberous sclerosis
      ·· Neurofibromatosis
      ·· Encephalitis
      ·· Skull injuries
      ·· Meningitis
      ·· Peptic arachnoiditis
- Pseudoprecocious puberty
  – No early secretion of gonadotropin
  – No maturation of the gonads
  – Early overproduction of sex hormones
    • Ovarian, testicular, and adrenocortical tumors
    • Adrenal cortical virilizing hyperplasia
    • Ingestion of estrogens or androgens
  – Development of secondary sex characteristics
  – Increased end-organ sensitivity to low levels of circulating sex hormones
    • Premature thelarche (breast development)
    • Premature pubarche (development of sexual hair)
    • Congenital adrenal hypoplasia
    • McCune-Albright syndrome
    • Chronic hypothyroidism

● Complications
- Behavioral problems
- Social difficulty related to age and appearance variance and mood swings

● Assessment findings
- Rapid growth spurt
- In females, before age 8, the following may occur independently or simultaneously
  – Thelarche
  – Pubarche
  – Menarche
- In males, pubarche before age 9

Characteristics of pseudoprecocious puberty

- No early secretion of gonado-tropin
- No maturation of the gonads
- Early overproduction of sex hormones
- Premature breast development
- Premature development of sexual hair

Assessment findings in precocious puberty

- Rapid growth spurt
- In females, thelarche, pub-arche, menarche before age 8
- In males, pubarche before age 9

● Diagnostic test findings

- X-rays of the hands, wrists, knees, and hips determine bone age and possible premature epiphyseal closure
- Tests that detect abnormally high hormonal levels for the patient's age
  - Vaginal smear for estrogen secretion
  - Urinary tests for gonadotropic activity and excretion of 17-ketosteroids
  - Radioimmunoassay for LH and FSH in females and testosterone in males
- Ultrasound, laparoscopy, or exploratory laparotomy may verify a suspected abdominal lesion
- EEG, CT scan, or angiography can detect CNS disorders
- Laboratory tests
  - LH, FSH, estradiol, testoterone, adrenal androgens, and thyroid function tests

● Medical management

- Medroxyprogesterone (Depo-Provera) to reduce secretion of gonadotropins and prevent menstruation
- Adrenogenital syndrome
  - Cortical or adrenocortical steroid replacement
- Abdominal tumors
  - Surgery to remove ovarian, testicular, and adrenal tumors
  - Regression of secondary sex characteristics may follow such surgery, especially in young children
- Choriocarcinomas
  - Surgery
  - Chemotherapy
- Hypothyroidism
  - Thyroid extract
  - Levothyroxine to decrease gonadotropic secretions
- Drug ingestion
  - Medication must be discontinued

● Nursing interventions

- Provide a calm, supportive atmosphere, and encourage the child and family to express their feelings about these changes
- Explain all diagnostic procedures, and tell the child and family that surgery may be necessary
- Explain the condition to the child in terms she can understand to prevent feelings of shame and loss of self-esteem
- Provide appropriate sex education
- Tell parents that, although their child seems physically mature, she isn't psychologically mature

---

Tests to detect hormone levels

- Vaginal smear
- Urinary tests
- Radioimmunoassay

TOP 3

Interventions for precocious puberty

1. Provide a calm, supportive atmosphere, and encourage the child and family to express their feelings about the changes.
2. Tell parents that, although their child seems physically mature, she isn't psychologically mature.
3. Suggest that parents continue to dress their child in clothes that are appropriate for her age and that don't call attention to physical development.

– The discrepancy between physical appearance and psychological and psychosexual maturation may create problems

– Warn them against expecting more of her than they would expect of other children her age

• Suggest that parents continue to dress their child in clothes that are appropriate for her age and that don't call attention to physical development

• Reassure parents that precocious puberty doesn't usually precipitate precocious sexual behavior

NCLEX CHECKS

It's never too soon to begin your NCLEX preparation. Now that you've reviewed this chapter, carefully read each of the following questions and choose the best answer. Then compare your responses to the correct answers.

1. An infant with congenital hypothyroidism shows which sign or symptom?

☐ **1.** Shrill cry
☐ **2.** Diaphoresis
☐ **3.** Hypothermia
☐ **4.** Diarrhea

2. A nurse administers oral thyroid hormone to an infant with hypothyroidism. The nurse should observe the infant for which signs of overdose?

☐ **1.** Tachycardia, fever, irritability, and sweating
☐ **2.** Bradycardia, cool skin temperature, and dry scaly skin
☐ **3.** Bradycardia, fever, hypotension, and irritability
☐ **4.** Tachycardia, cool skin temperature, and irritability

3. A nurse draws blood from the heel of an infant for a Guthrie screening test. The Guthrie screening test is used to diagnose which inborn error of metabolism?

☐ **1.** Glucose-6-phosphate dehydrogenase deficiency
☐ **2.** PKU
☐ **3.** Galactosemia
☐ **4.** Hypothyroidism

4. A nurse is teaching the mother of a child with diabetes how to recognize the signs and symptoms of hypoglycemia. Which signs and symptoms should the nurse discuss?

☐ **1.** Behavioral changes, increased heart rate, sweating, and tremors
☐ **2.** Nausea, fruity breath odor, headache, and fatigue
☐ **3.** Polydipsia, polyuria, polyphagia, and weight loss
☐ **4.** Enlarged tongue, hypotonia, easy weight gain, and cool skin temperature

TOP 7

Items to study for your next test on the endocrine and metabolic systems

1. Functions of the glands of the endocrine system

2. Signs and symptoms of Cushing's syndrome

3. Type 1 and type 2 diabetes mellitus

4. Signs and symptoms of hypoglycemia and hyperglycemia

5. Insulin administration

6. Role of thyroid hormones

7. Management of PKU, galactosemia, and MSUD

5. A nurse is assessing a child who might have diabetes. Which laboratory values help confirm a diagnosis of diabetes?

- ☐ **1.** A fasting plasma glucose level of 110 mg/dl
- ☐ **2.** A fasting plasma glucose level of 126 mg/dl
- ☐ **3.** A random plasma glucose level of 180 mg/dl
- ☐ **4.** A 2-hour glucose tolerance test of 140 mg/dl

6. A nurse is teaching the parents of a child with diabetes. Which agent should the nurse teach the parents to administer if their child suffers a severe hypoglycemic reaction?

- ☐ **1.** I.V. dextrose
- ☐ **2.** Subcutaneous insulin
- ☐ **3.** Subcutaneous glucagon
- ☐ **4.** Oral fast-acting carbohydrate

7. Which statement made by the caregiver of a child with insulin-dependent diabetes mellitus indicates a need for further teaching?

- ☐ **1.** "After each meal my child eats, I should count the carbohydrates and plan to give regular insulin accordingly."
- ☐ **2.** "After the child eats his meal, we should check his urine."
- ☐ **3.** "I should watch for my child to have symptoms of hypoglycemia about a half hour after I have given him his regular insulin."
- ☐ **4.** "I need to talk to his teacher each time he changes his grade level or if the teacher has any questions."

8. A nursing technician is being instructed about drawing a PKU test on a neonate. Which statement by the technician shows an understanding of PKU?

- ☐ **1.** "A Guthrie test should be done as soon as possible."
- ☐ **2.** "Urine needs to be collected to check for phenylpyruvic acid on every neonate."
- ☐ **3.** "I need to check when the baby had his first formula or breast-feeding."
- ☐ **4.** "I should plan on contacting the public health department."

9. An 8-year-old female was diagnosed with precocious puberty. Which teaching point is important for the nurse to review with the child and the mother?

- ☐ **1.** Teach the child to change her tampon at least every 8 hours to prevent toxic shock syndrome.
- ☐ **2.** The child should no longer be encouraged to play with dolls.
- ☐ **3.** The child shouldn't participate in active sports.
- ☐ **4.** Explain to the mother that the child may be physically maturing but isn't psychologically mature.

10. Which foods may be eaten by a child with galactosemia? Select all that apply.

- ☐ **1.** Instant potatoes
- ☐ **2.** Chicken
- ☐ **3.** Lima beans
- ☐ **4.** Whole wheat bread
- ☐ **5.** Apples
- ☐ **6.** 2% cow's milk

ANSWERS AND RATIONALES

1. CORRECT ANSWER: 3

Hypothermia is one common finding in congenital hypothyroidism. Other common findings in hypothyroidism include lethargy, poor feeding, prolonged jaundice, vomiting, constipation, mottling, coarse facial features, hoarse cry, large fontanels, and hypotonia. A shrill cry may indicate CNS damage. Diaphoresis is more common with hyperthermia (an abnormally high body temperature). Constipation, not diarrhea, is a common finding in hypothyroidism.

2. CORRECT ANSWER: 1

The infant experiencing an overdose of thyroid replacement hormone exhibits tachycardia, fever, irritability, and sweating. Bradycardia, cool skin temperature, and dry scaly skin are signs of hypothyroidism.

3. CORRECT ANSWER: 2

The Guthrie screening test is a bacterial inhibition assay that's used to diagnose PKU. Bacillus subtilis, present in the culture medium, grows if the blood contains an excessive amount of phenylalanine. Glucose-6-phosphate dehydrogenase deficiency isn't an inborn error of metabolism. Galactosemia is diagnosed by increased levels of galactose in the blood. Hypothyroidism isn't an inborn error of metabolism.

4. CORRECT ANSWER: 1

The nurse should instruct the mother of a child with diabetes to recognize such signs and symptoms of hypoglycemia as behavioral changes, increased heart rate, sweating, and tremors. Nausea, fruity breath odor, headache, and fatigue are present in hyperglycemia. Polydipsia, polyuria, polyphagia, and weight loss are classic signs of diabetes. Enlarged tongue, hypotonia, easy weight gain, and cool skin temperature are associated with hypothyroidism.

5. CORRECT ANSWER: 2

According to the American Diabetes Association, diabetes occurs when either there are: symptoms of diabetes plus a random plasma glucose level greater than or equal to 200 mg/dl, a fasting plasma glucose level greater than or equal to 126 mg/dl, or a 2-hour oral glucose tolerance test greater than or equal to 200 mg/dl.

6. CORRECT ANSWER: 3

The nurse should instruct the parents of a child with diabetes to administer subcutaneous glucagon if their child suffers a severe hypoglycemic episode. Subcutaneous insulin would worsen the child's condition. I.V. dextrose should only be administered by health care providers who are specially trained in I.V. drug administration. Oral administration of fast-acting carbohydrates is reserved for the conscious child who isn't suffering from a severe hypoglycemic reaction.

7. CORRECT ANSWER: 2

Urine ketone testing can be performed regardless of when the child ate. Counting carbohydrates, watching for hypoglycemia symptoms, administering insulin, and letting teachers know of the child's condition are all correct statements.

8. CORRECT ANSWER: 3

PKU testing ideally is done 48 hours after the neonate is given his first protein feeding. Phenylalanine levels don't rise without ingested protein. The technician need not contact the public health department because Guthrie testing for PKU is mandatory.

9. CORRECT ANSWER: 4

The mother should be taught not to equate physical maturity with psychological maturity. Playing with dolls is acceptable behavior for an 8-year-old. Tampons should be changed more frequently and may even be inappropriate for the child to manage. The child should be encouraged to be physically active.

10. CORRECT ANSWER: 2, 4, 5

The child with galactosemia must follow a lactose-free diet. Appropriate foods for his diet include fish and chicken, fresh fruits and vegetables (except for lima beans), and bread made from whole wheat. The child should avoid dairy products, such as 2% cow's milk, instant potatoes, and other lactose-containing foods.

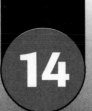

Altered dermatologic status

---

1. Which layer of the skin is rich in ribonucleic acid?

☐ 1. Stratum lucidum

☐ 2. Stratum basale

☐ 3. Stratum corneum

☐ 4. Stratum spinosum

CORRECT ANSWER: 4

2. Which glands located in the palms and soles are responsible for secreting fluid mainly in response to emotional stress?

☐ 1. Skene's

☐ 2. Sebaceous

☐ 3. Apocrine

☐ 4. Eccrine

CORRECT ANSWER: 1

3. Which type of burn extends into the subcutaneous tissue level?

☐ 1. Superficial partial-thickness

☐ 2. Deep partial-thickness

☐ 3. Full-thickness

☐ 4. Deep full-thickness

CORRECT ANSWER: 3

4. Which skin disorder causes honey-colored crusts surrounded by erythema?

☐ 1. Impetigo

☐ 2. Scabies

☐ 3. Acne

☐ 4. Contact dermatitis

CORRECT ANSWER: 1

5. Which disorder produces a papular rash in children?

☐ 1. Acne

☐ 2. Scarlet fever

☐ 3. Varicella

☐ 4. Impetigo

CORRECT ANSWER: 2

LEARNING OBJECTIVES

After studying this chapter, you should be able to:

● Assess and plan care for the child with a rash.

● Differentiate between contact dermatitis and infectious dermatitis.

● Discuss the nursing interventions for the child with burns.

CHAPTER OVERVIEW

Children with conditions involving altered dermatologic status typically present with some type of rash or skin manifestation. Assessment of the type of rash or manifestation is essential for determining its treatment. Nursing care centers on relieving itching, controlling inflammation and infection, and preventing infection transmission. Burns require close monitoring of all body functions to prevent complications.

KEY CONCEPTS

● **Structures and functions**
- Skin
  - Consists of two major layers plus a layer of subcutaneous tissue
    - Epidermis
      - The outermost layer
      - Varies in thickness from less than 0.1 mm on the eyelids to more than 1 mm on the palms and soles
      - Composed of avascular, stratified, squamous (scaly or plate-like) epithelial tissue
      - Divided into five layers (see *A view of the skin*)
        - Stratum corneum — outermost layer consisting of tightly arranged layers of cellular membranes and keratin
        - Stratum lucidum — clear layer
        - Stratum granulosum — granular layer
        - Stratum spinosum — spiny layer rich in ribonucleic acid
        - Stratum basale — basal layer; the innermost layer that produces new cells to replace outer cells that are shed away
    - Dermis
      - Also called the *corneum*
      - The skin's second layer
      - An elastic system
      - Made up of extracellular material called matrix
        - Collagen — a protein that gives strength to the dermis
        - Elastin — makes the skin pliable
        - Reticular fibers — bind the collagen and elastin fibers together
      - Divided into two layers
        - Papillary dermis — connects the dermis to the epidermis with fingerlike projections called papillae and contains characteristic ridges that on the fingers are known as *fingerprints*
        - Reticular dermis — covers a layer of subcutaneous tissue
  - Functions of the skin
    - Protects the inner body's structures
      - Migrates
      - Sheds

Layers of the skin

- Epidermis – the outermost layer that varies in thickness
- Dermis – the second layer that's also called the corneum
- Subcutaneous tissue

Layers of the epidermis

- Stratum corneum – outermost layer consisting of tightly arranged layers of cellular membranes and keratin
- Stratum lucidum – clear layer
- Stratum granulosum – granular layer
- Stratum spinosum – spiny layer rich in ribonucleic acid
- Stratum basale – the innermost layer that produces new cells

Layers of the dermis

- Papillary dermis – connects the dermis to the epidermis
- Reticular dermis – covers a layer of subcutaneous tissue

A view of the skin

Major components of the skin include the epidermis, dermis, and epidermal appendages.

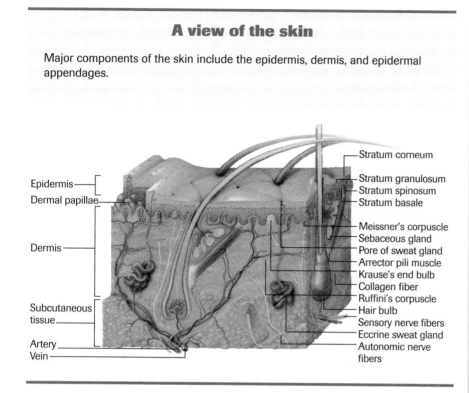

Epidermis
Dermal papillae
Dermis
Subcutaneous tissue
Artery
Vein

Stratum corneum
Stratum granulosum
Stratum spinosum
Stratum basale
Meissner's corpuscle
Sebaceous gland
Pore of sweat gland
Arrector pili muscle
Krause's end bulb
Collagen fiber
Ruffini's corpuscle
Hair bulb
Sensory nerve fibers
Eccrine sweat gland
Autonomic nerve fibers

- Repairs surface wounds by intensifying normal cell replacement mechanisms
- The top layer of the skin protects the body against noxious chemicals and invasion from bacteria and microorganisms
  - Langerhans' cells enhance the body's immune response by helping lymphocytes to process antigens entering the skin
  - Melanocytes protect the skin by producing the brown pigment melanin
- Helps filter ultraviolet light (irradiation)
– Involved in sensory perception
  - Sensory nerve fibers
    - Originate in the nerve roots along the spine
    - Supply specific areas of the skin known as dermatomes
    - Transmit various sensations from the skin to the central nervous system
      ·· Temperature
      ·· Touch
      ·· Pressure
      ·· Pain
      ·· Itching
  - Autonomic nerve fibers carry impulses to various destinations, such as the smooth muscle in the walls of the skin's blood vessels, and the muscles around the hair roots

Functions of the skin

- Protects the inner body's structures
- Involved in sensory perception
- Regulates body temperature
- Excretes some body fluids
- Helps prevent dehydration

Sensations the skin transmits

- Temperature
- Touch
- Pressure
- Pain
- Itching

How the skin responds to temperature changes

- Exposure to cold or a decrease in internal body temperature
- Blood vessels constrict
- Blood flow decreases
- Body heat is conserved
- Exposure to heat or an increase in internal body temperature
- Small arteries within the skin dilate
- Blood flow increases
- Body heat is dissipated or dispelled

Spotlight on sebaceous glands

- Occur on all parts of the skin except the palms and soles
- Prominent at the base of hair follicles on the scalp, face, upper torso, and genitalia
- Produce sebum, which is a mixture of keratin, fat, and cellulose debris; sebum combines with sweat to form a moist, oily, acidic film

Spotlight on sweat glands

- These include the eccrine glands and apocrine glands.
- The eccrine glands produce an odorless, watery fluid.
- The eccrine glands in the palms and soles respond to emotional stress; others respond to thermal stress.
- The apocrine glands are located chiefly in the underarms and groin.
- The aprocrine glands begin to function at puberty.

– Regulates body temperature
  • Performed by abundant nerves, blood vessels, and eccrine glands within the skin's deeper layer
  • When the skin is exposed to cold or the internal body temperature falls
    - Blood vessels constrict
    - Blood flow is decreased
    - Body heat is conserved
  • If the skin becomes too hot or the internal body temperature rises
    - Small arteries within the skin dilate
    - Blood flow is increased
    - Body heat is dissipated or dispelled
– Excretes some body fluids
  • Sweat (excreted by sweat glands)
    - Water
    - Electrolytes
    - Urea
    - Lactic acid
  • Body wastes (through skin's more than 2 million pores)
– Prevents dehydration caused by loss of internal body fluids by preventing body fluids from escaping
• Glands
  – Sebaceous glands
    • Occur on all parts of the skin except the palms and soles
    • Prominent at the base of hair follicles on the scalp, face, upper torso, and genitalia
    • Produce sebum
      - A mixture of keratin, fat, and cellulose debris
      - Exits through the hair follicle opening to reach the skin surface
      - Combines with sweat to form a moist, oily, acidic film
        ·· Antibacterial
        ·· Antifungal
        ·· Protects the skin's surface
  – Sweat glands
    • Eccrine glands
      - Widely distributed throughout the body
      - Contain a coiled duct comprising the secretory portion which passes through the dermis and epidermis, opening onto the skin surface
      - Produce an odorless, watery fluid with a sodium concentration equal to that of plasma
      - Glands in the palms and soles secrete fluid mainly in response to emotional stress

- Other eccrine glands respond to thermal stress and effectively regulate temperature
- Apocrine glands
  - Located chiefly in the axillary (underarm) and anogenital (groin) areas
  - The coiled secretory portion lies deeper in the dermis than that of the eccrine glands
  - Ducts connect apocrine glands to the upper portion of hair follicles
  - Begin to function at puberty
  - No known biological function
  - As bacteria decompose the fluids produced by these glands, body odor occurs

DIAGNOSTIC TESTS

● Diascopy
- Purpose
  - To observe a lesion under a microscope to determine whether dilated capillaries or extravasated blood is causing the redness of a lesion
- Nursing interventions
  - Explain the procedure to the child and parents

● Sidelighting
- Purpose
  - Shows minor elevations or depressions in lesions
  - Helps to determine the configuration and degree of eruption
- Nursing interventions
  - Explain the procedure to the child and parents

● Subdued lighting
- Purpose
  - Highlights the difference between normal skin and circumscribed lesions that are hypopigmented or hyperpigmented
- Nursing interventions
  - Explain the procedure to the child and parents

● Microscopic immunofluorescence
- Purpose
  - Helps to identify immunoglobulins and elastic tissue in detecting skin manifestations of immunologically mediated disease
- Nursing interventions
  - Explain the procedure to the child and parents

● Gram stains and exudate cultures
- Purpose

Quick guide to diagnostic tests for dermatologic disorders

- **Diascopy** – allows observation of a lesion by microscope to determine the cause of redness
- **Sidelighting** – shows minor elevation or depression of a lesion to determine degree of eruption
- **Subdued lighting** – shows the pigmented difference between normal skin and circumscribed lesions
- **Microscopic immunofluorescence** – identifies immunoglobulins and elastic tissue
- **Gram stains and exudate cultures** – help identify infectious organisms
- **Patch tests** – help identify contact sensitivity
- **Skin biopsy** – used to determine the histology of cells and help confirm the diagnosis of a disorder
- **Potassium hydroxide preparations** – used to detect mycelia in fungal infections

– Help to identify organisms responsible for underlying infections
* Nursing interventions
    – Explain the procedure to the child and parents
    – Obtain cultures as directed by facility policy

● **Patch tests**
* Purpose
    – Identify contact sensitivity (usually with dermatitis)
* Nursing intervention
    – Explain the procedure to the child and parents

● **Skin biopsy**
* Purpose
    – To determine the histology of cells
    – To diagnose or confirm a disorder
* Nursing interventions
    – Before the procedure
        · Explain the procedure to the child and parents
    – After the procedure
        · Tell the parents that the child should avoid wool or rough clothing
        · Prevent secondary infections by cutting the child's nails and applying mittens and elbow restraints
        · Suggest the child wear light, loose, nonirritating clothing
        · Teach the parents signs and symptoms of infection

● **Potassium hydroxide preparations**
* Purpose
    – Examine for mycelia in fungal infections
* Nursing interventions
    – Explain the procedure to the child and parents

NURSING DIAGNOSES

● **Probable nursing diagnoses**
* Impaired skin integrity
* Risk for infection
* Disturbed body image
* Impaired tissue integrity
* Ineffective tissue perfusion: All
* Ineffective protection
* Hyperthermia
* Hypothermia
* Acute pain

● **Possible nursing diagnoses**
* Chronic pain

What to do before any diagnostic test

● Explain the procedure to the child and his parents.

Probable nursing diagnoses for a patient with a dermatologic disorder

● Impaired skin integrity
● Risk for infection
● Disturbed body image
● Impaired tissue integrity
● Ineffective tissue perfusion: All
● Ineffective protection
● Hyperthermia
● Hypothermia
● Acute pain

- Bathing or hygiene self-care deficit
- Deficient knowledge (impetigo, scabies, acne, burns)
- Social isolation
- Situational low self-esteem
- Ineffective airway clearance
- Deficient fluid volume
- Imbalanced nutrition: Less than body requirements
- Anxiety
- Impaired gas exchange
- Risk for posttrauma syndrome

ACNE

● **Definition**
- An inflammatory disorder of the sebaceous gland contiguous with a hair follicle, known as the *pilosebaceous follicle*
- Acne lesions may be divided into inflammatory and noninflammatory lesions

● **Causes**
- Androgen-stimulated sebum production
- Follicular occlusion
- *Propionibacterium acnes*, a normal skin flora
- Predisposing factors
    - Androgen stimulation
    - Certain drugs
        · Corticosteroids
        · Corticotropin
        · Androgens
        · Iodides
        · Bromides
        · Trimethadione
        · Phenytoin
        · Isoniazid
        · Lithium
        · Halothane
    - Cobalt irradiation
    - Total parenteral nutrition
    - Cosmetics
    - Exposure to heavy oils, greases, or tars
    - Heredity
    - Hormonal contraceptives
    - Trauma or rubbing from tight clothing
    - Tropical climate
    - Menstrual cycle

Key facts about acne

- It's an inflammatory disorder of the sebaceous glands.
- Lesions may be inflammatory or noninflammatory.
- It's caused by androgen stimulation of sebum production, follicular occlusion, and normal skin flora.
- It isn't attributed to dietary influences.

Predisposing factors for acne

- Androgen stimulation
- Certain drugs
- Cobalt irradiation
- Total parenteral nutrition
- Cosmetics
- Exposure to heavy oils, greases, or tars
- Heredity
- Hormonal contraceptives
- Trauma or rubbing from tight clothing
- Tropical climate
- Menstrual cycle

Types of acne

- Noninflammatory—inflamed sebaceous gland ducts (comedones) that may be open (blackheads) or closed (whiteheads)
- Inflammatory—rupture of the follicular wall and inflammation of the surrounding dermis

TOP 2

Assessment findings in acne

1. Acne lesions, commonly located on the face, neck, shoulders, chest, and upper back
2. Acne plugs that appear as a closed or open comedone

- No longer attributed to dietary influences

● **Pathophysiology**
  - Acne begins with sebum accumulation that obstructs the pilosebaceous unit
  - The mass of accumulated keratinous sebaceous material and bacteria within the pilosebaceous follicle causes inflammation when it's exposed to the dermis with rupture of a follicle
  - The *Propionibacterium acnes* bacteria produce substances that promote inflammation
  - Two types of acne
    – Noninflammatory acne
      · Comedones (inflamed sebaceous gland ducts) develop
        - Blackheads—open comedones
        - Whiteheads—closed comedones
      · Accumulated material causes distention of the follicle and thinning of follicular canal and walls
    – Inflammatory acne
      · Develops in closed comedones when the follicular wall ruptures
      · Sebum is expelled into the surrounding dermis, causing inflammation
  - Pustules form when the inflammation is close to the surface; papules and cystic nodules can develop when the inflammation is deeper, causing mild to severe scarring
  - Most common among adolescents

● **Complications**
  - Deep cystic process
  - Gross inflammation
  - Abscess formation
  - Secondary bacterial infections
  - Acne scars

● **Assessment findings**
  - Pain and tenderness around the area of infected follicle
  - Acne lesions, commonly located on the face, neck, shoulders, chest, and upper back
  - Red and swollen area around the infected follicle
  - Acne plugs that appear as a closed comedone (whitehead) or an open comedone (blackhead)
  - Oily and thickened skin
  - Visible scars

● **Diagnostic test findings**
  - There's no diagnostic test for this disorder; diagnosis is made primarily by history and physical examination
  - Culture and sensitivity of pustules or abscesses show causative organism of secondary bacterial infection

● **Medical management**

- Well-balanced diet
- Exposure to ultraviolet light (but never when a photosensitizing agent, such as tretinoin, is being used)
- Medications
  - Intralesional corticosteroid injection
  - Oral isotretinoin (Accutane)
    - Limited to those with nodulocystic or recalcitrant acne who don't respond to conventional therapy
    - Contraindicated during pregnancy
  - Systemic therapy
    - Tetracycline to decrease bacterial growth
      - Contraindicated during pregnancy and childhood because it discolors developing teeth
    - Erythromycin (Ilotycin)
  - Topical medications
    - Benzoyl peroxide (Benzac)
    - Clindamycin (Cleocin)
    - Erythromycin antibacterial agents
    - Tretinoin (retinoic acid, Retin-A)
    - Keratolytics such as salicylic acid
  - Antiandrogenic agents
    - Estrogens
    - Spironolactone (Aldactazide)

● **Nursing interventions**

- Check the patient's drug history because some medications, such as hormonal contraceptives, may cause acne flare-ups
- Try to identify predisposing factors to determine those that can be eliminated or modified
- Explain the causes of acne to the patient and family
  - Make sure they understand the prescribed treatment is more likely to improve acne than a strict diet and fanatic scrubbing with soap and water
  - Assess the routine hygiene practices of the child and provide suggestions as needed
  - Provide written instructions regarding treatment to eliminate misconceptions
- If the patient is receiving tretinoin, provide him and his family with specific instructions
  - Apply it at least 30 minutes after washing the face and at least 1 hour before bedtime
  - Warn against using it around the eyes or lips to prevent damage

Managing acne

- Well-balanced diet
- Exposure to ultraviolet light
- Medications

Topical medications for acne

- Benzoyl peroxide (Benzac)
- Clindamycin (Cleocin)
- Erythromycin antibacterial agents
- Tretinoin (retinoic acid, Retin-A)
- Keratolytics such as salicylic acid

Key nursing interventions for acne

- Try to identify predisposing factors to determine those that can be eliminated or modified.
- If the patient is receiving tretinoin, provide him and his family with specific instructions.
- Advise the patient to avoid exposure to sunlight or to use a sunscreen to prevent a photosensitivity reaction.
- Inform the patient that acne takes a long time to clear.
- Explain the adverse effects of all medications to promote compliance.
- Pay special attention to the patient's perception of his physical appearance and self-esteem.

What to teach the patient taking isotretinoin

- Avoid taking vitamin A supplements
- Ways to deal with dry skin and mucous membranes
- The severe risk of teratogenesis in the female patient during child-bearing years
- The importance of monitoring liver function and lipid levels

---

TIME-OUT FOR TEACHING

Teaching about acne

Be sure to include these points in your teaching plan for the patient with acne:
- predisposing factors
- how acne develops
- stages of severity
- importance of adhering to treatment to improve acne and prevent scarring
- medications, such as benzoyl peroxide, tretinoin, antibiotics, and isotretinoin
- other care measures, including hygiene and cosmetic use.

  – After treatments, the skin should look pink and dry; if it appears red or starts to peel, the preparation may have to be weakened or applied less often
- Advise the patient to avoid exposure to sunlight or to use a sunscreen to prevent a photosensitivity reaction
- If the prescribed regimen includes tretinoin and benzoyl peroxide, tell the patient to use one preparation in the morning and the other at night to avoid skin irritation
- Instruct the patient to take tetracycline on an empty stomach and not to take it with antacids or milk because it interacts with their metallic ions and is then poorly absorbed
- Teach the patient who's taking isotretinoin the following:
  – To avoid vitamin A supplements, which can worsen adverse effects
  – Ways to deal with the dry skin and mucous membranes that usually occur during treatment
  – The severe risk of teratogenesis in the female patient during child-bearing years
  – The importance of monitoring liver function and lipid levels to avoid toxicity
- Inform the patient that acne takes a long time to clear — possibly even years for complete resolution (see *Teaching about acne*)
- Encourage continued local skin care even after acne clears
- Explain the adverse effects of all medications to promote compliance
- Pay special attention to the patient's perception of his physical appearance and self-esteem
- Offer emotional support to help the patient cope with the effects of his condition

Key facts about burns

- They may be caused by heat, electricity, or chemicals.
- Second- and third-degree burns occur more commonly in children.
- Children younger than age 3 are most commonly burned by hot liquids or electricity.
- Children older than age 3 are most commonly burned by flames.

BURNS

● **Definition**
- Thermal (heat), electrical, or chemical injury
- Most pediatric burns occur in children younger than age 5

Classification of burns by depth of injury

One method of classifying burns is to determine the burn's depth.

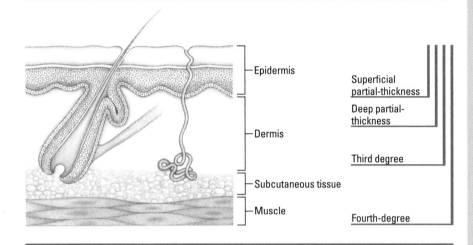

Types of burns

- Superficial partial-thickness — involve localized injury to the dermis
- Deep partial-thickness — involve destruction of epidermis and some dermis
- Third degree — extend into subcutaneous layer
- Fourth-degree — damage muscle, bone, and interstitial tissues

- Burns are the third leading cause of accidental death in children, after motor vehicle accidents and drowning
- Deep partial-thickness and full-thickness burns occur more commonly in children because their skin is thinner than that of adults, allowing for shorter penetration time

Causes

- Residential fires
- Motor vehicle accidents
- Improper use or handling of matches
- Improperly stored gasoline
- Space heater or electrical malfunctions
- Improper handling of firecrackers
- Scalding accidents
- Child or elder abuse
- Contact, ingestion, inhalation, or injection of acids, alkali, or vesicants
- Contact with faulty electrical wiring
- Contact with high-voltage power lines
- Chewing electric cords
- Friction or abrasion
- Sun exposure
- Contact with hot liquids or electricity (most common cause of burns in children younger than age 3)
- Older children are most commonly burned by flames

Pathophysiology

- Superficial partial-thickness burns (first-degree) (see *Classification of burns by depth of injury*)

Complications of burns

- Respiratory complications
- Sepsis
- Hypovolemic shock
- Anemia
- Malnutrition
- Multiple organ dysfunction syndrome

Findings for superficial partial-thickness (first-degree) burns

- Dry, painful, red skin with edema
- Sunburnlike appearance

Findings for deep partial-thickness (second-degree) burns

- Moist, weeping blisters with edema
- Very painful

Findings for full-thickness (third-degree) burns

- Avascular without blanching or pain
- Dry, pale, leathery skin
- Diuresis 2 to 5 days after the burn, as fluid shifts back
- Fluid shift from intravascular to interstitial compartments
- Hypovolemia and symptoms of shock from fluid shift, including renal failure
- Infection due to altered skin integrity

- Localized injury to epidermis
- Not life-threatening
- Deep partial-thickness burns (second-degree)
  - Destruction of epidermis and some dermis
  - Thin-walled and fluid-filled blisters
  - As blisters break, nerve endings exposed to air
  - Pain develops when blisters are exposed to air
  - Barrier function of the skin is lost
  - May cause scarring
- Third-degree and fourth-degree burns (full-thickness)
  - Affect every body system and organ
  - Third-degree extends into the subcutaneous tissue layer
  - Fourth-degree damages muscle, bone, and interstitial tissues
  - Interstitial fluids result in edema
  - Immediate immunologic response occurs
  - Wound sepsis threat
  - Painless
  - Scab forms

Complications
- Respiratory complications
- Sepsis
- Hypovolemic shock
- Anemia
- Malnutrition
- Multiple organ dysfunction syndrome

Assessment findings
- Superficial, partial-thickness (first-degree) burn
  - Dry, painful, red skin with edema
  - Looks like a sunburn
- Deep partial-thickness (second-degree) burn
  - Moist, weeping blisters with edema
  - Very painful
- Full-thickness (third-degree) burn
  - Avascular without blanching or pain
  - Dry, pale, leathery skin
  - Diuresis 2 to 5 days after the burn, as fluid shifts back
  - Fluid shift from intravascular to interstitial compartments
  - Hypovolemia and symptoms of shock from fluid shift, including renal failure
  - Infection due to altered skin integrity
- Major burns
  - More than 20% of a child's body surface area (BSA)
- Moderate burns
  - 10% to 20% of a child's BSA

- Minor burns
  - Less than 10% of a child's BSA

● **Diagnostic test findings**
- Arterial blood gas levels show evidence of smoke inhalation; may show decreased alveolar function, hypoxia
- Complete blood count shows decreased hemoglobin level and hematocrit if blood loss occurs
- Abnormal electrolytes due to fluid losses and shifts
- Increased blood urea nitrogen levels with fluid losses
- Decreased glucose levels in children due to limited glycogen storage
- Urinalysis showing myoglobinuria
- Increased carboxyhemoglobin levels
- Electrocardiogram may show ischemia, injury, or arrhythmias especially in electrical burns
- Fiber-optic bronchoscopy may show edema of the airways

● **Medical management**
- Stopping the burn source
- Securing an open airway
- Preventing hypoxia
- Wound care
- Diet
  - Nothing by mouth until severity of burn is established
  - High-protein, high-calorie
  - Increased hydration
  - Total parenteral nutrition if can't take food by mouth
- Physical therapy
- Medications
  - Booster of tetanus toxoid
  - Analgesics
  - Antibiotics
  - Antianxiety agents
  - Topical agents to prevent and treat bacterial or fungal infections
    · Mafenide (Sulfamylon)
    · Silver sulfadiazine (Silvadene)
  - Debriding agents
- Surgery
  - Loose tissue and blister debridement
  - Escharotomy
  - Skin grafting

● **Nursing interventions**
- Apply immediate, aggressive burn treatment
- Use sterile technique
- Remove clothing that's still smoldering

Diet for burn management
- Nothing by mouth until severity of burn is established
- High-protein, high-calorie
- Increased fluids
- Total parenteral nutrition if can't take food by mouth

Medications for burn management
- Booster of tetanus toxoid
- Analgesics
- Antibiotics
- Antianxiety agents
- Topical agents to prevent and treat bacterial or fungal infections
- Debriding agents

Surgery for burn management
- Loose tissue and blister debridement
- Escharotomy
- Skin grafting

- Remove the patient's rings and other constricting items
- Perform appropriate wound care
- Provide adequate hydration by administering lactated Ringer's solution through a large-bore I.V. line
- Weigh the patient daily
- Monitor urine output; for a child under 66 lb (30 kg), output should be 1 ml/kg/hour
- Assess for pain and provide medication as needed; medicate before dressing changes
- Encourage verbalization and provide support
- Monitor urine specific gravity, which is usually between 1.010 and 1.025; this helps detect dehydration
- Maintain a patent airway
- Care for the burn wound
  - Assist with debridement
  - Elevate the burned part
- Prevent heat loss
- Provide diversional, age-appropriate activities for the hospitalized child
- Assist with coping skills for disfiguring burns
  - Refer the family to support groups
  - Address parents' feelings of guilt
- Reassure the child that the pain isn't punishment; implement measures to decrease fear

CONTACT DERMATITIS: DIAPER RASH

● Definition
- A local skin reaction in the areas normally covered by a diaper

● Causes
- Body soaps and bubble baths
- Tight clothes, wool or rough clothing
- Clothing dyes or the soaps used to wash diapers
- Irritation due to acidic urine and stools or the formation of ammonia in the diaper
- Moist, warm environment contained by a plastic diaper lining
- Bacteria
- Candida

● Pathophysiology
- The skin of a full-term neonate serves as an effective barrier to disease, but the skin barrier may be broken down by a combination of factors
  - Dampness
  - Lack of air exposure
  - Acidic or irritant exposures
  - Increase in skin friction

Key facts about diaper rash

- It's a skin reaction in the areas covered by a diaper.
- It's caused by acidic urine and stools or the formation of ammonia in the moist, warm environment of a diaper, especially a plastic one.

- Prolonged exposure to moisture and diaper contents (urine and stools) causes a rash

Complications
- Pain
- Infection

Assessment findings
- Characteristic bright red, maculopapular rash in the diaper area
- Irritability because the rash is painful and warm

Diagnostic test findings
- Diagnostic testing isn't necessary
- Diagnosis is based on inspection

Medical management
- Cleaning the affected area with mild soap and water
- Leaving the affected area open to air
- Medications
  - Zinc oxide ointment or a barrier-type ointment to help the skin heal
  - Topical antibiotic ointment if secondary infection occurs
  - Topical antifungal ointment

Nursing interventions
- Keep the diaper area clean and dry to maintain skin integrity
- Change the diaper immediately after the child voids or defecates to prevent skin breakdown
- Wash the area with mild soap and water to promote healing
- Completely remove all previous ointments before reapplying
- Keep the area open to the air without plastic linings, if possible, to promote circulation and comfort
- Avoid using commercially prepared diaper wipes on broken skin; the chemicals and alcohol in commercially prepared wipes may be irritating
- Apply medication as ordered

CONTACT DERMATITIS: POISON IVY

Definition
- A severe allergic reaction caused by contact with any of several species of climbing vine of the genus *Rhus*

Causes
- Skin to vine contact with the shiny, three-pointed leaves

Pathophysiology
- Poisonous oil on the plant leaf causes a delayed hypersensitivity (T cell) response
- The rash appears 1 to 2 days after contact

Assessment findings in diaper rash
- Bright red, maculopapular rash in diaper area
- Irritability

Key facts about poison ivy
- It's a severe allergic reaction caused by contact with the climbing vine commonly called poison ivy.
- The poisonous oil on the plant leaf causes a 1- to 2-day delayed hypersensitivity response.
- The poisonous oil remaining on clothing, skin, and animals is contagious.

Assessment findings in poison ivy

- Pruritus
- Red, localized streaks that precede vesicles

Managing poison ivy

- Wash the oils from the skin with soap and water.
- Don't touch other body parts until the area has been cleaned.
- Carefully wash resin out of the clothes.
- Apply calamine lotion.
- Apply topical steroids.

Ways to discourage scratching and prevent secondary infection

- Trim fingernails short.
- Cover the child's hands if necessary.
- Cover the lesions.
- Encourage the patient not to scratch.
- Use meticulous hand-washing technique.

Key facts about head lice

- It's also known as *pediculosis capitis.*
- It's a contagious infestation with any of the small wingless insect or lice order of *Anoplura.*
- It's spread by close contact and by shared clothing and combs.
- The lice feed on human blood and lay their eggs in hair.
- The louse injects a toxin when it bites.
- The toxin causes inflammation.

- Oils that remain on the clothes and skin are contagious to others; the eruptions aren't a source of infection and won't spread the disease
- Animals may carry the oils to humans

● **Complications**
- Infection
- Scarring

● **Assessment findings**
- Pruritus
- Red, localized streaks that precede vesicles

● **Diagnostic test findings**
- Diagnostic testing isn't necessary
- Diagnosis is based on inspection

● **Medical management**
- Wash the oils from the skin with soap and water to prevent absorption through the skin and spread to other areas
- Don't touch other body parts until the area has been cleaned
- Carefully wash resin out of the clothes
- Apply calamine lotion
- Apply topical steroids to reduce inflammation and itching
- Oral steroids may be used if dermatitis is severe, especially on the face

● **Nursing interventions**
- Follow standard precautions
- Prevent secondary infection and spreading that may occur as a result of scratching
  - Trim fingernails short
  - Cover the child's hands if necessary
  - Cover the lesions
  - Encourage the patient not to scratch
  - Use meticulous hand-washing technique
- Teach the patient and family what the poison ivy plant looks like to prevent future reactions

HEAD LICE

● **Definition**
- Also known as *pediculosis capitis*
- A contagious infestation with any of the small wingless insect or lice order of *Anoplura*
- It's estimated that 6 to 10 million children per year are infested with lice

● **Causes**
- Sharing of clothing and combs
- Close personal contact with peers

Pathophysiology
- Lice feed on human blood and lay their eggs (nits) in body hairs
- After the nits hatch, the lice must feed within 24 hours or die; they mature in about 2 to 3 weeks
- When a louse bites, it injects a toxin into the skin that produces mild irritation and a purpuric spot
- Repeated bites cause sensitization to the toxin, leading to more serious inflammation
- Treatment can effectively eliminate lice

Complications
- Excoriation

Assessment findings
- Pruritus of the scalp
- Visual examination of lice eggs, which look like white flecks, firmly attached to hair shafts
- Black specks at the base of hair

Diagnostic test findings
- Diagnostic tests aren't necessary because diagnosis is based on visual examination

Medical management
- Removal of lice and eggs using a fine-toothed comb
- Medications
  - Pyrethrins (RID)
  - Permethrin (Elimite) shampoos
  - Lindane, in resistant cases
  - Preventive drug therapy for other family members and classmates

Nursing interventions
- Carefully follow the manufacturer's directions when applying medicated shampoo to avoid neurotoxicity
- Repeat treatment in 7 to 12 days to ensure that all the eggs have been killed
- Instruct the child's parents to wash bed linens, furniture, hats, combs, brushes, and anything else that came in contact with the hair to prevent reinfestation
- Explain the importance of refraining from exchanging combs, brushes, headgear, or clothing with other children
- Place stuffed toys in a sealed plastic bag for 2 weeks

IMPETIGO

Definition
- A contagious, superficial bacterial skin infection
- Most commonly appears on the face and extremities

Assessment findings in head lice

- Pruritus of the scalp
- Visual examination of lice eggs, which look like white flecks, firmly attached to hair shafts
- Black specks at the base of hair

Medications for head lice

- Pyrethrins (RID)
- Permethrin (Elimite) shampoos
- Lindane, in resistant cases

Key facts about impetigo

- Highly contagious bacterial skin infection
- Common on the face and extremities
- Spread by scratching
- Common in children ages 2 to 5

Types of impetigo

- Nonbullous
- Eruption occurs when bacteria inoculate traumatized skin cells.
- Lesions are small and rapidly erode.
- Honey-colored crusts form.
- Bullous
- Eruption occurs in nontraumatized skin via bacterial toxin or exotoxin.
- Lesions are thin-walled and contain clear to turbid yellow fluid.

Predisposing factors for impetigo

- Poor hygiene
- Anemia
- Malnutrition
- Warm climate

Causes
- Bacterial infection from group A beta-hemolytic streptococci; may also be due to staphylococci
- Spread by autoinoculation through scratching

Pathophysiology
- Two types
  - May occur simultaneously and be clinically indistinguishable
  - Nonbullous impetigo
    - Eruption occurs when bacteria inoculate traumatized skin cells
    - Lesions begin as small vesicles, which rapidly erode
    - Honey-colored crusts surrounded by erythema are formed
  - Bullous impetigo
    - Eruption occurs in nontraumatized skin via bacterial toxin or exotoxin
    - Lesions begin as thin-walled bullae and vesicles
    - Lesions contain clear to turbid yellow fluid; some crusting exists
- May complicate chickenpox, eczema, and other skin disorders marked by open lesions
- Predisposing factors
  - Poor hygiene
  - Anemia
  - Malnutrition
  - Warm climate
    - Most outbreaks occur in the late summer and early fall
    - In the United States, impetigo occurs most commonly in the southern states
- Highly contagious until all lesions are healed
  - The infection is spread by direct contact
  - The incubation period is 2 to 5 days after contact
- Common in children ages 2 to 5

Complications
- Acute glomerulonephritis
  - More likely to occur when many members of the same family have impetigo
- Ecthyma (an infection that occurs usually as a result of untreated impetigo; may be followed by pigmentation and scarring of the skin)
- Exfoliative eruption (staphylococcal scalded-skin syndrome) in neonates, infants, and children younger than age 5

Assessment findings
- Painless itching
- Nonbullous impetigo
  - Small, red macule or vesicle that becomes pustular within a few hours

Recognizing impetigo

In impetigo, when the vesicles break, crust forms from the exudate. This infection is especially contagious among young children.

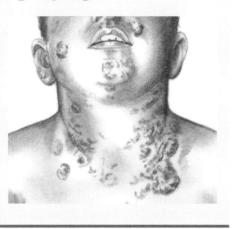

Assessment findings in nonbullous impetigo

1. Lesions on the face around the mouth and nose
2. Thick, honey-colored crust formed from the exudates
3. Pruritus

- Lesions can occur anywhere, but usually occur on the face around the mouth and nose
- Characteristic thick, honey-colored crust formed from the exudates
- Satellite lesions caused by autoinoculation
- Pruritus
- Burning
- Regional lymphadenopathy
- Infants and children develop aural impetigo or otitis externa; lesions usually clear without treatment in 2 to 3 weeks, unless there is an underlying disorder such as eczema
- Bullous impetigo
  - Thin-walled vesicle
  - Thin, clear crust formed from exudates (see *Recognizing impetigo*)
  - Lesions that appear as a central clearing circumscribed by an outer rim
  - Most commonly appear on the face or other exposed areas

● Diagnostic test findings
- Gram stain of vesicular fluid showing infecting organism
- Culture and sensitivity testing of exudates or denuded crust showing infecting organism
- Elevated white blood cell count

● Medical management
- Removal of exudates by washing the lesions 2 to 3 times per day with soap (or antibacterial soap) and water
- Warm soaks or compresses of normal saline or a diluted soap solution for stubborn crusts
- Prevention by using benzoyl peroxide soap

Assessment findings in bullous impetigo

- Thin-walled vesicle
- Thin, clear crust formed from exudates
- Lesions appear as a central clearing surrounded by an outer rim
- Commonly appear on the face or other exposed areas

Medications for impetigo

- Antibiotics for 10 days
- Topical antibiotics for minor infections
- Antihistamines

- Medication
  - Antibiotics for 10 days
    - Penicillinase-resistant penicillins such as dicloxacillin
    - Cephalosporins such as cephalexin (Keftab)
    - Azithromycin (Zithromax)
    - Clarithromycin (Biaxin)
    - Retapamulin (Altabax) a new class of antibiotics called pleuro-mutilins, inhibit bacteria from making protein and has been approved to treat impetigo. It's prescribed twice per day for 5 days in children age 9 months or older
  - Topical antibiotics for minor infections such as mupirocin ointment (Bactroban)
  - Antihistamines
- Therapy shouldn't be delayed for laboratory results, which can take up to 3 days

● **Nursing interventions**
- Follow standard precautions
- Prevent secondary infection and the spread of impetigo
  - Trim fingernails short
  - Cover the child's hands if necessary
  - Cover the lesions
  - Encourage the patient not to scratch
  - Use meticulous hand-washing technique
- Remove crusts by gently washing with bactericidal soap and water
- Soften stubborn crusts with warm compresses
- Administer medications as ordered
- Remember to check for penicillin allergy
- Encourage verbalization of feelings about body image
- Comply with local public health standards and guidelines
- Review the importance of not sharing towels, washcloths, or bed linens with other family members

RASHES

● **Definition**
- A temporary skin eruption

● **Causes**
- Allergic reactions
- Environmental causes
- Viral, fungal, or bacterial infestations

● **Pathophysiology**
- Three types
  - Papular
    - Small, well-circumscribed, raised, solid lesions

Ways to prevent secondary infection and the spread of impetigo

- Trim fingernails short.
- Cover the child's hands if necessary.
- Cover the lesions.
- Encourage the patient not to scratch.
- Use meticulous hand-washing technique.

Causes of rashes

- Allergic reactions
- Environmental causes
- Viral, fungal, or bacterial infestations

- May erupt anywhere on the body in various configurations
- May be acute or chronic
- The result of various disorders
  - Allergic reaction or drug reaction
  - Infectious disorders
    -- Molluscum
    -- Scarlet fever
    -- Scabies
    -- Insect bites
    -- Malaria
  - Neoplastic disorders
  - Systemic disorders
- Pustular
  - Crops of raised lesions that contain lymph or pus
  - Lesions vary greatly in size and shape
  - Can be generalized or localized to the hair follicles or sweat glands
  - Disorders that produce a pustular rash in children
    - Erythema toxicum neonatorum
    - Candidiasis
    - Impetigo
    - Acne vulgaris
    - Folliculitis
- Vesicular
  - A scattered or linear distribution of vesicles (small, blisterlike lesions of raised skin that contain serous fluid)
  - May be mild or severe
  - May be temporary or permanent
  - In children, vesicular rashes are caused by
    - Staphylococcal infections
    - Hand-foot-mouth disease
    - Malaria
    - Varicella
    - Herpes simplex, herpes zoster
- The child has thinner and more sensitive skin than the adult
- Apparent birthmarks in the neonate result from the sensitivity of the infant's skin, the incomplete migration of skin cells, or clogged pores

● **Complications**
- Infection
- Scarring
- Sepsis

● **Assessment findings**
- Papular rash
  - Solid lesions with color changes in circumscribed areas

Types of rashes

- Papular — small, well-circumscribed, raised, solid lesions that can erupt anywhere on the body
- Pustular — raised lesions that contain lymph or pus
- Vesicular — scattered or linear distribution of vesicles

Assessment findings for rashes

- Papular — solid lesions with color changes in circumscribed areas
- Pustular — vesicles and bullae that fill with purulent exudates
- Vesicular — small, raised, circumscribed lesions filled with clear fluid

- Pustular rash
  - Vesicles and bullae that fill with purulent exudates
- Vesicular rash
  - Small, raised, circumscribed lesions filled with clear fluid

● **Diagnostic test findings**
- Aspirate from lesions may reveal cause
- Patch test may identify cause

● **Medical management**
- Antibacterial, antifungal, or antiviral agent (depending on cause)
- Antihistamines if the rash is from an allergy

● **Nursing interventions**
- Keep the area cool
  - Heat aggravates most skin rashes and increases pruritus
  - Coolness decreases pruritus
- Keep the affected area clean and pat it dry to promote healing
- Don't apply powder or cornstarch because these agents encourage bacterial growth
- Maintain standard precautions to prevent transmission
- Teach the parent and child
  - Sanitary techniques
  - Importance of not sharing combs or hats with others
  - Importance of avoiding scratching
  - Application of topical medications
  - Adverse effects of topical medications
- Apply cool, soothing soaks of Burow's solution (aluminum acetate)
- Give baths with added baking soda, or dab site with calamine lotion
- Administer antipruritics; give antihistamines if the rash is from an allergy
- Distract the child and provide projects that make use of the hands
- Don't use commercially prepared diaper wipes on broken skin; the chemicals and alcohol in them may be irritating

SCABIES

● **Definition**
- Transmissible skin infestation with *Sarcoptes scabiei* var. *hominis* (itch mite)
- Characterized by burrows, severe pruritus, and excoriations

● **Causes**
- Transmissible by direct (skin to skin) contact or contact with contaminated articles for up to 48 hours

---

Topics to teach the parents and child about rashes

- Sanitary techniques
- Importance of not sharing combs or hats with others
- Importance of avoiding scratching
- Application of topical medications
- Adverse effects of topical medications

Key facts about scabies

- Transmissible skin infestation with itch mite
- Characterized by burrows, severe pruritus, and excoriations
- Transmitted by direct contact
- Itching occurs after sensitization to the mite develops
- Sensitization requires several weeks after initial infestation

Pathophysiology

- Mites burrow into the skin on contact, progressing 2 to 3 mm per day
- Females live about 4 to 6 weeks and lay about 40 to 50 eggs, which hatch in 3 to 4 days
- Pruritus occurs only after sensitization to the mite develops
  - With initial infestation, sensitization requires several weeks
  - With reinfestation, sensitization develops within 24 hours
- Dead mites, eggs, larvae, and their excrement trigger an inflammatory eruption of the skin in infested areas

Complications

- Excoriations
- Secondary bacterial infection
- Abscess formation
- Septicemia

Assessment findings

- May be asymptomatic initially
- Intense pruritus that's more severe at night
- Characteristic gray-brown threadlike burrows (0.5 to 1 cm long) with tiny papule or vesicle at one end
- Common sites include flexor surfaces of wrists, elbows, axillary folds, waistline, nipples (in females), and genitalia; in infants, the burrows may appear on the head and neck
- Papules, vesicles, crusting, abscess formation, and cellulitis with secondary infection

Diagnostic test findings

- Wound culture demonstrating secondary bacterial infection
- Mineral oil burrow-scraping reveals mites, nits, or eggs, and feces or scybala
- Punch biopsy may help to confirm the diagnosis
- Resolution of infestation with therapeutic trial of a pediculicide confirms the diagnosis

Medical management

- Bathing with soap and water before treatment and after medication has been applied for the required time frame
- Scabicides or pediculicide in a thin layer over the entire skin surface; application should be repeated in 1 week to ensure thorough treatment
  - Permethrin, left on for 8 to 12 hours
  - Lindane cream, left on for 8 to 12 hours
    - Shouldn't be used if the skin is raw or inflamed
    - Applied from the neck down, covering the entire body
  - Crotamiton (Eurax), left on for 5 days
- 6% to 10% sulfur solution

TOP 3
Assessment findings in scabies

1. Intense pruritus that's more severe at night
2. Characteristic gray-brown threadlike burrows with tiny papule or vesicle at one end
3. Signs of infestation on flexor surfaces of wrists, elbows, axillary folds, waistline, nipples (in females), and genitalia; in infants, burrows may appear on the head and neck

Medications for scabies

- Permethrin
- Lindane cream
- Crotamiton
- 6% to 10% sulfur solution
- Systemic antibiotics
- Antipruritics

- Systemic antibiotics
- Antipruritics
- In infants, include the head in treatment
- Avoid the use of topical steroids, which may potentiate the infection

● **Nursing interventions**
- Prevent secondary infection and the spread of scabies
  – Trim fingernails short
  – Isolate the child until treatment is completed
  – Use meticulous hand-washing technique
  – Have blood pressure cuffs sterilized in gas autoclave before using on others
  – Decontaminate linens, towels, clothing, and personal articles
  – Disinfect the room after discharge
- Administer medications as ordered
- Notify a child's school of infestation
- Encourage verbalization of feelings
- Observe wound and skin precautions for 24 hours after treatment with a scabicide
- Anticipate treating family members and close contacts because parasite is transmitted by close personal contact and through clothes and linens

NCLEX CHECKS

It's never too soon to begin your NCLEX preparation. Now that you've reviewed this chapter, carefully read each of the following questions and choose the best answer. Then compare your responses to the correct answers.

1. During the assessment of a 2-year-old child, the nurse notes gray-brown burrows primarily on the hands and wrists. Which condition does the nurse suspect?

☐ **1.** Atopic dermatitis
☐ **2.** Poison ivy
☐ **3.** Pediculosis
☐ **4.** Scabies

2. A 3-year-old child is brought to the clinic with sores on his arms and legs. The mother says the child had numerous insect bites and scratched them. They now have honey-colored exudate. The child has no fever, and vital signs are stable. The child most likely has which disorder?

☐ **1.** Impetigo
☐ **2.** Ringworm
☐ **3.** Rubella
☐ **4.** Scabies

Ways to prevent secondary infection and the spread of scabies

- Trim fingernails short.
- Isolate the child until treatment is completed.
- Use meticulous hand-washing technique.
- Have blood pressure cuffs sterilized in gas autoclave before using on others.
- Decontaminate linens, towels, clothing, and personal articles.
- Disinfect the room after discharge.
- Anticipate treating family members and close contacts.
- Notify a child's school of infestation.

TOP 8

Items to study for your next test on the dermatologic system

1. Layers of the skin
2. Functions of the skin
3. Types of acne
4. Teaching for the patient taking isotretinoin
5. Types of burns
6. Nursing interventions for the patient with burns
7. Assessment findings in impetigo and scabies
8. Types of rashes

3. Which instruction about relieving the pruritus associated with a rash should a nurse give the parents of a 6-year-old child?
- ☐ **1.** Apply a heating pad to the area.
- ☐ **2.** Use tight clothing to prevent rubbing.
- ☐ **3.** Give the child cool baths.
- ☐ **4.** Have the child wear mittens to scratch.

4. Deep partial-thickness and full-thickness burns occur most commonly in children because:
- ☐ **1.** children take risks.
- ☐ **2.** children have thinner skin.
- ☐ **3.** children aren't aware of danger.
- ☐ **4.** children may experiment with dangerous objects.

5. A child is admitted to the hospital with major burns. What's the nurse's first priority?
- ☐ **1.** Give pain medication.
- ☐ **2.** Stop the burning process.
- ☐ **3.** Maintain an open airway.
- ☐ **4.** Start I.V. fluids to maintain hydration.

6. A skin biopsy is performed on the leg of a 16-year-old adolescent suspected of having systemic lupus erythematosus. Which action should the nurse take?
- ☐ **1.** Wear nylon stockings to hold the dressing in place.
- ☐ **2.** Wear loose, baggy cotton slacks until the lesion has healed.
- ☐ **3.** Wear tights with metallic designs to disguise the biopsy site.
- ☐ **4.** Wear wool leg warmers to increase circulation to her legs.

7. Which activity is right for an 18-year-old adolescent with acne vulgaris on her face and back who has been prescribed oral isotretinoin (Accutane) by a physician?
- ☐ **1.** Expose her face to sunlight or ultraviolet light for 3 to 6 hours per day.
- ☐ **2.** Scrub her face with benzoyl peroxide then apply oil-based lotion.
- ☐ **3.** Consult her physician before using any makeup or astringents.
- ☐ **4.** Seek hormonal contraception from her practitioner to avoid pregnancy.

8. A 6-month-old infant has a bright red, maculopapular rash in her diaper area. She cries when the nurse touches it as part of a rash evaluation. The mother should be advised to take which action?
- ☐ **1.** Expose the infant's buttocks to the air.
- ☐ **2.** Scrub any zinc oxide ointment off.
- ☐ **3.** Change the infant's diaper every 3 hours.
- ☐ **4.** Clean the diaper area with commercial diaper wipes.

9. A 3-year-old child played around his family's summer campsite. Two days later, his mother notices that the skin around his hands, arms, knees, face, and neck have many red, localized streaks, and he has been constantly scratching. What should the child's mother should do first?

☐ **1.** Wash his skin with soap and water.
☐ **2.** Launder his clothes and bed sheets.
☐ **3.** Give the child an oral antihistamine.
☐ **4.** Trim his nails and wrap his hands.

10. Eccrine sweat glands are widely distributed throughout the body. Identify the eccrine gland in this illustration.

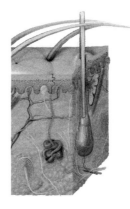

ANSWERS AND RATIONALES

1. CORRECT ANSWER: 4
Scabies results in linear, gray-brown burrows, usually seen on the hands and wrists. Atopic dermatitis is characterized by erythematous, weepy lesions that eventually become scaly and lichenified. Poison ivy appears as red, localized streaks that ultimately progress to vesicles. Pediculosis (head lice) is characterized by tiny white eggs attached to the hair shaft.

2. CORRECT ANSWER: 1
Multiple sores with a honey-colored exudate are typical of impetigo. This skin infection is common in infants and toddlers. Areas where a previous lesion, such as an insect bite, has occurred are common sites of impetigo infection. Ringworm is caused by a group of fungi that invade the stratum corneum, hair, and nails. The lesion is scalelike and round. Rubella (measles) is a virus that results in a fine, maculopapular exanthema. It first begins on the face, then rapidly spreads downward toward the neck, arms, trunk, and legs. Scabies exhibits a minute whitish-gray brown, threadlike lesion and is caused by the scabies mite that burrows under the skin.

3. CORRECT ANSWER: 3

Cooling the affected areas with cool baths or compresses can prevent itching by decreasing irritation. Heat to the area will aggravate the itching and make it worse. Tight clothing will rub and cause irritation. Soft, loose clothing should be worn. The child should wear mittens to prevent scratching if she's uncooperative; she shouldn't wear them to scratch.

4. CORRECT ANSWER: 2

Children have thinner skin than adults, which means burns can penetrate the second and third layers faster. Although children may take risks, experiment with dangerous objects, and be unaware of danger, these factors don't account for the depth of burn injuries.

5. CORRECT ANSWER: 2

When a child has been burned, the nurse's first priority is to stop the burning process and then establish and maintain an open airway. Pain medication and I.V. fluids are important but these should be given after the burning has been stopped and the airway has been opened.

6. CORRECT ANSWER: 2

The skin surrounding a skin biopsy will be sensitive and, for a time, possibly itchy due to the healing process. Healing is best promoted by allowing air to circulate around the wound and by minimizing any scratching, local irritation, or localized heat. Wearing nylon stockings, tights with metallic designs, or wool leg warmers are likely to increase heat and cause irritation.

7. CORRECT ANSWER: 4

Accutane may cause teratogenic effects on a fetus so any female taking the drug should be especially vigilant to not become pregnant. Hormonal contraception is an effective birth-control method. Exposure to sunlight or ultraviolet rays should be minimized when taking Accutane to avoid a photosensitivity reaction. Scrubbing acne-inflamed skin causes infected sebum to rise to the skin surface and inflame surrounding debrided skin. Many sunscreens, astringents, and cosmetics contain substances that provoke acne.

8. CORRECT ANSWER: 1

The infant's skin needs to be cleaned with a gentle soap, patted dry, and then left open to the air. Zinc oxide is used to form a barrier between urine or feces and the healing skin. Scrubbing it off would further irritate the newly healing skin and remove the protective barrier. Diapers should be changed as soon as the infant voids or has a bowel movement. Commercial diaper wipes commonly contain chemicals and alcohol, which could further damage the skin.

9. CORRECT ANSWER: 1

Washing poison ivy oils from the skin with soap and water as soon as possible prevents absorption through the skin and subsequent spreading of the oils to other areas. Laundering clothes, providing antihistamines, and trimming nails are important measures but all can be done after the soapy wash.

10. CORRECT ANSWER:

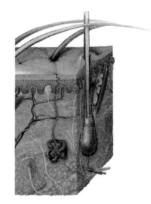

The eccrine gland is located between the dermis and the subcutaneous tissue.

15

Cancer

---

1. What are the usual sites of metastasis for Ewing's sarcoma?

☐ 1. Brain and lungs

☐ 2. Liver and bone

☐ 3. Lungs and bone

☐ 4. Liver and lungs

CORRECT ANSWER: 3

2. Which stage of Hodgkin's lymphoma involves two or more lymph nodes on the same side of the diaphragm and in the extra-lymphatic region?

☐ 1. I

☐ 2. II

☐ 3. III

☐ 4. IV

CORRECT ANSWER: 2

3. In a child with acute lymphocytic leukemia, which white blood cell count at the time of diagnosis has the best prognosis?

☐ 1. Less than 10,000/μl
☐ 2. Less than 20,000/μl
☐ 3. More than 20,000/μl
☐ 4. More than 40,000/μl

CORRECT ANSWER: 1

4. What's the most common extracranial solid tumor diagnosed in children?

☐ 1. Ependymoma
☐ 2. Medulloblastoma
☐ 3. Astrocytoma
☐ 4. Neuroblastoma

CORRECT ANSWER: 4

5. In what stage of Wilms' tumor has the tumor metastasized to the lung, liver, bone, and brain?

☐ 1. II
☐ 2. III
☐ 3. IV
☐ 4. V

CORRECT ANSWER: 3

LEARNING OBJECTIVES

After studying this chapter, you should be able to:

● Assess and plan care for the major types of pediatric cancer.

● Describe the staging protocols for the various solid tumors.

● Anticipate the psychosocial needs of the child with cancer and the needs of the child's family.

● Assess the child's perception of death at various stages of development, and plan appropriate interventions when death is imminent.

CHAPTER OVERVIEW

Various coping strategies are used by the child with a chronic life-threatening disease. Most of these chronic problems are associated with cancer. Regardless of the problem, supportive, informative nursing care is crucial before, during, and after diagnosis. In addition, the nurse must consider the child's stage of development, especially when dealing with the possibility of death.

KEY CONCEPTS

● Definition
- An alteration in cell function resulting from the overproduction of immature and nonfunctional cells; tissues enlarge for no physiologic function
- Can be life-threatening
- Can invade and destroy healthy tissues
- Pediatric cancers
  - Second to accidents as the leading cause of death in children between ages 1 and 14
  - Occur primarily in rapidly differentiating tissues such as bone marrow
  - Most solid tumors are sarcomas
  - In order of frequency: leukemia, neurologic tumors, neuroblastomas, lymphomas, Wilms' tumors, bone tumors
  - Any tumor in a child is considered malignant until histologically identified, even if it's encapsulated
  - Childhood cancers grow faster because body tissues are normally in a state of rapid growth and high metabolic rate
  - The incidence of cancer increases with age

● Causes
- Unknown
- Mutations within the genes of cells
- Specific agents that cause mutations
  - Ionizing radiation
  - Asbestos
  - Electromagnetic fields
  - Vinyl chloride
  - Tobacco
- Some forms of cancer result from genetic predisposition
- Children who are immunosuppressed, such as those infected with human immunodeficiency virus (HIV) and those with acquired immunodeficiency syndrome (AIDs) or Wiskott-Aldrich syndrome, children on immunosuppressive therapy, and children with chromosomal abnormalities, such as those with Down syndrome, are more prone to developing certain types of cancer

TOP 6

Types of pediatric cancers

1. Leukemia
2. Neurologic tumors
3. Neuroblastomas
4. Lymphomas
5. Wilms' tumors
6. Bone tumors

Specific agents that cause cell mutations

- Ionizing radiation
- Asbestos
- Electromagnetic fields
- Vinyl chloride
- Tobacco

Children prone to certain types of cancer

- Children who are immunosuppressed
  - Those with HIV infection or AIDS
  - Those with Wiskott-Aldrich syndrome
  - Those on immunosuppressive therapy
- Children with chromosomal abnormalities

GO WITH THE FLOW

How cancer metastasizes

Cancer usually spreads through the bloodstream to other organs and tissues, as shown here.

Cancer cells secrete enzymes and motility factors.

↓

Basement membrane in blood vessels is disrupted.

↓

Cancer cells escape into circulation.

↓

Undetected cells move out of blood.

↓

Enzymes are secreted.

↓

Cell wall is cut.

↓

New tissue is invaded downstream.

↓

Chemical attraction occurs.

↓

Malignant cells target specific site.

↓

New site is invaded.

↓

Cells multiply.

↓

Metastatic tumor appears.

Pathophysiology

- Rapid, uncontrollable proliferation of cells
- Independent spread from a primary site (site of origin) to other tissues where it establishes secondary foci (metastasis)
- Cancer cells metastasize via circulation through the blood or lymphatics, by unintentional transplantation from one site to another during surgery, and by local extension (see *How cancer metastasizes*)
- A particular concern with pediatric cancer is the increased risk of development of secondary cancer after successful treatment of the primary cancer

Complications

- May arise from therapy as well as the disease
- Anemia
- Leukopenia
- Thrombocytopenia
- Nausea and vomiting
- Alopecia
- Fluid and electrolyte imbalances
- Death

Assessment findings

- Signs and symptoms vary with the type and location of cancer
- Pain, including headache and bone pain
- Abnormal skin lesions, such as petechiae or bruising
- Fatigue
- Fever
- Weight loss
- Eye or vision changes

Diagnostic test findings

- Biopsy (the removal of a portion of the suspicious tissue) for direct histologic study of tumor tissue
    - The only definitive method to diagnose cancer
    - Can also provide information about the stage and grade of the cancer
        - The TNM staging system (tumor size, nodal involvement, and metastatic progress) allows comparison of treatments and survival rates among large population groups
        - Grading compares tumor tissue to normal cells and estimates the tumor's growth rate
- Imaging studies, such as X-rays, computed tomography (CT) scanning, ultrasonography, and magnetic resonance imaging (MRI), are useful in detecting tumors
- Bone scans can detect bony lesions, but aren't definitive because they don't distinguish between inflammation and malignancy

Complications of cancer in children

- Anemia
- Leukopenia
- Thrombocytopenia
- Nausea and vomiting
- Alopecia
- Fluid and electrolyte imbalances
- Death

TNM staging system

- Categorizes tumor size, nodal involvement, and metastatic progress
- Allows comparison of treatments and survival rates among large population groups

Tumor grading

- Compares tumor tissue to normal cells
- Estimates the tumor's growth rate

Quick guide to chemotherapeutic agents

- **Alkylating agents** – inhibit cell growth and division by reacting with DNA
- **Antimetabolites** – prevent cell growth by competing with metabolites in the production of nucleic acid
- **Antitumor antibiotics** – block cell growth by binding with DNA and interfering with DNA-dependent RNA synthesis
- **Plant alkaloids** – prevent cellular reproduction by disrupting cell mitosis
- **Steroid hormones** – inhibit the growth of hormone-susceptible tumors by changing their chemical environment

● **Medical management**
- Goal of treatment is to achieve remission; a 5-year remission is considered a cure
- Surgery
  - Typically combined with other therapies
  - May be performed for various reasons
    - Biopsy to obtain tissue for histologic study
    - Debulking of the tumor
    - Relieve pain and alleviate pressure
    - Correct obstruction
- Radiation therapy
  - Normal cells recover from radiation faster than malignant cells
  - Approaches
    - External beam radiation
    - Interstitial implants
- Chemotherapy
  - Induces regression of the tumor and its metastasis
  - Particularly useful in controlling residual disease and relieving pain
  - Alkylating agents — inhibit cell growth and division by reacting with deoxyribonucleic acid (DNA)
  - Antimetabolites — prevent cell growth by competing with metabolites in the production of nucleic acid
  - Antitumor antibiotics — block cell growth by binding with DNA and interfering with DNA-dependent ribonucleic acid (RNA) synthesis
  - Plant alkaloids — prevent cellular reproduction by disrupting cell mitosis
  - Steroid hormones — inhibit the growth of hormone-susceptible tumors by changing their chemical environment
- Biotherapy
  - Interferons have antiviral and antiproliferative effects
  - Interleukins exert their effects on the T-lymphocytes
  - Monoclonal antibodies selectively bind to tumor cell surfaces
  - Hematopoietic growth factors increase the patient's blood counts when chemotherapy or radiation causes a decrease
- Bone marrow transplant
  - For children for whom other treatments haven't been or are unlikely to be successful
  - Complications may include graft-versus-host disease, veno-occlusive disease, complications from immunosuppressant medications

● **Nursing interventions**
- Anticipate the need for pain relief, and provide it on a schedule that doesn't allow pain to break through

TIME-OUT FOR TEACHING

Teaching about chemotherapy

Be sure to include these points in your teaching plan for the parents of a child receiving chemotherapy:
- signs and symptoms of fluid and electrolyte imbalances
- signs and symptoms of possible adverse effects, such as nausea, vomiting, and infection
- oral hygiene measures
- nutritional status measures, including possible nutritional supplements or parenteral nutrition
- relaxation techniques, diversional activities, play therapy
- methods and measures to deal with possible adverse reactions
- compliance with follow-up diagnostic tests and physician visits
- signs and symptoms to report to the physician.

- Assist with I.V. and intrathecal chemotherapy
    - Be aware that chemotherapy may include such drugs as cyclophosphamide (Cytoxan), methotrexate, vincristine (Oncovin), prednisone (Deltasone), and asparaginase (Elspar)
    - Monitor for and help the child deal with chemotherapeutic adverse effects (see *Teaching about chemotherapy*)
        - Alopecia
        - Nausea and vomiting
        - Infection
        - Anemia
        - Stomatitis
        - Bleeding
    - Provide care for the venous access device as necessary
    - Take special protective precautions when administering or disposing of chemotherapeutic drugs because they're easily absorbed through the skin and mucous membranes
- Assist with radiation and help the child deal with its adverse effects
    - Vomiting
    - Dry mouth and sore throat
    - Diarrhea
    - Desquamation (scaling) of the skin
    - May be site specific (dependent upon the site being irradiated)
- Prepare for possible surgery, performed for biopsy, tumor removal, determination of the disease's severity, and palliation
- Anticipate aftereffects years after treatments and counsel parents accordingly
    - Genetic changes
    - Learning disabilities
    - Secondary cancers

Adverse effects of chemotherapy

- Alopecia
- Nausea and vomiting
- Infection
- Anemia
- Stomatitis
- Bleeding

Adverse effects of radiation therapy

- Vomiting
- Dry mouth and sore throat
- Diarrhea
- Scaling of the skin

Long-term effects of cancer therapy

- Genetic changes
- Learning disabilities
- Secondary cancers
- Altered function of specific organ systems

Key facts about Ewing's sarcoma

- Nonosseous tumor
- Arises from cells within the bone marrow
- Usually occurs in the diaphysis of long bones in males ages 10 to 20
- Highly malignant to the lungs and bones

TOP 2

Findings in Ewing's sarcoma

1. Pain and swelling at the site that become increasingly severe and persistent
2. "Moth-eaten" or "onionskin" appearance of bones on X-ray

– Altered function of specific organ systems
- Ensure adequate hydration and nutrition
- Use coping strategies, such as play therapy, relaxation techniques, and imagery, to deal with the pain and disability

EWING'S SARCOMA

Definition
- Nonosseous tumor arising from cells within the bone marrow
- Usually affects lower extremities
- Occurs between ages 4 and 25, usually in males ages 10 to 20
- Highly malignant to lungs and bones with a poor prognosis

Causes
- Unknown

Pathophysiology
- Malignant cells originate in the bone marrow and invade the shafts of the long and flat bones
- Occurs most commonly in the diaphysis (midshaft) of long bones
- Metastasis usually occurs to the lungs and bones

Complications
- Metastasis to other organs
- Death

Assessment findings
- Pain and swelling at the site becoming increasingly severe and persistent
- Pain may become so severe that the child can't sleep at night
- Fever

Diagnostic test findings
- Biopsy (by incision or by aspiration) confirms the diagnosis
- Bone X-rays have a "moth-eaten" or "onionskin" appearance
- Blood tests show mild anemia, leukocytosis, and an elevated sedimentation rate
- MRI provides accurate information on tumor size and delinates the extent of the neuroblastoma

Medical management
- Radiation
- Chemotherapy to slow growth using dactinomycin (Actinomycin D), doxorubicin (Adriamycin), cyclophosphamide, ifosfamide (Ifex), vincristine, and etoposide (VP-16)
- Amputation only if there's no evidence of metastasis or the tumor appears unresectable

Nursing interventions
- Assist with radiation and chemotherapy

- Note that amputation isn't routine because the tumor spreads easily through the bone marrow

HODGKIN'S LYMPHOMA

● Definition
- A malignant neoplasm of the lymphoid tissue
- Commonly seen in adolescents and young adults
- Prognosis is excellent

● Causes
- Although the cause is unknown, a viral etiology is suspected, with the Epstein-Barr virus as a leading candidate
- Environmental and immunologic factors may also contribute

● Pathophysiology
- Usually originates in a localized group of lymph nodes
- Proliferates by way of lymphocytes to other sites including the bone marrow, liver, lungs, mediastinum, and spleen

● Complications
- Recurrence of the disease after a period of remission
- A second malignancy located in another part of the body, such as the bone, breast, or blood
- Hypothyroidism from irradiation of the neck area during the treatment phase
- Sterility
- Death

● Assessment findings
- Painless, firm, persistently enlarged lymph nodes
  - Appear insidiously
  - Most common in the lower cervical region
- Night sweats and pruritus
- Recurrent fever
- Weight loss
- Fatigue

● Diagnostic test findings
- Lymph node and bone marrow biopsies confirm diagnosis by revealing Reed-Sternberg cells (enlarged, abnormal histiocytes)
- Detection of lymph node or organ involvement
  - Chest X-ray
  - CT of abdomen, chest, and pelvis
  - Ultrasound
  - Lymphangiogram
    - Dye is injected I.V. into the feet

Staging Hodgkin's lymphoma

Treatment of Hodgkin's lymphoma depends on the stage it has reached — that is, the number, location, and degree of involved lymph nodes.

STAGE I
Hodgkin's lymphoma appears in a single lymph node region or a single extralymphatic organ.

STAGE II
The disease appears in two or more nodes on the same side of the diaphragm and in an extralymphatic organ.

STAGE III
Hodgkin's lymphoma spreads to lymph node regions on both sides of the diaphragm and perhaps to an extralymphatic organ, the spleen, or both.

STAGE IV
The disease disseminates, involving one or more extralymphatic organs or tissues, with or without associated lymph node involvement.

- X-rays track the dye as it travels up the body and is absorbed by the lymphatic system (cancerous nodes have a different appearance from normal lymph nodes)
- Blood tests
  - Show mild to severe normocytic anemia
  - Elevated serum alkaline phosphatase indicates liver or bone involvement
- Positron emission tomography scan helps find malignant tumor cells

● Medical management

- Depends on the number, location, and degree of involved lymph nodes (see *Staging Hodgkin's lymphoma*)
- Radiation therapy, chemotherapy, or a combination may be used for stages I and II
- Chemotherapy is used for stages III and IV, sometimes inducing a complete remission
  - MOPP protocol — mechlorethamine (Mustargen), vincristine (Oncovin), procarbazine (Matulane), and prednisone
  - ABVD protocol — doxorubicin (Adriamycin), bleomycin (Blenoxane), vinblastine (Vira-A), and dacarbazine (DTIC)
  - High-dose chemotherapy with autologous bone marrow transplant or autologous peripheral blood stem cell transfusions for a patient who's unresponsive to radiation therapy or chemotherapy

● Nursing interventions

- Assess for adverse effects of radiation and chemotherapy including anorexia, nausea, vomiting, diarrhea, fever, and bleeding
- Control pain and bleeding of stomatitis by using a soft toothbrush, applying petroleum jelly to the lips, and avoiding astringent mouthwashes

How to control pain and bleeding of stomatitis

- Use a soft toothbrush.
- Apply petroleum jelly to the lips.
- Avoid astringent mouthwashes.

• Offer appropriate emotional support including information on the local chapter of the American Cancer Society

LEUKEMIA

● **Definition**
- Leukemia is the abnormal, uncontrolled proliferation of white blood cells (WBCs)
- Acute lymphocytic leukemia (ALL) is the most common type of leukemia and cancer in children
  - Peak age is 2 to 5 years
  - 90% to 95% of children with ALL achieve a first remission
  - Almost 80% live 5 years
  - The child between ages 3 and 7 with ALL and an initial WBC count of less than 10,000/µl at the time of diagnosis has the best prognosis
- Acute myeloblastic (myelogenous) leukemia (AML) is more common than ALL in adolescents
  - 50% to 70% of adolescents with AML achieve a first remission
  - 40% live 5 years

● **Causes**
- The exact cause of most leukemias remains unknown
- Increasing evidence suggests a combination of contributing factors
- Predisposing factors
  - Familial tendency
  - Monozygotic twin with leukemia
  - Congenital disorders, such as Down syndrome, Bloom syndrome, and ataxia-telangiectasia
  - Viruses
  - Ionizing radiation
  - Exposure to the chemical benzene and cytotoxins such as alkylating agents

● **Pathophysiology**
- WBCs are produced so rapidly that immature cells (blast cells) are released into the circulation
- Blast cells are nonfunctional, can't fight infection, and multiply continuously without respect to the body's needs
- Blast cells appear in the peripheral blood, where they normally don't appear
- Blast cells may be as high as 95% in the bone marrow (they're normally less than 5%) as measured by marrow aspiration in the posterior iliac crest (the sternum can't be used in children)
- The increased proliferation of WBCs robs healthy cells of nutrition
- Bone marrow first undergoes hypertrophy, possibly resulting in patho-

logic fractures
- Bone marrow then undergoes atrophy, resulting in a decrease in all blood cells, which leads to anemia, bleeding disorders, and immuno-suppression

Complications
- Organ malfunction, especially the spleen and liver
- Anemia
- Infection
- Bleeding (petechiae)
- Death

Assessment findings
- High fever
- Thrombocytopenia
- Abdominal or bone pain
- Pallor, chills, and recurrent infections
- Petechiae and ecchymosis
- Abnormal bleeding, such as nosebleeds, poor wound healing, and oral lesions
- Confusion, lethargy, and headache if the blood-brain barrier has been crossed
- Fatigue
- Painless lumps in neck, underarm, stomach, and groin

Diagnostic test findings
- Bone marrow aspirate showing a proliferation of immature WBCs (greater than 25% blasts)
- Bone marrow biopsy of the posterior superior iliac spine can help confirm diagnosis
- Blood counts show thrombocytopenia, neutropenia, and anemia
- Differential leukocyte count determines cell type
- Lumber puncture detects meningeal involvement (if central nervous system [CNS] is involved)
- Cytogenetic analysis shows a "Philadelphia chromosome" in ALL

Medical management
- Systemic chemotherapy aims to eradicate leukemic cells and induce remission
    - ALL — combination therapy that may include vincristine, prednisone, high-dose cytarabine (Cytosar-U), asparaginase (Elspar), amsacrine (AMSA), and daunorubicin (Cerubidine)
    - AML — combination of I.V. daunorubicin and cytarabine; combination of cyclophosphamide, vincristine, prednisone, or methotrexate; high-dose cytarabine alone or with other drugs; amsacrine; etoposide; and azacitidine (5-azacytidine) and mitoxantrone (Novantrone)

Medical management of leukemia

- Systemic chemotherapy to eradicate leukemic cells and induce remission
- Intrathecal chemotherapy to prevent or treat CNS infiltration by leukemic cells
- Anti-infectives and granulocyte injections to control infection
- Transfusions of platelets to prevent bleeding
- Transfusion of RBCs to prevent anemia
- Possible bone marrow transplant

- Intrathecal chemotherapy to prevent or treat CNS infiltration by leukemic cells
- Antibiotic, antifungal, and antiviral drugs and granulocyte injections to control infection
- Transfusions of platelets to prevent bleeding and of red blood cells to prevent anemia
- Possible bone marrow transplant (especially in children with the Philadelphia chromosome)

● **Nursing interventions**
  - Prevent infection by placing the patient in a private room, giving special attention to mouth care, and screening staff and visitors for contagious diseases
  - Inspect the skin frequently; avoid taking a rectal temperature or administering rectal medications
  - Use interventions for anemia and thrombocytopenia
  - Give increased fluids to flush chemotherapy through the kidneys
  - Provide a high-protein, high-calorie, bland diet
  - Provide pain relief
  - Monitor the CNS for involvement (confusion, lethargy, and headache)
  - Gear nursing measures toward easing the adverse effects of radiation and chemotherapy
  - Help the child and the family verbalize their fears and guilt; allow the family to participate in the child's care, as appropriate
  - Help the child adjust to changes in body image
  - Refer parents and adolescents with cancer to support groups

MALIGNANT BRAIN TUMORS

● **Definition**
  - Growths within the intracranial space
  - Tumors of the brain tissue, meninges, pituitary gland, and blood vessels
  - Second most prevalent type of cancer in children
  - Most common tumor types in children
    – Astrocytomas
    – Medulloblastomas
    – Ependymomas
    – Brain stem gliomas (see *Common brain tumors in children,* page 412)
  - Most occur in children before age 1 or between ages 2 and 12
  - The most common cause of cancer death in children

● **Causes**
  - Unknown
  - Risk factors include preexisting cancer, radiation exposure, and exposure to industrial or chemical toxins

Most common types of malignant brain tumors in children

- Astrocytomas
- Medulloblastomas
- Ependymomas
- Brain stem gliomas

Secondary effects of malignant brain tumors

- Compression of the brain, cranial nerves, and cerebral vessels
- Cerebral edema
- Increased ICP

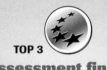

TOP 3

Assessment findings in malignant brain tumors

1. Headache
2. Vomiting
3. Behavioral changes

Common brain tumors in children

This illustration shows the locations of common brain tumors in children.

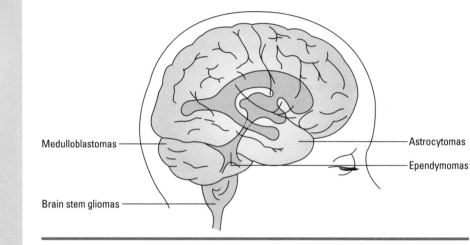

Pathophysiology
- Classified based on histology or grade of cell malignancy
- Brain tumor effects
  - CNS changes—tumor invades and destroys tissues and causes secondary effects
    - Compression of the brain, cranial nerves, and cerebral vessels
    - Cerebral edema
    - Increased intracranial pressure (ICP)
    - Increased head circumference while anterior fontanel closes

Complications
- Coma
- Respiratory or cardiac arrest
- Brain herniation

Assessment findings
- Difficult to diagnose in an infant or a young child because of the elasticity of the skull and normally poor coordination; be alert for signs and symptoms and investigate parental observations that may indicate a brain lesion or increased ICP
- Headache (most common symptom)
  - Intermittent
  - Most common after the child wakes up
- Vomiting
  - Unrelated to food or fluid consumption
  - Typically occurs as the child wakes up

– Because the vomiting is unrelated to nausea, the child can usually eat immediately after vomiting
- Behavioral changes
- Signs and symptoms of increased ICP
    – Vision disturbances
    – Weakness or paralysis
    – Aphasia or dysphagia
    – Ataxia and incoordination
    – Seizures
- Loss of previously attained developmental skills
- Decline in school performance

● **Diagnostic test findings**
- Tissue biopsy via stereotactic surgery provides a definitive diagnosis
- Skull X-rays, brain scan, CT scan, MRI, and cerebral angiography confirm presence of a tumor
- Lumbar puncture shows increased protein levels, decreased glucose levels and, occasionally, tumor cells in cerebrospinal fluid (CSF); not done if the child has increased ICP

● **Medical management**
- Prognosis varies based on the type and location of the tumor
- Treatments vary with the tumor's histologic type, radiosensitivity, and location
- Reducing the size of a nonresectable tumor with surgery, radiation therapy, or chemotherapy
- Decreasing ICP
    – Diuretics
    – Corticosteroids
    – Ventriculoatrial or ventriculoperitoneal shunting of CSF
- Anticonvulsants to control seizures
- Surgery
    – For astrocytoma
        · Repeated surgeries
        · Radiation therapy
        · Shunting of fluid from obstructed CSF pathways
    – For medulloblastoma
        · Surgical resection
        · Possibly, intrathecal infusion of methotrexate or another antineoplastic drug
    – For ependymoma
        · Surgical resection
        · Radiation therapy
    – For glioma
        · Resection by craniotomy
        · Radiation therapy and chemotherapy following resection

Signs and symptoms of increased ICP
- Vision disturbances
- Weakness or paralysis
- Aphasia or dysphagia
- Ataxia and incoordination
- Seizures

Ways to reduce ICP
- Diuretics
- Corticosteroids
- Ventriculoatrial or ventriculoperitoneal shunting of CSF

● **Nursing interventions**
- Monitor the child's neurologic status, vital signs, and wound site
- Prepare the child and parents for surgery
  - Preoperative head shaving
  - Orientation to the intensive care unit
  - Child's appearance after surgery
    - Large, bulky head dressing
    - Drowsy or unconscious
    - Facial edema
- Provide postoperative care
  - Monitor neurologic status, vital signs, and wound site, as well as for postoperative complications (infection, bleeding, seizures)
  - Monitor for signs of increased ICP, indicating cerebral edema
  - Elevate the head to promote venous drainage and prevent edema, and position the child on the nonoperative side to minimize pressure on the operative site
  - Relieve eye edema with cold compresses; lubricate the eyes
  - Prevent increased ICP by telling the child to avoid coughing forcefully and straining during bowel movements
  - Administer medications as ordered, including analgesics for headaches
  - Teach the child and his family signs of recurrence; urge compliance with the treatment regimen

NEUROBLASTOMA

● **Definition**
- Most common extracranial solid tumor diagnosed in the infant years
- Tumors usually arise from the adrenal gland but can also arise at multiple other sites usually within the abdomen
- The cancer usually metastasizes before it's diagnosed
  - Highly malignant
  - Poor prognosis (less than 50% chance of survival) for the child older than age 1; prognosis approaches 75% survival for children diagnosed younger than age 1
- If a tumor is in the abdomen, manifestations resemble Wilms' tumor

● **Causes**
- Unknown

● **Pathophysiology**
- Tumors start from embryonic cells in the neural crest that give rise to the adrenal medulla and the sympathetic nervous system
- Tumors occur most commonly in the abdomen near the adrenal gland or spinal ganglia

- Most common sites of metastasis include the bone marrow, liver, and subcutaneous tissue
- Stages
  - In stage I, the tumor is confined to the organ or structure of origin and is completely removable by surgery
  - In stage II, continuity extends beyond the primary site but not across the midline; tumor can't be completely removed by surgery
  - In stage III, the tumor extends beyond the midline, with bilateral regional lymph node involvement
  - In stage IV, the tumor metastasizes

● **Complications**
- Neurologic impairment
- Obstruction of the airway
- Spinal paralysis

● **Assessment findings**
- Be aware that the symptoms vary and typically result from compression of the tumor on adjacent structures
- Firm abdominal mass crossing the midline
- Urinary frequency or urine retention
- Bone pain
- Weakness and lethargy
- Anorexia and weight loss

● **Diagnostic test findings**
- Ultrasound and CT scan allow for a definite diagnosis
- 24-hour urine collection to measure catecholamines, preceded by a vanillylmandelic acid diet for 3 days (eliminate bananas, nuts, chocolate, vanilla)
- MRI allows for the evaluation of the extent of the neuroblastoma

● **Medical management**
- Complete surgical removal for stages I and II
- Radiation for stage III may not improve survival rate but may alleviate pain from metastasis
- Chemotherapy for treatment of extensive disease, including vincristine, doxorubicin, cyclophosphamide, and cisplatin (Platinol)
- Bone marrow stem cell transplantation, when the marrow is completely destroyed by chemotherapy

● **Nursing interventions**
- Explain treatment options to the patient and his family including possible adverse effects from radiation and chemotherapy
- Prepare the patient and his family for operative procedures
- Offer emotional support to the family because of the high degree of mortality associated with the disease

Quick guide to staging neuroblastoma

- **Stage I** – Tumor confined to organ or structure of origin; completely removable by surgery
- **Stage II** – Continuity extends beyond primary site but not across midline; can't be completely removed by surgery
- **Stage III** – Tumor extends beyond midline, with bilateral regional lymph node involvement
- **Stage IV** – Tumor metastasizes

Medical management of neuroblastoma

- Complete surgical removal for stages I and II
- Radiation for stage III
- Chemotherapy for treatment of extensive disease, including vincristine, doxorubicin, cyclophosphamide, and cisplatin
- Bone marrow stem cell transplantation

Key facts about non-Hodgkin's lymphoma

- Includes lymphosarcoma, reticulum cell sarcoma, and Burkitt's lymphoma
- Also known as *malignant lymphoma*
- Survival rate in aggressively treated localized disease approaches 90%
- Survival rate in advanced disease is greater than 60%
- Cause is unknown

What happens in non-Hodgkin's lymphoma

- Primary tumor arises in lymphoid tissue
- Spreads beyond nodes into neighboring tissues
- Metastasizes faster than Hodgkin's lymphoma

Signs and symptoms of non-Hodgkin's lymphoma

- Symptoms depend on the organ involved
- Enlarged lymph nodes, most commonly in the lower cervical lymph node region, including tonsils and adenoids
- Dyspnea and coughing
- Night sweats, fatigue, malaise, weight loss, fever

NON-HODGKIN'S LYMPHOMA

● **Definition**
- Includes lymphosarcoma, reticulum cell sarcoma, and Burkitt's lymphoma
- Also known as *malignant lymphoma*
- Prognosis for aggressively treated localized disease approaches 90% survival; for those with advanced disease, survival is greater than 60%

● **Causes**
- Cause is unknown although some theories suggest a viral source for some cases

● **Pathophysiology**
- The primary tumor arises in any lymphoid tissue
- The lymphoma spreads beyond nodes into neighboring tissue
- Metastasizes faster than Hodgkin's lymphoma

● **Complications**
- Metastasis to other organs including the bone marrow or CNS
- Obstruction of the airway or GI tract
- Cranial nerve palsies
- Spinal paralysis
- Death

● **Assessment findings**
- The symptoms depend on the organ involved
- Enlarged lymph nodes, most commonly in the lower cervical lymph node region, including tonsils and adenoids
- Dyspnea and coughing
- Night sweats, fatigue, malaise, weight loss, and fever

● **Diagnostic test findings**
- Biopsy of lymph nodes confirms diagnosis
- Detection of organ involvement is made with bone and chest X-rays, lymphangiography, liver and spleen scan, abdominal CT scan, and excretory urography
- Blood tests show anemia, increased uric acid, and an elevated calcium level if bone lesions are present

● **Medical management**
- Radiation therapy is used mainly in the early localized stage of the disease
- Chemotherapy is most effective with multiple combinations of drugs
  - CHOP—cyclophosphamide, doxorubicin (also known as *hydroxydaunorubicin*), vincristine (Oncovin), and prednisone
  - M-BACOP—methotrexate, bleomycin, doxorubicin (Adriamycin), cyclophosphamide, vincristine (Oncovin), and prednisone

Nursing interventions
- Assess for adverse effects of radiation and chemotherapy including anorexia, nausea, vomiting, diarrhea, fever, and bleeding
- Instruct the patient to keep irradiated skin dry

OSTEOGENIC SARCOMA

Definition
- The most common bone cancer in children
- Peak age is late adolescence; rare in young children
- Usually involves the diaphyseal long bones; about 50% of cases are in the femur but may also occur in tibia, humerus, fibula, ileum, vertebra, or mandible
- Highly malignant; metastasizes quickly to the lungs
- Survival rate is about 60%; increases to 85% if nonmetastasized

Causes
- Unknown
- Theories point to heredity, trauma, and excessive radiotherapy

Pathophysiology
- Tumor arises from bone-forming osteoblast and bone-digesting osteoclast

Complications
- Metastasis to other organs, especially the lungs

Assessment findings
- Impaired mobility
- Pain and swelling at the site
  - Pain more intense at night and isn't usually associated with mobility
- Absence of infection or trauma at the site preceding the pain
- Pathologic fractures, which may result from bone marrow involvement

Diagnostic test findings
- A biopsy (by incision or by aspiration) confirms the diagnosis
- Body CT scan determines the extent of the lesion
- Sunburst appearance noted on X-ray because new bone formations grow at right angles to one another
- Elevated alkaline phosphatase level
- Lung tomography reveals any lung metastasis

Medical management
- Amputation at the joint proximal to the tumor; some institutions remove only the bone and salvage the limb
- Chemotherapy agents either alone or in combination with one another
  - Dactinomycin, doxorubicin, bleomycin, cyclophosphamide, and high-dose methotrexate
  - May be infused intra-arterially into the long bones of the legs

- A thoracotomy is performed followed by chemotherapy if lung metastasis is present

● **Nursing interventions**
- Reinforce the fact that the child didn't cause the tumor
- Provide psychological support and reinforcement of the child's strengths
- Provide support through phantom limb pain
- Provide stump care and help the child prepare for a prosthesis
- Assist with chemotherapy

WILMS' TUMOR

● **Definition**
- Malignant mixed tumor of the kidney
- Also called *nephroblastoma*
- The most common intra-abdominal tumor in children; the average age at diagnosis is 2 to 4 years
- The tumor favors the left kidney and is usually unilateral
- The tumor remains encapsulated for a long time
- The prognosis is excellent if metastasis hasn't occurred

● **Causes**
- Genetic inheritance
- Associated with several other congenital anomalies including hypospadias, cryptorchidism, Beckwith-Wiederman syndrome, and Denys-Drash syndrome

● **Pathophysiology**
- Wilms' tumor is an embryonal cancer of the kidney originating during fetal life
- In early stages the tumor is well encapsulated, but it may later spread into the lymph nodes, renal vein, or vena cava; metastasis may occur to the lungs or other sites
- Staging
  - In stage I, the tumor is limited to one kidney
  - In stage II, the tumor extends beyond the kidney but can be completely excised
  - In stage III, the tumor spreads but is confined to the abdomen and lymph nodes
  - In stage IV, the tumor metastasizes to the lung, liver, bone, and brain
  - In stage V, the tumor involves both kidneys

● **Complications**
- Metastasis to other organs
- Symptoms of metastasis including shortness of breath, coughing, chest pain, and weight loss

---

Key facts about Wilms' tumor

- Malignant mixed tumor of the kidney that originates during fetal life
- Also called *nephroblastoma*
- Remains well encapsulated for a long time
- Most common intra-abdominal tumor in children
- Average age at diagnosis is 2 to 4 years
- Genetic inheritance
- Prognosis excellent if metastasis hasn't occurred

Quick guide to staging Wilms' tumor

- **Stage I** – tumor limited to one kidney
- **Stage II** – tumor extends beyond kidney but can be completely excised
- **Stage III** – tumor spreads but is confined to abdomen and lymph nodes
- **Stage IV** – tumor metastasizes to lung, liver, bone, and brain
- **Stage V** – tumor involves both kidneys

● **Assessment findings**
- Nontender abdominal mass (most common), usually midline near the liver; commonly identified by the parent while bathing or dressing the child
- Enlarged abdomen
- High blood pressure
- Vomiting
- Hematuria
- Anemia
- Constipation

● **Diagnostic test findings**
- Abdominal ultrasound and CT scan to view tumor size, location, and possible metastasis
- Excretory urography assesses kidney function of the normal-functioning kidney
- Blood tests reveal polycythemia if tumor secretes erythropoietin

● **Medical management**
- Nephrectomy—surgery to remove the tumor and affected kidney in stage I and II
- Radiation is indicated with large tumors or those that weren't completely surgically resected
- Chemotherapy with dactinomycin and vincristine

● **Nursing interventions**
- Preoperative
  – Don't palpate the abdomen, and prevent others from doing so; it may disseminate cancer cells to other sites
  – Handle and bathe the child carefully
  – Loosen clothing near the abdomen
  – Prepare the family for a nephrectomy within 24 to 48 hours of diagnosis
- Postoperative
  – Provide routine care as for a patient who has had a nephrectomy
  – Be aware that chemotherapy and radiation will follow

THE CHILD'S VIEW OF DEATH

● **Language and cognitive development affect perceptions of death**
- Ask what the child knows, give the child facts, and elicit the child's feelings; allow the child to hope
- Use language appropriate to the child's cognitive age
  – Don't substitute clichés, such as "passed away," for the word "death"
  – Don't refer to death as sleep; the child may be afraid to go to bed
- The child may seem unresponsive to the information at first; allow

Developmental stages and the perception of death

- Toddler — fears death only as an extension of the primary fear of separation from parents
- Preschooler — perceives death as only a temporary departure
- School-age child — understands death's permanence; views death as something that happens only to adults
- Adolescent — expresses anger because of inability to be independent and plan future; may feel immune to death

When death is imminent

- Ensure that a parent, relative, or health care provider remains with the child at all times.
- Discuss everyday life events or even death itself.
- Encourage touching and hugging.
- Encourage quiet, passive play that provided satisfaction in the past.
- Provide emotional support to the parents.
- Be aware of the parents' responses to the potential death of their child.
- Include siblings and grandparents in the dying process.

time for the information to be processed
- Reassure the child that he won't be alone

● **Death is viewed differently at different stages of development**
- Toddler
  - Has no concept of time or space other than the here-and-now
  - Fears death only as an extension of the primary fear of separation from the parents
  - Can sense the feelings of others
- Preschooler
  - Perceives death as only a temporary departure
  - May relate death to sleep
  - May believe that illness and death are punishment
  - May fear separation from parents; may worry about who will provide care after death
  - Possesses a rudimentary concept of time
- School-age child
  - Understands the past, present, and future; understands death's permanence
  - Views death as something that happens only to adults
  - Engages in games that play-act death; perceives death as immobility
  - Possesses a concrete understanding of causality; may construe illness as a punishment for a misdeed
  - Fears pain and abandonment
  - Is curious about the rituals of death; may ask directly about own death
- Adolescent
  - Expresses anger because of inability to be independent or plan future goals
  - May feel immune to death and engage in risk-taking behaviors
  - May want to plan own funeral
  - May want to complete projects, make tapes to loved ones, or give belongings to others as a way of keeping part of self alive

● **Take the following steps when death is imminent**
- Ensure that a parent, relative, or health care provider remains with the child at all times to diminish fears of abandonment
- Discuss everyday life events or even death itself; encourage touching and hugging
- Encourage quiet, passive play that provided satisfaction in the past
- Help the parents do all that they can do emotionally
- Be aware of the parents' responses to the potential death of their child
  - Fear of the unexpected
  - Anger

– Guilt at the thought that they caused the problem by not observing the symptoms earlier, not seeking health care earlier, or not providing a safe environment for their child
- Include siblings and grandparents in the dying process

NCLEX CHECKS

It's never too soon to begin your NCLEX preparation. Now that you've reviewed this chapter, carefully read each of the following questions and choose the best answer. Then compare your responses to the correct answers.

1. A 19-year-old student comes to the college health center with multiple painless, enlarged lymph nodes in the cervical neck region. The nurse suspects:
- ☐ **1.** leukemia.
- ☐ **2.** sickle cell anemia.
- ☐ **3.** Hodgkin's disease.
- ☐ **4.** AIDS.

2. A 5-year-old child is admitted to the hospital with a tentative diagnosis of leukemia. The child's grandmother asks the nurse to explain how leukemia is diagnosed. Which diagnostic procedure should the nurse discuss?
- ☐ **1.** Bone marrow aspiration
- ☐ **2.** Peripheral lymph node biopsy
- ☐ **3.** Blood studies
- ☐ **4.** CT scanning

3. A child diagnosed with Wilms' tumor is admitted to the hospital. What's the most common presenting sign?
- ☐ **1.** Abdominal mass
- ☐ **2.** Hematuria
- ☐ **3.** Fever
- ☐ **4.** Lethargy

4. In a child with leukemia, which condition increases the risk of infection?
- ☐ **1.** Thrombocytopenia
- ☐ **2.** Leukopenia
- ☐ **3.** Anemia
- ☐ **4.** Vitamin K deficiency

5. Which child would be considered to be at highest risk for cancer?
- ☐ **1.** 2-year-old with cystic fibrosis
- ☐ **2.** 10-year-old with juvenile rheumatoid arthritis
- ☐ **3.** 8-year-old with Down syndrome
- ☐ **4.** 4-year-old with chickenpox

TOP 7

Items to study for your next test on pediatric cancer

1. Most common types of pediatric cancer
2. Complications of cancer in children
3. Types of chemotherapeutic agents
4. Adverse reactions to chemotherapy and radiation therapy
5. Types of leukemia
6. Signs and symptoms of malignant brain tumors
7. Views of death at developmental stages

6. Which blood value would be expected after a child has received chemotherapy?

- [ ] **1.** Platelet count of 20,000/μl
- [ ] **2.** Hemoglobin level of 14.5%
- [ ] **3.** WBC count of 10,000/μl
- [ ] **4.** Hematocrit of 42%

7. What nursing intervention should be instituted in a child with cancer?

- [ ] **1.** Instruct the parent to take only rectal temperatures on the child.
- [ ] **2.** Encourage the child to brush his teeth with a hard toothbrush and floss three times per day.
- [ ] **3.** Advise the parent that the child shouldn't receive the oral poliovirus and varicella vaccines.
- [ ] **4.** Advise the parents that the child should be isolated from the rest of the family.

8. What leukemia-related condition does intrathecal chemotherapy prevent or treat?

- [ ] **1.** Mucositis
- [ ] **2.** Increased ICP
- [ ] **3.** Alopecia
- [ ] **4.** CNS infiltration

9. In the developmental stages of death, children in which stage perceive death as something that only happens to adults?

- [ ] **1.** Toddler
- [ ] **2.** Preschooler
- [ ] **3.** School-age
- [ ] **4.** Adolescent

10. Place in chronological order the stages of neuroblastoma. Use all of the options.

1. Extends beyond midline	
2. Involves the liver	
3. Confined to organ	
4. Not across midline	

ANSWERS AND RATIONALES

1. CORRECT ANSWER: 3

Hodgkin's disease is a malignancy that originates in the lymphoid system. In its early stages, it results in painless, enlarged lymph nodes. These enlarged nodes are firm, nontender, movable, and especially common in the cervical lymph node region. Leukemia is characterized by the uncontrolled proliferation of immature WBCs. Findings in leukemia include anorexia, irritability, lethargy, anemia, infection, and bleeding tendencies. The major symptom of sickle cell anemia is sickle cell crisis, and it's most commonly diagnosed in infants, toddlers, or young school-age children. AIDS is typically accompanied by recurrent infections.

2. CORRECT ANSWER: 1
Bone marrow aspiration reveals the immature and abnormal lymphoblasts and hypercellular marrow that characterize leukemia. A peripheral lymph node biopsy establishes a diagnosis of Hodgkin's disease. Blood studies, and imaging studies such as radiography, bone scans, and CT scans are used to diagnose other childhood cancers.

3. CORRECT ANSWER: 1
The most common sign of Wilms' tumor is an abdominal mass that's firm and nontender, confined to one side, and deep within the flank. Hematuria occurs in less than one-fourth of children with Wilms' tumor. Lethargy is a late sign and is due to anemia caused by hemorrhage in the tumor. Fever is an effect of the tumor, but isn't a common presenting sign.

4. CORRECT ANSWER: 2
Leukemia can result in leukopenia (decreased WBC count), which increases the risk of infection. Thrombocytopenia results in bleeding. Anemia results in fatigue and hypoxia. Vitamin K deficiency has no direct relationship to leukemia.

5. CORRECT ANSWER: 3
Children with chromosomal abnormalities such as Down syndrome are prone to develop childhood cancer. Children with juvenile rheumatoid arthritis, cystic fibrosis, or chickenpox aren't at high risk for cancer.

6. CORRECT ANSWER: 1
A platelet count of 20,000 µl in a child is abnormal but expected after chemotherapy. Decreased hemoglobin level, hematocrit, WBC count, and platelet count are to be expected after treatment with chemotherapy.

7. CORRECT ANSWER: 3
Children with cancer are immunosuppressed and shouldn't receive any live virus vaccines, such as oral poliovirus and varicella vaccines. Children with cancer shouldn't have rectal temperatures taken due to the risk of bleeding. Soft swab toothbrushes should be used and flossing should be avoided, also because of a risk of bleeding and mucositis. Children with cancer should have frequent family contact.

8. CORRECT ANSWER: 4

Intrathecal chemotherapy is given to prevent or treat CNS infiltration with leukemic cells. Intrathecal chemotherapy doesn't prevent or treat mucositis, alopecia, or increased ICP.

9. CORRECT ANSWER: 3

A school-age child perceives death as something that can happen only to adults. A toddler fears death only as an extension of the primary fear of separation from parents. A preschooler perceives death as only a temporary departure. An adolescent expresses anger because of the inability to be independent and plan his future and may feel more immune to death.

10. CORRECT ANSWER:

3. Confined to organ
4. Not across midline
1. Extends beyond midline
2. Involves the liver

In stage I neuroblastoma, the tumor is confined to the organ or structure of origin. In stage II, continuity extends beyond the primary site but not across the midline. In stage III, the tumor extends beyond the midline with bilateral regional lymph node involvement. In stage IV, the tumor metastasizes.

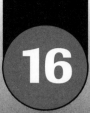

16

Altered psychosocial functioning

---

1. Which psychosocial disorder is suggested in a client who misses at least three consecutive expected menstrual cycles?

- [ ] 1. Failure to thrive
- [ ] 2. Bulimia
- [ ] 3. Anorexia nervosa
- [ ] 4. Functional encopresis

CORRECT ANSWER: 3

2. In which psychosocial disorder does a child use peripheral vision rather than central vision?

- [ ] 1. Anorexia nervosa
- [ ] 2. Tourette syndrome
- [ ] 3. Attention deficient hyperactivity disorder
- [ ] 4. Autistic disorder

CORRECT ANSWER: 4

3. Which disorder would be indicated by the presence of Russell's sign?

☐ 1. Bulimia

☐ 2. Anorexia nervosa

☐ 3. Failure to thrive

☐ 4. Functional enuresis

CORRECT ANSWER: 1

4. Which classification of a tic disorder includes facial gestures and hitting or biting oneself?

☐ 1. Simple verbal

☐ 2. Complex verbal

☐ 3. Simple motor

☐ 4. Complex motor

CORRECT ANSWER: 4

5. Which stress disorder is a normal developmental event in 2- and 3-year-old children?

☐ 1. Stuttering

☐ 2. Sleep terrors

☐ 3. Functional enuresis

☐ 4. Functional encopresis

CORRECT ANSWER: 2

LEARNING OBJECTIVES

After studying this chapter, you should be able to:

● Describe the nursing interventions for the child with an eating disorder.

● Identify the criteria used to diagnose autism.

● List appropriate nursing interventions for an autistic child.

● Explain the differences between organic and nonorganic failure to thrive.

● Identify the criteria used to diagnose attention deficit hyperactivity disorder.

● Recognize Tourette syndrome.

● List appropriate nursing interventions for tic disorders.

CHAPTER OVERVIEW

Conditions involving altered psychiatric or psychological functioning require consistent, supportive nursing care. Thorough assessment of the patient's condition provides the basis for this care. Realistic goal setting and the family's participation are essential for a positive outcome.

ANOREXIA NERVOSA

● **Definition**
- A voluntary refusal to eat accompanied by a loss of more than 15% of body weight without an organic cause
- Results from a distorted, unrealistic attitude toward body size, body weight, and intake that overrides feelings of hunger, threats by family, or accurate knowledge

● **Causes**
- Exact cause unknown
- Social attitudes that equate slimness with beauty
- Subconscious effort to exert personal control over life or to protect oneself from dealing with issues surrounding sexuality
- Achievement pressure
- Dependence and independence issues
- Stress due to multiple responsibilities
- History of sexual abuse
- Risk factors include a low self-esteem, a compulsive personality, perfectionism, and high academic achievement goals

● **Pathophysiology**
- Decreased caloric intake depletes body fat and protein stores
- Estrogen deficiency occurs (in women) due to lack of lipid substrate for synthesis, causing amenorrhea
- Testosterone levels fluctuate (in men) and decreased erectile function and sperm count occur
- Ketoacidosis occurs from increased use of fat as energy fuel

● **Complications**
- Electrolyte imbalances
- Malnutrition
- Dehydration
- Esophageal erosion, ulcers, tears, and bleeding
- Tooth and gum erosion and dental caries
- Decreased left ventricular muscle mass and chamber size
- Decreased cardiac output and hypotension
- Electrocardiogram (ECG) changes
- Increased susceptibility to infection
- Anemia

Risk factors for anorexia nervosa
- Low self-esteem
- A compulsive personality
- High achievement goals

TOP 7
Complications of anorexia nervosa
1. Electrolyte imbalances
2. Malnutrition
3. Dehydration
4. Esophageal erosion, ulcers, tears, and bleeding
5. Decreased cardiac output and hypotension
6. ECG changes
7. Death

TOP 8

Assessment findings in anorexia nervosa

1. Body image disturbance
2. Compulsive behavior
3. Excessive exercising
4. Emaciated appearance
5. Obsessive rituals concerning food
6. Perfectionist attitude
7. Hypotension
8. Delayed secondary sex characteristics

DSM-IV-TR criteria for anorexia nervosa

- Refusal to maintain or achieve normal weight
- Intense fear of gaining weight
- Disturbed perception of body
- Absence of menstrual cycles (females)

Key diagnostic findings in anorexia nervosa

- Eating attitude test suggests eating disorder.
- ECG reveals nonspecific ST interval, prolonged PR interval, and T-wave changes.
- Females exhibit low estrogen levels; males exhibit low testosterone levels.
- Elevated BUN levels and electrolyte imbalances.

- Thyroid gland deficiencies
- Osteoporosis
- Death

● **Assessment findings**
- Amenorrhea, fatigue, loss of libido, infertility
- Body image disturbance
- Cognitive distortions, such as overgeneralization, dichotomous thinking, or ideas of reference
- Compulsive behavior
- Excessive exercising
- Dependency on others for self-worth
- Muscle weakness, seizures, or cardiac arrhythmias
- Emaciated appearance
- Hypotension
- Delayed secondary sex characteristics
- GI complications, such as constipation or laxative dependence
- Guilt associated with eating
- Impaired decision making
- Need to achieve and please others
- Obsessive rituals concerning food
- Overly compliant attitude
- Perfectionist attitude
- Refusal to eat
- Depression

● **Diagnostic test findings**
- All of the criteria of the American Psychiatric Association's *Diagnostic and Statistical Manual of Mental Disorders*, Fourth Edition, Text Revision *(DSM-IV-TR)*, are present
  - Refusal to maintain or achieve normal weight for age and height
  - Intense fear of gaining weight or becoming fat, even though underweight
  - Disturbance in perception of body weight, size, or shape
  - In females, absence of at least three consecutive menstrual cycles when otherwise expected to occur
- Eating attitude test suggests eating disorder
- ECG reveals nonspecific ST interval, prolonged PR interval, and T-wave changes
- Females exhibit low estrogen levels, and males exhibit low testosterone levels
- Low hemoglobin level, platelet count, and white blood cell (WBC) count
- Leukopenia and anemia
- Elevated blood urea nitrogen (BUN) levels and electrolyte imbalances

---

TIME-OUT FOR TEACHING

Teaching about anorexia nervosa

Be sure to include these points in your teaching plan for the parents of an adolescent with anorexia:
- avoidance of power struggles around food
- need for realistic goals
- need for adolescent's positive self-image
- follow-up counseling
- compliance with medical follow-up.

Medical management
- Behavioral modification
- Curtailed activity for cardiac arrhythmias
- Group, family, or individual psychotherapy
- Balanced diet with a normal eating pattern and vitamin supplements
- Medications
  - Antianxiety agents
    - Lorazepam (Ativan)
    - Alprazolam (Xanax)
  - Antidepressants
    - Amitriptyline (Elavil)
    - Imipramine (Tofranil)
  - Selective serotonin reuptake inhibitors
    - Paroxetine (Paxil)
    - Fluoxetine (Prozac)

Nursing interventions
- Monitor parenteral nutrition and I.V. administration, if necessary, to replace protein and electrolytes
- Provide a specific goal-oriented plan that's followed consistently; behavior modification may help decrease the adolescent's manipulative behavior
- Support the adolescent's efforts to achieve target weight (see *Teaching about anorexia nervosa*)
- Negotiate an adequate food intake with the adolescent
- Supervise the adolescent one-on-one during meals and for 1 hour afterward
- Help the adolescent identify coping mechanisms for dealing with anxiety and encourage verbal expression of feelings
- Weigh adolescent once or twice per week at the same time of day using the same scale

---

Medications used to treat anorexia nervosa
- Antianxiety agents
- Antidepressants
- Selective serotonin reuptake inhibitors

Key nursing interventions for anorexia nervosa
- Monitor parenteral nutrition and I.V. administration.
- Provide a goal-oriented plan that's followed consistently.
- Support the adolescent's efforts to achieve target weight.
- Supervise the adolescent one-on-one during meals and for 1 hour afterward.

Criteria for diagnosing ADHD

- Behaviors must be present in two or more settings.
- Behaviors must be present before age 7.
- Behaviors must result in significant impairment in social or academic functioning.

TOP 5
Assessment findings in ADHD

1. Excessive climbing, running, or talking
2. Decreased attention span
3. Easily distracted
4. Failure to give close attention to schoolwork or failure to finish activity
5. Impulsive behavior

ATTENTION DEFICIT HYPERACTIVITY DISORDER

● Definition
- Behavior problem characterized by difficulty focusing attention, engaging in quiet passive activities, or both
- Can have attention deficit without hyperactivity
- Behaviors must be present in two or more settings, must be present before age 7, and must result in significant impairment in social or academic functioning

● Causes
- Underlying causes of attention deficit hyperactivity disorder (ADHD) are unknown
- Limited evidence of a genetic component
- Some studies indicate that it may result from altered neurotransmitter levels in the brain

● Pathophysiology
- Alleles of dopamine genes may alter dopamine transmission in the neural networks
- During fetal development, bouts of hypoxia and hypotension could selectively damage neurons located in some of the critical regions of the anatomical networks

● Complications
- Emotional and social complications
- Poor nutrition
- Poor self-image and self-worth
- Weight loss

● Assessment findings
- Excessive climbing, running, or talking
- Decreased attention span
- Difficulty organizing tasks and activities
- Difficulty waiting for turns or playing quietly
- Easily distracted
- Failure to give close attention to schoolwork or failure to finish activity
- Failure to listen when spoken to directly
- Fidgeting or squirming in seat
- Frequent forgetfulness; frequent loss of things needed for tasks; carelessness
- Impulsive behavior
- Inability to follow directions

● Diagnostic test findings
- Complete psychological, medical, and neurologic evaluations rule out other problems

- Findings are combined with data from several sources, including parents, teachers, and the child

● **Medical management**
  - Behavior modification and psychological therapy
  - Interdisciplinary interventions, including pathologic assessment and diagnosis of specific learning needs
  - Elimination of sugar, dyes, and additives from the diet
  - Medications
    - Stimulants
      - Amphetamines (Adderall)
      - Methylphenidate (Ritalin, Concerta)
      - Pemoline (Cylert)
      - Dextroamphetamine (Dexedrine)
    - Nonstimulants
      - Bupropion (Wellbutrin)
      - Atomoxetine (Strattera)

● **Nursing interventions**
  - Monitor growth; if the child is receiving methylphenidate, growth may be slowed
  - Give one simple instruction at a time so the child can successfully complete the task, which promotes self-esteem
  - Give medications in the morning and at lunch to avoid interfering with sleep
  - Ensure adequate nutrition; medications and hyperactivity may cause increased nutrient needs
  - Reduce environmental stimuli to decrease distraction
  - Formulate a schedule for the child to provide consistency and routine

AUTISTIC DISORDER

● **Definition**
  - A pervasive developmental disorder
  - Usually apparent before the child reaches age 30 months but may not be recognized until child enters school
  - Affects 1 in 500 children
  - Four to five times more common in males than females, usually the firstborn male
  - Must be differentiated from mental retardation, deafness, and childhood schizophrenia
  - Poor prognosis

● **Causes**
  - No specific cause has been fully supported
  - Some children show abnormal but nonspecific EEG findings that suggest brain dysfunction

Managing ADHD

- Behavior modification
- Psychological therapy
- Diagnosis of specific learning needs
- Dietary modifications
- Medications

Key facts about autistic disorder

- It's a pervasive developmental disorder that affects 1 in 500 children.
- It's usually apparent before the child reaches age 30 months but may not be recognized until the child enters school.
- It's four to five times more common in males than females.

Conditions associated with autistic disorder

- Maternal rubella
- Phenylketonuria
- Tuberous sclerosis
- Anoxia during birth
- Encephalitis
- Infantile spasms
- Fragile X syndrome
- Brain dysfunction

TOP 5

Behavioral assessment findings in a child with autistic disorder

1. Doesn't relate to or interact with others
2. Doesn't cuddle or mold body to that of a caretaker
3. Doesn't appear to be comforted by the parent's touch after an injury
4. Avoids eye contact
5. Performs repetitive motions and self-stimulating behaviors, such as rocking or head banging, and appears hyperactive

- Autistic disorder has also been associated with maternal rubella, untreated phenylketonuria, tuberous sclerosis, anoxia during birth, encephalitis, infantile spasms, and fragile X syndrome
- Linked with abnormalities in neurotransmitters, including increased dopamine and increased serotonin
- Nutritional deficiency
- 10% to 20% risk of recurrence in families with one affected child

● **Pathophysiology**
- Defects in the central nervous system (CNS) that may arise from prenatal complications

● **Complications**
- Seizure disorder
- Depression
- Catatonic phenomena and undifferentiated psychotic state during periods of stress

● **Assessment findings**
- The child doesn't relate to or interact with others
- The child doesn't cuddle or mold body to that of a caretaker
- The child doesn't demonstrate anticipatory behaviors as the parent approaches, such as lifting his arms in anticipation of being picked up
- The child doesn't appear to be comforted by the parent's touch after an injury
- The child uses peripheral vision rather than central vision; the child looks past you and avoids eye contact
- The child may not have meaningful speech
  - Uses inappropriate noises and responses
  - Appears deaf but isn't
  - Uses pronoun reversal ("you go walk" when he means "I want to go for a walk")
- If speech is present, the child rarely refers to self and uses echolalia (meaningless repetition of words or phrases addressed to him)
- The child appears fascinated by objects that spin, reflect light, sparkle, or are smooth; the child prefers inanimate objects but may relate to pets
- The child performs repetitive motions and self-stimulating behaviors, such as rocking or head banging, and appears hyperactive
- The child doesn't appear to be anxious when separated from the parents
- The child demonstrates inappropriate fears of harmless items
- The child resists a change in routines
- The child may exhibit cognitive impairment (IQ scores typically fall within the moderate to severe range)
- Seizures develop in one in four children

Other pervasive developmental disorders

Although autistic disorder is the most severe of the pervasive developmental disorders, other similar disorders exist in this class.

For example, the *Diagnostic and Statistical Manual of Mental Disorders,* Fourth edition, Text Revision (*DSM-IV-TR*), category *pervasive developmental disorder not otherwise specified* refers to those patients who don't meet the criteria for autistic disorder but who *do* exhibit impaired development of reciprocal social interaction and of verbal and nonverbal communication skills.

Some patients with this diagnosis exhibit a markedly restricted repertoire of activities and interests, but others don't. Research suggests that these disorders are more common than autistic disorder.

● Diagnostic test findings
- According to the *DSM-IV-TR,* at least 6 of these 12 characteristics must be present, including at least 2 items from the first category, 1 from the second category, and 1 from the third category
  - Qualitative impairment in social interaction
    - Marked impairment of nonverbal behavior, such as facial expression, body posture, and eye-to-eye contact
    - Absence of peer relationships
    - Failure to spontaneously seek or share enjoyment, interests, or achievements
    - Lack of social or emotional reciprocity
  - Qualitative impairment in communication
    - Delay or lack of language development
    - Inability to initiate or sustain conversation
    - Idiosyncratic or repetitive language
    - Lack of appropriate imaginative play
  - Restricted, repetitive, and stereotyped patterns of behavior, interests, and activities
    - Abnormal preoccupation with a restricted pattern of interest
    - Inflexible routines or rituals
    - Repetitive motor mannerisms
    - Preoccupation with parts of objects
- The diagnostic criteria also include delays or abnormal functioning in at least one of these areas before age 3 (see *Other pervasive developmental disorders*)
  - Social interaction and language skills
  - Symbolic or imaginative play

● Medical management
- Must begin early and continue for years (through adolescence)
- May take place in psychiatric institutions, in a specialized school, or in a day-care program, but the current trend is toward home treatment

Diagnostic findings in autistic disorder
- Impaired social interaction
- Impaired communication
- Repetitive patterns of behavior, interests, and activities
- Delays in language skills
- Abnormal symbolic or imaginative play

Behavioral management techniques in autistic disorder

- Positive reinforcement
- System of rewards for good behavior
- Pleasurable sensory and motor stimulation
- Increase social awareness of others

Key facts about bulimia nervosa

- Characterized by recurrent episodes of binge eating followed by feelings of guilt, humiliation, and self-deprecation
- Involves self-induced vomiting or the use of laxatives or diuretics after binging
- May also involve strict dieting or fasting
- Unknown cause

Complications of bulimia nervosa

- Dental problems, such as enamel erosion and gum infections
- Dehydration and electrolyte imbalances
- Digestive system problems such as esophageal tears
- Cardiac problems such as arrhythmias
- Anemia

- Behavioral techniques are used to decrease symptoms and increase the child's ability to respond
  - Positive reinforcement using a system of rewards for good behavior
  - Pleasurable sensory and motor stimulation
  - Increased social awareness of others
- Drug therapy with an agent such as haloperidol (Haldol) may be helpful
- Speech, occupational therapy, and physical therapy

● **Nursing interventions**
- Work with child on a one-to-one relationship
- Give the child specific directions to follow, initially without rationales
- Reduce self-destructive behaviors such as hitting and biting
- Minimize handling to prevent upsetting the child
- Decrease stimulation in the environment
- Initiate a goal of getting the child to be aware of others
- Provide the family with support and refer them to the Autism Society of America

BULIMIA NERVOSA

● **Definition**
- Recurrent episodes of binge eating followed by feelings of guilt, humiliation, and self-deprecation
- Self-induced vomiting, the use of laxatives or diuretics, strict dieting or fasting, or strenuous exercise to overcome the effects of the binges
- Seldom incapacitating

● **Causes**
- Exact cause is unknown
- Contributing factors include family disturbance or conflict, history of sexual abuse, low self-esteem, neurochemical changes, and a family history of eating disorders, affective disorders, or substance abuse

● **Pathophysiology**
- Decreased caloric intake depletes body fat and protein stores
- Estrogen deficiency occurs (in women) due to lack of lipid substrate for synthesis, causing amenorrhea
- Testosterone levels fluctuate (in men) and decreased erectile function and sperm count occur
- Ketoacidosis occurs from increased use of fat as energy fuel
- Increased carbohydrate intake triggers increased insulin production

● **Complications**
- Dental caries, erosion of tooth enamel, and gum infections
- Dehydration and electrolyte imbalances

- Esophageal tears, gastric rupture, and mucosal damage to intestine
- Arrhythmias, cardiac failure, and sudden death
- Suicide
- Anemia

Assessment findings

- Alternating episodes of binge eating and purging (both behaviors occur on average at least two times per week for 3 months)
- Thin or slightly overweight with use of diuretics, laxatives, vomiting, and exercise
- Abdominal and epigastric pain
- Amenorrhea
- Painless swelling of the salivary glands
- Hoarseness
- Throat irritation or lacerations
- Calluses of the knuckles or abrasions and scars on the dorsum of the hand (Russell's sign) due to induced vomiting
- Anxiety, avoidance of conflict, extreme need for approval, guilt and self-disgust
- Constant preoccupation with food and possible use of amphetamines to control hunger

Diagnostic test findings

- Beck Depression Inventory may reveal depression
- Eating Attitudes test suggests eating disorder
- Metabolic acidosis may occur from diarrhea caused by enemas and excessive laxative use
- Metabolic alkalosis (the most common metabolic complication) may occur from frequent vomiting
- Elevated bicarbonate, decreased potassium, and decreased sodium levels
- Decreased hematocrit

Medical management

- Inpatient or outpatient therapy to identify triggers for binge eating and purging
- Self-help groups
- Drug therapy, including selective serotonin reuptake inhibitors such as Paxil, Prozac, and sertraline (Zoloft)

Nursing interventions

- Monitor parenteral nutrition and I.V. administration, if necessary, to replace protein and electrolytes
- Supervise mealtimes and for a specified time period after meals, usually up to 1 hour, to help the adolescent avoid purging behavior
- Set a time limit for each meal
- Use behavior modification techniques

TOP 4

Assessment findings in bulimia nervosa

1. Alternating episodes of binge eating and purging
2. Thin or slightly overweight with use of diuretics, laxatives, vomiting, and exercise
3. Throat irritation or lacerations
4. Calluses of the knuckles or abrasions and scars on the dorsum of the hand

Managing bulimia nervosa

- Therapy to identify triggers
- Self-help groups
- Drug therapy

- Establish a food contract, specifying the amount and type of food to be eaten at each meal
- Encourage verbalization and provide support

FAILURE TO THRIVE

● **Definition**
- Chronic, potentially life-threatening condition characterized by failure to maintain weight and height above the 5th percentile on age-appropriate growth charts
- Most children are diagnosed before age 2

● **Causes**
- Organic: acute or chronic illness such as GI reflux, malabsorption syndrome, congenital heart defect, or cystic fibrosis
- Nonorganic: psychological problem between child and primary caregiver such as failure to bond
- Mixed: combination of physical (organic) and emotional (nonorganic) causes

● **Pathophysiology**
- Organic type is dependent on the physical disorder responsible
- The nonorganic and mixed types represent a complex dynamic between parent and child
  - Parent may feel little emotional attachment to the child
  - Parent may offer insufficient food
  - Child may sense parental detachment
  - Child may contribute by being irritable, fussy, or colicky

● **Complications**
  - Below-normal intellectual development
  - Poor language development and reading skills
  - Social immaturity
  - Increased incidence of behavioral disturbances

● **Assessment findings**
- Altered body posture; child is stiff or floppy; doesn't cuddle
- Delayed psychosocial behavior; for example, reluctance to smile or talk
- Disparities between chronological age and height and weight
- History of inadequate feeding techniques, such as bottle propping or insufficient burping
- History of insufficient stimulation and inadequate parental knowledge of child development
- History of medical problems
- History of sleep disturbances
- Psychosocial family problems

Causes of failure to thrive

- Organic — acute or chronic illness such as GI reflux, malabsorption syndrome, congenital heart defect, or cystic fibrosis
- Nonorganic — psychological problem between child and primary caregiver such as failure to bond
- Mixed — combination of organic and nonorganic causes

Complications of failure to thrive

- Poor intellectual, language, and reading skills
- Social immaturity
- Behavioral disturbances

Key assessment findings in failure to thrive

- Delayed psychosocial behavior
- Disparities between chronological age and height and weight
- History of inadequate feeding techniques
- History of insufficient stimulation and inadequate parental knowledge of child development
- History of medical problems

- Regurgitation of food after almost every feeding, part being vomited and the remainder swallowed (rumination of food)

● **Diagnostic test findings**
- Negative nitrogen balance indicates inadequate intake of protein or calories
- Associated physiologic causes may be detected
- Reduced creatinine-height index reflects muscle mass and estimates muscle protein depletion
- Other tests may be performed to rule out any organic cause

● **Medical management**
- High-calorie diet with vitamin and mineral supplements
- Parent counseling
- Respite care for the child
- Structured feeding regime with specified volume needed per feeding

● **Nursing interventions**
- Weigh the child on admission to determine baseline weight; continue to weigh daily during treatment
- Measure intake and output carefully
- Assess growth and development using an appropriate tool such as the Denver Developmental Screening Test
- Properly feed and interact with the child to promote nutrition and growth and development
- Establish specific times for feeding, bathing, and sleeping to establish and maintain a structured routine
- Provide the child with visual and auditory stimulation to promote normal sensory development
- Assess interaction of parent with child to determine if failure to thrive is due to parent's inability to form emotional attachment to child
- Teach the parent effective parenting skills to increase the parent's knowledge of routine child care practices
  – Comfort measures
  – Age-appropriate developmental tasks
  – Play activities
- Serve as role model for parent

TIC DISORDERS

● **Definition**
- Involuntary, spasmodic, recurrent, and purposeless motor movements or vocalizations
- Classifications
  – Motor

TOP 4

Interventions for children who fail to thrive

1. Weigh the child on admission to determine baseline weight.
2. Properly feed and interact with the child to promote nutrition and growth and development.
3. Establish specific feeding, bathing, and sleeping times
4. Teach the parent effective parenting skills, such as comfort measures, age-appropriate developmental tasks, and play activities to increase the parent's knowledge of routine child care practices.

Key facts about tic disorders

- Involve spasmodic, recurrent, and purposeless motor movements or vocalizations
- Begin between ages 9 and 13
- Three times more common in boys than girls
- Occur more in certain families, suggesting a genetic cause
- May be precipitated or exacerbated by the use of phenothiazines or CNS stimulants or by head trauma

Classifications of tic disorders

- Motor — simple (such as blinking) and complex (such as jumping)
- Verbal — simple (such as coughing) and complex (such as using socially unacceptable words)

- Simple: Eye blinking, neck jerking, shoulder shrugging, head banging, head turning, tongue protrusion, lip or tongue biting, nail biting, hair pulling, facial grimacing
  - Complex: Facial gestures, grooming behaviors, hitting or biting oneself, jumping, hopping, touching, squatting, retracing steps, twirling when walking, stamping, smelling an object, and imitating the movements of someone who's being observed (echopraxia)
  – Verbal
  - Simple: Coughing, throat clearing, grunting, sniffing, snorting, hissing, clicking, yelping, and barking
  - Complex: Repeating words out of context; using socially unacceptable words, many of which are obscene (coprolalia); repeating the last-heard sound, word, or phrase of another (echolalia); or repeating own sounds or words (palilalia)
- Include Tourette syndrome, chronic motor or verbal tic disorder, and transient tic disorder
- Begin between ages 9 and 13
- Three times more common in boys than girls

Causes
- Exact cause unknown
- Occur more in certain families, suggesting a genetic cause
- May be precipitated or exacerbated by the use of phenothiazines or CNS stimulants or by head trauma

Pathophysiology
- Develop when a child experiences overwhelming anxiety, usually associated with normal maturation

Complications
- Obsessive-compulsive behaviors
- Disruptive behaviors
- Learning disabilities

Assessment findings for tic disorders

- Specific motor or vocal patterns
- Specific frequency, complexity, and precipitating factors
- Exacerbated by stress
- Diminish during sleep

Assessment findings
- Vary according to the type of tic disorder
- Inspection, coupled with the patient's history, may reveal the specific motor or vocal patterns that characterize the tic as well as the frequency, complexity, and precipitating factors
- Tic disorders are exacerbated by stress and usually diminish markedly during sleep (see *Stress disorders with physical signs*)

Diagnostic test findings
- Based on *DSM-IV-TR* criteria
- Tourette syndrome
  – The patient has had multiple motor tics and one or more vocal tics at some time during the illness, but not necessarily concurrently

Stress disorders with physical signs

Besides tic disorders, stress-related disorders that produce physical signs in children include stuttering, functional enuresis, functional encopresis, sleepwalking, and sleep terrors.

STUTTERING

Characterized by abnormal speech rhythms with repetitions and hesitations at the beginning of words, stuttering may involve movements of the respiratory muscles, shoulders, and face. It may be associated with mental dullness, poor social background, and a history of birth trauma. However, this disorder most commonly occurs in children of average or superior intelligence who fear they can't meet expectations. Related problems may include low self-esteem, tension, anxiety, humiliation, and withdrawal from social situations.

About 80% of stutterers recover after age 16. Evaluation and treatment by a speech pathologist teaches the stutterer how to place equal weight on each syllable in a sentence, how to breathe properly, and how to control anxiety.

FUNCTIONAL ENURESIS

Functional enuresis is characterized by intentional or involuntary voiding of urine, usually during the night (nocturnal enuresis). Considered normal in young children, functional enuresis occurs in about 40% of children until age 4. It persists in 10% of children to age 5, in 5% to age 10, and in 1% of boys to age 18. Enuresis is more common in boys than girls.

Causes may be related to stress, such as the birth of a sibling, the move to a new home, divorce, separation, hospitalization, faulty toilet training (inconsistent, demanding, or punitive), and unrealistic responsibilities. Associated problems include low self-esteem, social withdrawal from peers because of ostracism and ridicule, and anger, rejection, and punishment by caregivers.

Advise parents that a matter-of-fact attitude helps the child learn bladder control without undue stress. If enuresis persists into late childhood, treatment with imipramine (Tofranil) may help. Dry-bed therapy may include the use of an alarm (wet bell pad), social motivation, self-correction of accidents, and positive reinforcement.

FUNCTIONAL ENCOPRESIS

Denoted by evacuation of feces into the child's clothes or inappropriate receptacles, functional encopresis is associated with low intelligence, cerebral dysfunction, or other developmental symptoms such as language lag. Some children also show inefficient and ineffective gastric motility. Related problems may include repressed anger, withdrawal from peer relationships, and loss of self-esteem.

Treatment involves encouraging the child to come to his parents when he has an "accident." Advise parents to give the child clean clothes without criticism or punishment. Medical examination should rule out any physical disorder. Child, adult, and family therapy may help reduce anger and disappointment over the child's development and improve parenting techniques.

SLEEPWALKING AND SLEEP TERRORS

In sleepwalking, the child calmly rises from bed in a state of altered consciousness and walks around with no subsequent recollection of any dreams. In sleep terrors, he awakes terrified, in a state of clouded consciousness, commonly unable to recognize parents and familiar surroundings. Visual hallucinations are common.

Sleepwalking is usually a response to an emotional concern. Tell parents to gently "talk" the child back to his bed. If he wakes, they should comfort and support him — not tease him.

Sleep terrors are a normal developmental event in 2- and 3-year-old chil-
(continued)

Quick guide to other stress disorders with physical signs

- **Stuttering** – characterized by abnormal speech rhythms with repetitions and hesitations at the beginning of words
- **Functional enuresis** – intentional or involuntary voiding of urine
- **Functional encopresis** – evacuation of feces into the child's clothes or inappropriate receptacles
- **Sleepwalking** – walking around in a state of altered consciousness with no subsequent recollection of dreams
- **Sleep terrors** – awakening in terror in state of clouded consciousness that may be accompanied by visual hallucinations

Key findings in Tourette syndrome

- Multiple motor tics
- One or more vocal tics
- Bouts occurring many times per day nearly every day for more than 1 year

Key findings in chronic motor or vocal tic disorder

- Single or multiple motor or vocal tics, but not both
- Bouts occurring nearly every day for more than 1 year
- Criteria don't meet those for Tourette syndrome

Key findings in transient tic disorder

- Single or multiple motor or vocal tics, or both
- Bouts occurring nearly every day for at least 4 weeks, but for no longer than 12 months
- Criteria don't meet those for Tourette syndrome or chronic motor or vocal tic disorder

Stress disorders with physical signs (continued)

dren, usually occurring within 30 minutes to 3½ hours of sleep onset. Tachycardia, tachypnea, diaphoresis, dilated pupils, and piloerection are associated with sleep terrors. The child may also fear being alone.

Tell parents to make sure the child has access to them at night. Sleep terrors usually are self-limiting and subside within a few weeks. Sleep terrors need to be distinguished from seizure activity.

- The tics occur many times per day (usually in bouts) nearly every day or intermittently for more than 1 year
- The disturbance causes marked distress or significant impairment in social, occupational, or other important areas of functioning
- Onset occurs before age 18
- The disturbance isn't the direct physiologic effect of a substance or a general medical condition
- Chronic motor or vocal tic disorder
  - The patient has had single or multiple motor or vocal tics, but not both, at some time during the illness
  - The tics occur many times per day nearly every day or intermittently for more than 1 year; during this time, the person has never had a tic-free period exceeding 3 consecutive months
  - The disturbance causes marked distress or significant impairment in social, occupational, or other important areas of functioning
  - Onset occurs before age 18
  - The disturbance isn't the direct physiologic effect of a substance or a general medical condition
  - Criteria have never been met for Tourette syndrome
- Transient tic disorder
  - The patient has single or multiple motor or vocal tics, or both
  - The tics occur many times per day nearly every day for at least 4 weeks, but for no longer than 12 consecutive months
  - The disturbance causes marked distress or significant impairment in social, occupational, or other important areas of functioning
  - Onset occurs before age 18
  - The disturbance isn't the direct physiologic effect of a substance or a general medical condition
  - Criteria have never been met for Tourette syndrome or chronic motor or vocal tic disorder

● **Medical management**
- Most tic disorders resolve by early adolescence without treatment
- Behavior modification and operant conditioning
- Psychotherapy helps the patient uncover underlying conflicts and issues as well as deal with the problems caused by the tics

- Tourette syndrome is best treated with medication (haloperidol [Haldol], pimozide [Orap], clonidine [Catapres]) and resperiodone (Risperdol) and psychotherapy
- Antianxiety agents may be useful in dealing with secondary anxiety, but they don't reduce the severity or frequency of the tics

● **Nursing interventions**

- Offer emotional support and help the patient prevent fatigue
- Suggest the patient with Tourette syndrome and his family contact the Tourette Syndrome Association to obtain information and support
- Help the patient identify and eliminate avoidable stress and learn positive new ways to deal with anxiety
- Encourage the patient to verbalize his feelings about his disorder
  - Help him to understand the movements are involuntary
  - Tell him he shouldn't feel guilty or blame himself for them
- Encourage parents to foster feelings of self-esteem in the child

NCLEX CHECKS

It's never too soon to begin your NCLEX preparation. Now that you've reviewed this chapter, carefully read each of the following questions and choose the best answer. Then compare your responses to the correct answers.

1. A school nurse is teaching a class of high school students about anorexia nervosa. Which statement by one of the students reveals an early sign of anorexia nervosa?

- ☐ **1.** "I have my menstrual period every 28 days."
- ☐ **2.** "I go out to eat with my friends at least three times per week."
- ☐ **3.** "I jog three times per day for a total of 5 hours per day."
- ☐ **4.** "I try to maintain my weight around 115 lb for my height of 5 feet."

2. The mother of an 11-month-old infant brings her child to the pediatrician's office for a checkup. The nurse assesses the infant and finds that the infant falls below the third percentile for height and weight. The infant may be suffering from:

- ☐ **1.** failure to thrive.
- ☐ **2.** Munchausen syndrome by proxy.
- ☐ **3.** physical neglect.
- ☐ **4.** physical abuse.

3. A 15-year-old adolescent tells the nurse that she engages in binge eating. Which eating disorder is this patient likely to have?

- ☐ **1.** Anorexia nervosa
- ☐ **2.** Bulimia
- ☐ **3.** Munchausen syndrome
- ☐ **4.** Gastroesophageal reflux

TOP 2

Interventions for tic disorders

1. Help the patient identify and eliminate avoidable stress and learn positive new ways to deal with anxiety.

2. Encourage the patient to verbalize his feelings about his disorder.

TOP 6

Items to study for your next test on psychosocial disorders in children

1. Differences between anorexia nervosa and bulimia nervosa

2. Key nursing interventions for a child with an eating disorder

3. Medications used to treat ADHD

4. Assessment findings in autism

5. Types of failure to thrive

6. Interventions for a child with failure to thrive

4. A 7-year-old child is diagnosed with ADHD. Which medication should a nurse anticipate administering to the child?

☐ **1.** Amitriptyline (Elavil)
☐ **2.** Dextroamphetamine (Adderall)
☐ **3.** Paroxetine (Paxil)
☐ **4.** Phenytoin (Dilantin)

5. Which statement about Tourette syndrome is true?

☐ **1.** Children with Tourette syndrome frequently display obsessive-compulsive behaviors.
☐ **2.** Manifestations are stable and rarely change once displayed.
☐ **3.** Medications aren't effective in the treatment of Tourette syndrome.
☐ **4.** Tics result in physical debilitation and shorten the child's life expectancy.

6. If failure to thrive has been a long-standing problem for an infant, what physical measurement should be expected?

☐ **1.** Height noted to be less than the 10th percentile
☐ **2.** Height and weight below the 5th percentile
☐ **3.** Head circumference stays at 50th percentile
☐ **4.** Height, weight, and head circumference at the 10th percentile

7. An adolescent with bulimia must be monitored by the nurse for medical complications. To which finding must the nurse respond with immediate intervention?

☐ **1.** Anemia from malabsorption of nutrients from laxative abuse
☐ **2.** Chronic esophagitis from selfinduced vomiting
☐ **3.** Erosion of teeth enamel from self-induced vomiting
☐ **4.** Potassium depletion from diuretic abuse

8. Which behavior would a nurse recognize as a common finding among adolescent girls with anorexia nervosa?

☐ **1.** Has strong peer relationships with classmates and several best friends
☐ **2.** Has poor schoolwork performance and displays little interest in academics
☐ **3.** Is present at meals, selects foods, and appears to family and friends as eating appropriately
☐ **4.** Wears form-fitting clothing and has a healthy body image

9. A nurse is caring for an autistic child in the hospital. Which nursing intervention would be most appropriate?

☐ **1.** Encouraging the child to tell you where he hurts
☐ **2.** Keeping the noise level to a minimum in the child's room
☐ **3.** Making eye contact with the child while administering his medications
☐ **4.** Stroking and holding the child to comfort him

10. A nurse is reviewing laboratory results for several adolescents on the eating disorder unit. Which abnormal findings should be expected in a bulimic adolescent? Select all that apply.

☐ **1.** Elevated bicarbonate level

☐ **2.** Low red blood cell (RBC) count

☐ **3.** Decreased potassium level

☐ **4.** Decreased sodium level

☐ **5.** Suppressed WBC count

☐ **6.** Increased hematocrit

ANSWERS AND RATIONALES

1. CORRECT ANSWER: 3

Excessive exercise, consumption of very small amounts of food, and food rituals are all signs of anorexia nervosa. Menstruation commonly stops, and the adolescent's weight is below normal.

2. CORRECT ANSWER: 1

An infant with failure to thrive falls below the 5th percentile for weight and height on a standard growth chart. This condition may have an organic cause, such as heart disease, or a nonorganic cause, such as a disturbance in the parent-child relationship. In Munchausen syndrome by proxy, a parent repeatedly brings a child to a health care facility reporting symptoms of illness when the child is well. Physical neglect is typically subtle. The neglected child may appear unwashed or be improperly dressed for the weather. The physically abused child may have peculiar lacerations or bruises such as curved imprints from a belt buckle.

3. CORRECT ANSWER: 2

Bulimia is an eating disorder characterized by binge eating. The binge behavior consists of secretive, frenzied consumption of large amounts of high-calorie foods during a brief period. Anorexia nervosa is characterized by extreme control of food intake. In Munchausen syndrome, the adolescent feigns symptoms. Gastroesophageal reflux is the passive transfer of gastric contents into the esophagus. It isn't an eating disorder.

4. CORRECT ANSWER: 2

Adderall is a pharmacologic treatment modality for ADHD, serving as a CNS stimulant which, in children with ADHD, helps them focus better. Elavil and Paxil are both antidepressants and have no effect on treating ADHD. Dilantin is a seizure medication.

5. CORRECT ANSWER: 1

Tourette syndrome is expressed as nonvoluntary movements and vocalizations, and children with the condition commonly exhibit obsessive-compulsive behavior. Tourette syndrome often changes in its physical expression and isn't stable. Medications such as neuroleptics (haloperidol [Haldol] and pimozide [Orap]) and an atypical neuroleptic agent risperidone (Risperdal) can help in the management of Tourette syndrome. Although tics are frustrating and can be embarrassing to the child, they don't appear to affect the child's life span or lead to debilitation.

6. CORRECT ANSWER: 2

To be considered failure to thrive, an infant's height and weight must fall below the 5th percentile in the standardized growth chart. A height less than the 10th percentile and a decreased head circumference don't indicate failure to thrive. There are many factors that can cause these findings. Microcephaly could result in a decreased head circumference but isn't failure to thrive.

7. CORRECT ANSWER: 4

A potassium level below 3.5 mEq/L can have serious consequences, such as cardiac arrhythmias, so depleted potassium must be treated immediately. Although anemia from malabsorption of nutrients from laxative abuse, chronic esophagitis from self-induced vomiting, and erosion of teeth enamel from self-induced vomiting are all important medical problems that require prompt intervention, they aren't life-threatening, so a low potassium level takes priority.

8. CORRECT ANSWER: 3

Most anorexic adolescents outwardly appear to be eating and show no nutritional problems to friends and family. Families are commonly surprised when the initial diagnosis occurs. Adolescents with anorexia nervosa rarely have strong peer relationships and close friends. Their academic performance is usually strong. Many wear loose clothing to hide weight loss or to conceal perceived poor body image of being fat even though they're severely malnourished and emaciated.

9. CORRECT ANSWER: 2

Autistic children don't like to be touched or surrounded by stimulation. When caring for the autistic child, the nurse must keep the room quiet and the lighting low to minimize stimulation. Communication difficulties are common in children with autism and these children would have problems verbalizing their pain. Children with autism won't make eye contact; it's a hallmark sign of the disease.

10. CORRECT ANSWER: 1, 3, 4

A bulimic adolescent has complications that include fluid and electrolyte disturbances (decreased potassium and sodium levels) and metabolic alkalosis (elevated bicarbonate level). Low RBC count, suppressed WBC count, and increased hematocrit aren't commonly seen with bulimia.

Glossary
Selected references
Index

Glossary

accessory muscles: thoracic and abdominal muscles used during respiratory distress to help expand and contract the chest so the patient can inhale and exhale

allergic salute: pushing up and out on the base of the nose to relieve stuffiness

allergic shiners: dark circles under the eyes from edema and congestion related to histamine

allergy: hypersensitivity to normal environmental antigens

anemia: decrease in the number or quality of circulating red blood cells due to hemorrhage, hemolysis, or lack of production

anorexia: lack or loss of appetite for food

anorexia nervosa: voluntary control of hunger characterized by a refusal to eat and a loss of 15% of body weight without an organic cause

antigen: foreign substance that stimulates the body to produce antibodies

astrocytoma: benign, slow-growing tumor in the cerebellum

atelectasis: failure of a portion of the lung to expand, preventing respiratory exchange in that area

atresia: termination or absence of a normal anatomic passageway

autism: psychiatric disorder characterized by a lack of interest in reality, especially in relating to others

bulimia: multiple episodes of compulsive overeating followed by forced emesis; also called *the binge-purge cycle*

cancer: multiple and varying alterations in cell function resulting from overproduction of immature and nonfunctional cells or tissue enlargement for no physiologic reason

chemotherapy: medical treatment with highly toxic doses of medications aimed at interfering with the mitotic division of cancerous cells

chorea: purposeless, rapid, involuntary movements seen as a consequence of rheumatic fever and lasting for months

debridement: removal of eschar (dead skin) to allow granulation

dehydration: deficiency in body fluid due to decreased intake, output greater than intake, or loss of fluids caused by vomiting, diarrhea, or diaphoresis

developmental assessment: measurement of physical (motor), cognitive, psychosocial, and psychosexual parameters compared to norms for one's chronological age

diaphoresis: excessive sweating

echolalia: verbal pattern of one who repeats whatever is said

enuresis: involuntary urination after the age at which control should have been attained

ependymoma: ventricular tumor that results in a noncommunicating hydrocephalus; usually benign, but pressure can damage vital organs

fontanel: space covered by membranous tissue at the juncture of cranial sutures

glioma: slow-growing tumor that's usually inoperable because of its location in the brain stem

hemarthrosis: bleeding into a joint

human leukocyte antigen: genetically transferred antigenic marker on the cell surface of all nucleated cells that allows the body to recognize self and non-self

hypertrophy: increase in the size of a body organ or structure, sometimes due to an increase in cell size

hypoxia: deficiency of oxygen to the tissue

immunotherapy: using specially treated white blood cell immunopotentiators to replace immunocompetent lymphoid tissue, such as bone marrow and thymus

incubation period: time between the reception of an antigen and initiation of clinical symptoms

infratentorial: below the plate that's under the cerebellum

interstitial compartments: spaces between tissues

intravascular compartments: spaces within blood vessels

left-to-right shunt: pressure from the left side of the heart pushing blood through a septal defect to the right side, thereby increasing blood flow to the lungs

medulloblastoma: highly malignant, fast-growing tumor in the cerebellum

metastasize: growing and spreading of malignant cells from the primary site to other tissues

neurogenic bladder: dribbling of urine from the lack of spontaneous bladder emptying

nystagmus: involuntary, rapid, jerky movement of the eye

object permanence: awareness that objects exist while not in view

opisthotonos: spasmodic body posturing in which the back arches and the head and heels bend back

polycythemia: overproduction of red blood cells, resulting in increased blood viscosity and hematocrit

priapism: painful, prolonged, and abnormal erection of the penis, usually unrelated to sexual desire

pruritus: itching

puberty: physical changes resulting in reproductive maturity

rumination: voluntary regurgitation and reswallowing

steatorrhea: more than normal amounts of fat in the feces resulting in foamy, light-colored, bulky, foul-smelling, greasy stools

strabismus: condition in which the eyes are misaligned when fixating on the same object, from a muscle imbalance

subluxation: partial dislocation of any joint

supratentorial: within the cerebrum and above the tentorial plate

surfactant: phospholipid that lines the alveoli, preventing them from collapsing during exhalation

talipes: clubfoot; inability of the foot or ankle to attain correct alignment from twisting in any of multiple directions

toxoid: toxin that's rendered nontoxic

transitional object: object or comfort measure that represents parental security

Selected references

Chung, E.K., et al. *Visual Diagnosis in Pediatrics.* Philadelphia: Lippincott Williams & Wilkins, 2006.

Davids, J.R., et al. "Indications for Orthoses to Improve Gait in Children with Cerebral Palsy," *Journal of the American Academy Orthopaedic Surgery* 15(3):178-88, March 2007.

Doring, G., et al. "Clinical Trials in Cystic Fibrosis," *Journal of Cystic Fibrosis* 6(2):85-99, April 2007.

Garg, A., et al. "Primary Ewing's Sarcoma of the Occipital Bone Presenting as Hydrocephalus and Blindness," *Pediatric Neurosurgery* 43(2):170-73, 2007.

Geller, D.E., et al. "Novel Tobramycin Inhalation Powder in Cystic Fibrosis Subjects: Pharmacokinetics and Safety," *Pediatric Pulmonology* 42(4):307-13, April 2007.

Hay, W.W., et al. *Essentials of Pediatrics.* Philadelphia: McGraw-Hill, 2007.

Hockenberry, M.J. *Wong's Essentials of Pediatric Nursing,* 7th ed. St. Louis: Mosby, 2005.

Huh, J.S., et al. "Lateral Ventricular Diverticulum Extending into Supracerebellar Cistern from Unilateral Obstruction of the Foramen of Monro in a Neonate," *Pediatric Neurosurgery* 43(2):115-20, 2007.

Londhe, V.A, et al. *Blueprints Clinical Cases in Pediatrics,* 2nd ed. Philadelphia: Lippincott Williams & Wilkins, 2006.

McGahren, E.D., and Wilson, W.G. *Pediatrics Recall,* 3rd ed. Philadelphia: Lippincott Williams & Wilkins, 2007.

Mori, K., et al. "Myocardial Strain Imaging for Early Detection of Cardiac Involvement in Patients with Duchenne's Progressive Muscular Dystrophy," *Echocardiography* 24(6):598-608, July 2007.

Powers, J.H. "Diagnosis and Treatment of Acute Otitis Media: Evaluating the Evidence," *Infectious Disease Clinics of North America* 21(2):409-426, June 2007.

Sabella, C., and Cunningham, R.J. *The Cleveland Clinic Intensive Review of Pediatrics,* 2nd ed. Philadelphia: Lippincott Williams & Wilkins, 2006.

Vrijlandt, E.J., et al. "Respiratory Health in Prematurely Born Preschool Children With and Without Bronchopulmonary Dysplasia," *Journal of Pediatrics* 150(3):256-61, March 2007.

Wilmott, R.W. "Cystic Fibrosis Foundation Guidelines for Diagnostic Sweat Testing," *Journal of Pediatrics* 151(1):A2, July 2007.

Index

---

i refers to an illustration; t refers to a table.

i refers to an illustration; t refers to a table.

i refers to an illustration; t refers to a table.

i refers to an illustration; t refers to a table.

i refers to an illustration; t refers to a table.

i refers to an illustration; t refers to a table.

ABOUT THE CD-ROM

The enclosed CD-ROM is just one more reason why the *Straight A's* series is at the head of its class. The more than 250 additional NCLEX-style questions contained on the CD provide you with another opportunity to review the material and gauge your knowledge. The program allows you to:

- take tests of varying lengths on subject areas of your choice
- learn the rationales for correct and incorrect answers
- print the results of your tests to measure progress over time.

Minimum system requirements

To operate the *Straight A's* CD-ROM, we recommend that you have the following computer equipment:

- Windows XP-Home
- Pentium 4
- 512 MB RAM
- 10 MB of free hard-disk space
- SVGA monitor with High Color (16-bit)
- CD-ROM drive
- mouse.

Installation

Before installing the CD-ROM, make sure that your monitor is set to High Color (16-bit) and your display area is set to 800 × 600. If it isn't, consult your monitor's user's manual for instructions about changing the display settings. (The display settings are typically found in Start/Settings/Control Panel/Display/Settings tab.)

To run this program, you must install it onto the hard drive of your computer, following these three steps:

1. Start Windows XP-Home (minimum).
2. Place the CD in your CD-ROM drive. After a few moments, the install process will automatically begin. *Note:* If the install process doesn't automatically begin, click the Start menu and select Run. Type *D:\setup.exe* (where *D:* is the letter of your CD-ROM drive) and then click OK.
3. Follow the on-screen instructions for installation.

Technical support

For technical support, call toll-free 1-800-638-3030, Monday through Friday, 8:30 a.m. to 5 p.m. Eastern Time. You may also write to Lippincott Williams & Wilkins Technical Support, 351 W. Camden Street, Baltimore, MD 21201-2436, or e-mail us at *wkhealth-support@wolterskluwer.com*.
